ABORTION

ABORTION

MALCOLM POTTS

Consultant to International Pregnancy Advisory Services
International Fertility Research Program

PETER DIGGORY

Senior Consultant Gynaecologist to the
Kingston and Richmond Group of Hospitals

JOHN PEEL

Head of Department of Social Studies, Teesside Polytechnic

CAMBRIDGE UNIVERSITY PRESS

CAMBRIDGE

LONDON · NEW YORK · MELBOURNE

Published by the Syndics of the Cambridge University Press
The Pitt Building, Trumpington Street, Cambridge CB2 1RP
Bentley House, 200 Euston Road, London NW1 2DB
32 East 57th Street, New York, NY 10022, USA
296 Beaconsfield Parade, Middle Park, Melbourne 3206, Australia

First published 1977

Printed in Great Britain at the
University Press, Cambridge

Library of Congress Cataloguing in Publication Data

Potts, Malcolm.
Abortion.

Includes index.

1. Abortion. 2. Abortion – Great Britain.
I. Diggory, Peter, joint author. II. Peel, John, joint author.
III. Title. [DNLM: 1. Abortion, Induced. HQ767 P871a]
HQ767. P.69   301   76–27907
ISBN 0 521 21442 4
ISBN 0 521 29150 X pbk

To Vera Houghton and the late Alan Guttmacher, who, on opposite sides of the Atlantic and in different ways, have changed the attitudes of society and professional groups towards the difficult problem of abortion.

CONTENTS

PREFACE

The unique nature of abortion is apparent even when writing a book
on the subject. We have gathered data from a great many sources.
Much insight has been obtained by direct conversations with women
seeking abortions and through other medical practitioners whose
anonymity must be respected. We contacted abortionists acting
illegally in Britain before 1967 and in several contemporary countries
with restrictive laws. Sometimes, we have come to respect the
illegal abortionists, on other occasions we have had feelings of
contempt or sorrow. But we have only reported events that we have
seen ourselves or that have been described by trustworthy witnesses.
During the time when this book was being written one or more of
the authors has visited Afghanistan, Australia, Bangladesh, Barbados, Belgium, Brazil, Canada, Colombia, Czechoslovakia, Eire,
Egypt, El Salvador, Ethiopia, France, Finland, German Federal
Republic, Ghana, Hong Kong, Hungary, Iceland, India, Indonesia,
Italy, Jamaica, Japan, Kenya, Khmer Republic (Cambodia),
Korea (South), Laos, Mexico, Nepal, Netherlands, New Zealand,
Nigeria, Norway, Pakistan, Philippines, Poland, Sri Lanka, Sing-
apore, Sudan, Sweden, Switzerland, Taiwan, Thailand, Trinidad,
Tunisia, Turkey, USA, USSR, Venezuela, Vietnam (South) and
Yugoslavia. For countries that we have been unable to visit we have
had discussions with friends and colleagues who know both the
countries concerned and the problem of abortion well.

We are especially grateful for the friendship, opportunities to
learn, and instant supply of information from Anna Marie Dourlen-
Rollier, Merle Goldberg, Sarah Lewit, Emily Moore-Čavar, Madeleine Simms, Jean van der Tak, Henry David, Geoffrey Davis and
Christopher Tietze. Numerous facts and insights were supplied by

Rebecca Cook, Pamela David, Alice Gubaya, Phyllis Piotrow, Margaret Sparrow, Leslie Vick, Daniel Ampofo, G. Arjoon, Ben Branch, Roger Bernard, Berislav Beric, Tim Black, George Cenarda, Don Casey, Don Collins, Lloyd Cox, Ian Craft, Teddy Cummins, Robert Gillespie, Lessel David, Denhanom Muangman, Marcus Filshie, James Grieg, Harold Francis, A. A. Haspels, Song-Bong Hong, Peter Huntingford, Jorgen Jenk, Edmund Kellogg, Elton Kessel, Philip Kestleman, Len Laufe, Doug Larson, Torben Larsen, Harry Lean, Luke Lee, Luigi de Marchi, K.-H. Mehlan, Bahram Mohit, Tegualda Monreal, Isam Nazer, Datta Pai, Minoru Muramatsu, I. S. Puvan, Ismail Ragab, Ferdinand Rath, Mario Raquena, Hamid Rushwan, Fred Sai, Trevor Saver, H. Stamm, Alistair Service, Demos Taliadores, Mechai Viravaidya, Benjamin Viel, T. Wagatsuma, Nicholas Wright and Timor Ethesham Zadeh. These personal sources of observation and information cover many details of our subject, which, because of its unusual nature, could not be referenced in the conventional academic way. (We can, of course, supply details of unpublished sources, on request).

We are grateful to Derek Waite of Hull University, who prepared many of the illustrations, to Ramon Bloomfield for the design of Fig. 29 and to Mavis Warnes, Evelyn Kerr, Peggy Lehman, Beryl Hales and Judy Chu who typed successive drafts of the manuscript.

Introduction

Abortion may be defined as the loss of a pregnancy before the fetus or fetuses are potentially capable of life independent of the mother. In most mammals this period extends roughly over the first two-thirds of the pregnancy. Loss subsequent to this is regarded as premature birth. In Britain and the USA there is a legal definition of abortion as loss before the twenty-eighth week of menstrual age. Before this date the conception, when delivered, is disposed of by incineration or any other convenient method, whereas once this date has passed a stillbirth certificate must be issued, and disposal by burial or cremation must follow the same registration and certification procedures as for adult deaths. This arbitrary distinction between abortion and premature stillbirth, made by society, is usually mirrored by the woman's own reaction. Sorrow for the abortion is non-specific and few women lament the loss of early pregnancy; the stillborn child is generally felt as loss of a personified individual and is a subject for mourning.

Abortion is a ubiquitous and important medical, demographic and sociological event. Both individually and culturally it takes time to learn effective birth control. As soon as either an individual or a society comes to accept the need for restricting reproduction it is likely that first attempts at contraception will be relatively ineffective and initially the resort will be primarily to abortion. Following the recent explosive growth of world population there is nowadays an extremely high proportion of young and fertile people. It appears likely that at the present time the number of fetuses deliberately aborted throughout the world is at least equal to the number of adult deaths.

Both spontaneous and induced abortion are poorly understood

conditions. Like malignant disease, abortion is endemic in all communities and although the incidence and complications of both conditions can be reduced by health education and by preventive and curative medicine they cannot be eliminated.

Termination of pregnancy is one of the oldest and commonest forms of fertility control. No human community has ever shown a marked fall in its birth rate without a significant recourse to induced abortion and it is unlikely that contraceptive procedures alone will provide a sufficient measure of population control in developing nations wishing to lower their birth rate. In problems of world population growth, the logistics of induced abortion services will become increasingly significant.

Observation suggests that abortion is an acceptable form of fertility control for the individual, although it is frequently condemned by the community. Many people find it easier to initiate action to deal with the concrete reality of a pregnancy than to take precautions against the possibility of such an event. We can now show that within a community a woman who has had an abortion is more likely to accept contraception thereafter, but it is also true that she will be more willing, if necessary, to accept a second abortion. The majority of women will resort to the operation in the face of religious and legal sanctions and will accept considerable pain, danger and expense to achieve their aims.

All over the world, legal, medical and public opinion on therapeutic abortion is changing rapidly. At the same time a revolution is taking place in abortion techniques and in the involvement of doctors with the problem. Unfortunately, confusion and contradictions remain and even family planners have sometimes found it difficult to adopt a balanced approach to induced abortion. On the one hand, the opponents of planned parenthood have tried to blur the distinction between contraception and abortion while, on the other, the protagonists of family planning have overestimated the potential of contraceptive methods in cutting down the induced abortion rate and have been reluctant to recognise that there will continue to be an unavoidable role for abortion within their speciality.

Attitudes

It has been assumed that individual opinion is against abortion wherever the cultural milieu condemns it. But perhaps the world-wide common usage of criminal abortion should be recognised as a truer more reliable indicator of feelings. In a sample survey of the United States in 1965, only a minority favoured the possibility of allowing therapeutic abortion for social reasons. Women proved even more restrictive than men in their views, although it was estimated that, at that time, 30–50 per cent of married American women had had an abortion for social reasons between their thirtieth and fiftieth birthdays. In Great Britain public opinion changed rapidly during the course of the campaign that preceded the passing of the 1967 Abortion Act, and during that time a majority of the public came to demand consideration of social, as well as medical, grounds when deciding upon termination. Some subgroups in society remained opposed to the new law; in particular, Roman Catholics and members of the medical 'establishment'. Experience has shown, however, that it is precisely these two groups who prove particularly liable to seek induced abortion for themselves. The conflicts found in some cultures are well illustrated by a sample of residents of Melbourne, Australia, including recent immigrants from Europe.[1] Thirty per cent of the Greek- and 11 per cent of the Italian-born immigrants could envisage, given the choice, having an *illegal* abortion rather than a legal one. The West is not alone in tortuous thinking. In Japan 50 per cent of a group of college students, when questioned about their attitude to abortion, wanted to see their country's laws made more strict, although many of them will certainly resort to abortion to achieve their own fertility goals.

Abortion is unlike all other human problems, in that an individual may sincerely condemn the procedure until that one brief occasion when he, or his wife, is faced with what appears to be an overwhelming reason for termination. The paradox is completed in some cases by the couple who, having had their abortion, then revert, sometimes quite strongly, to condemnatory attitudes.

We know of a staunchly Catholic nurse who sought special assurances regarding privacy for her abortion because she is publicly known to be a prominent member of the right-to-life movement in her town. Such behaviour has been confirmed elsewhere and the daughters of men who publicly condemn abortion in hysterical tones seek legal abortions from responsible services in private.

Theology

The sad confusion which often surrounds public and private decision-making about abortion should not be allowed to erode the crucial nature of the basic question of assigning a status to the early embryo and the later fetus. It is a genuine, immediate and continuing problem for individuals and society, which a great many adults have to face in practice and which it is reasonable for others to attempt to answer in theory. At this point we intend to summarise briefly the attitude of the main world religions. In the final conspectus (Chapter 15) we return to the same topic and present our own best judgement, based on the facts we have assembled, on striking a balance between the status of the embryo and the needs of the mother and her family.

Christian

Abortion ethics have been the subject of many moral statements, numerous clashes of opinion, but relatively little careful constructive thought. Slogans have been more common than analysis. Twentieth-century biology has not been merged with nineteenth-century theology, and there have been powerful social pressures not to discuss the topic of abortion, even inside ivory towers. Where the process has begun, it is of recent origin. The relatively small amount of philosophical and objective analysis of the ethical problems of abortion is nearly all of the last decade, much of it of the past few years,[2-4] and all of it coinciding with the splitting open of the intellectual straitjacket which, for two millennia, the Western world has worn when discussing the topic of abortion.

ROMAN CATHOLIC

The Catholic position on abortion is not as absolutist as is commonly believed. Many of the Latin Fathers of the Church did not believe in the immediate animation of the embryo. Gratianus in a codification of Canon Law in 1140 held that abortion was not murder before infusion of the soul.[5] It was only in 1869 that Pius IX dropped any reference to the 'ensouled fetus' when condemning abortion.[6] At that time the understanding of the biology of human reproduction was limited. For example, the 'safe period' was thought to coincide with menstruation. Even in 1930, when Pius XI condemned abortion in the encyclical *Casti connubii*, the biological context of the pronouncement was vague, it spoke of 'the offspring

hidden in the maternal breast'. The Second Vatican Council exhorted, 'Life from its conception is to be guarded with the greatest
care. Abortion and infanticide are horrible crimes.' Pope Paul VI
in *Humanae vitae* (1968) reiterated the condemnation of abortion.
As with contraception, papal pronouncements in the present century
have given theologians a hard time in trying to find escape routes
– but few things are truly impossible! For one thing, an exception
to the Catholic condemnation of abortion already exists, which has
interesting implications. In 1902 the Holy Office rejected arguments
justifying operation for ectopic pregnancy, but subsequently such
operations have been judged licit by invoking the principle of
'double effect' – i.e. it is the diseased fallopian tube which is being
removed.[7]

Ectopic pregnancy occurs in about one in 300 pregnancies and,
untreated, it is nearly always fatal, because of internal haemorrhage
as the placenta erodes the ill-prepared tube. However, in extremely
rare cases, ectopic pregnancy can go to term.[8] Live-born deliveries
have taken place of babies that have not grown in the mother's womb,
although the chances of survival may well be less than one in 100000.
Clearly, both the compassionate theologian and the hardest Church
politician appreciate that it would be impossible to reverse the
exception that permits the remote possibility of ectopic fetal viability
to be sacrificed in order to save the mother from virtually certain
death. Yet, as long as the exception remains, the outside observer
will conclude that the Catholic differs from others in his social and
clinical arithmetic, not in the way he does his sums.

The Catholic lay theologian, Daniel Callahan has argued the
essentially human quality of abortion decision in his book *Abortion:
Law, Choice and Mortality*.[9] He seeks for a meaningful abortion ethic
within a pluralistic society. He warns how 'the abortion debate
prepared the ground for deception on all sides. Those opposed to
abortion, particularly on the grounds that it is the taking of human
life, may well be tempted to sacrifice other values – truth-telling,
open discussion, freedom of choice – for the sake of protecting that
life. Those in favour of abortion, and convinced that an embryo or
fetus is not human life, may be subject to exactly the same
temptation.' He quotes Father Kell to point out the problem of
identifying a common starting point, '"to those who really believe
in creation and the supreme dominion of God, the principle (the
sanctity of life) is too obvious to need proof; whereas for those who

do not believe in creation there is no basis on which to build proof'".
Then Callahan goes on to quote from Norman St John-Stevas,
another Catholic layman, and Sir Peter Medawar, a Humanist, to
demonstrate the philosophical similarities and limitations of arguments from first principles:

> 'ultimate justification' will always, in an important sense, seem
> circular, if not to ourselves then to others. The logical
> conundrum here is that it is always necessary to justify any
> 'ultimate justification' as indeed 'ultimate'. In the end, we are
> forced as individual persons to break out through this
> circularity or infinite regress (in practice if not in theory) by an
> existential choice. We decide, for motivations both rational and
> irrational that we must push the issue no further, that we have
> reached a point of diminishing intellectual return. At that
> stage, we choose our final (or first) starting point, hoping that it
> will express all that our limited wisdom has been able to
> achieve.

Callahan continues elsewhere:

> the key dilemma for Christian ethics, placing in conflict a
> commitment to stand back where God's lordship seems to hold
> sway and a practical realisation that man himself must judge
> when these situations occur. To say, for instance, that God
> forbids the taking of 'innocent' life, while conceding – as I
> think we must – that it is left up to man to define what an
> 'innocent' life is, is to fail to see that the only possible *meaning*
> this rule could have is the meaning human beings *choose* to give
> it.

Finally, he concludes,

> Contraception, abortion, euthanasia, medical experimentation
> and the prolongation of human life, are all problems which fall
> *totally* within the sphere of human rules and human
> judgements. To place the solution on these problems 'in the
> hands of God' is to misjudge God's role and misuse human
> reason and freedom.

The theology of the soul is that a spiritual quality enters the
physical body either slowly, like the maturing of wine, or in an
instant, like some coffees, at some undetermined stage of pregnancy.
It is generally held that the soul cannot enter before fertilisation and,
as souls are individuals, some theologians now hold that it cannot

enter before the chance of twinning has passed (that is, after the primitive streak formation at about 16 days post fertilisation).[10] Such thinking would lead to the classification of menstrual regulation as a contraceptive measure. The soul could enter at some much later stage of pregnancy, but as long as the stage is indeterminable, then some theologians argue that the only infallibly safe decision is to offer total protection at all stages of gestation (or at all stages beyond approximately 16 days). In other words, the right to life is asserted at all times because of lack of alternative arguments. However, even this restrictive argument requires a second theological assumption that is an essential, although often overlooked, element in Catholic teaching on abortion. Abortion only becomes anathema when a second doctrine is introduced, namely that of Original Sin. In Taussig's words, 'the fetus as the inheritor of original sin was certain of eternal damnation if it perished without baptism'.[6]

PROTESTANT

Protestant thinking allows considerable variation of approach to abortion. Lord Fisher, the former Archbishop of Canterbury, has written in a letter to *The Times*:

> In Church and State the unit of moral respect is the human person. When does the human embryo become a person?
>
> The Abbot of Downside (November 24) holds that there is no determinable point, other than conception, at which it is biologically or philosophically reasonable to suppose that human life begins. Even so I find it hard to believe that in any real sense personal life begins at that point.
>
> Lord Soper (November 26) holds that there is no convenient dividing line in human development at which the embryo instantly acquires a special worth. But does it not in plain fact do so in the moment of birth when the new born child draws its first breath, utters its first cry and begins its own separate and distinct life as a person already possessing rights and soon to learn duties?
>
> On the other hand all agree that at the time of conception the mother acquires all the personal rights and duties which belong to motherhood. She is bound to carry, care for, and nourish the embryo from the moment of conception to the moment of birth. At the same time the doctor has his direct duty to the mother as a person which requires him, if a choice has to be made, always to prefer the life of the mother to the life of the

embryo. That medical responsibility no one can share with him.

However, there are mothers who wish for one reason or another to be relieved of their moral responsibility for the embryo, and there are doctors who find it in conscience possible to meet the personal wishes of such mothers. So there has grown up in our society a state of affairs morally so unhappy as to demand fresh regulation. Many, including the doctors themselves, feel that further advice is needed as to what is or may be owed to the mother as a person so as to satisfy the medical and moral requirements of each situation. A new law must state the conditions under which a doctor might legitimately relieve the mother of her moral duty towards the embryo which she carries.

All of us, including especially the medical profession, must be reasonably satisfied that these conditions are medically and morally justifiable and can be accepted as wise even when not physically inevitable. Discussion should be about the moral responsibilities of mother and doctor and, I suggest, is not helped by introducing ideas of infanticide which attribute to the embryo personal rights which it cannot be shown to possess.[11]

ORTHODOX

The Orthodox Church embraces 100–130 million baptised Christians. Like the Roman Church, it claims to be the only infallible Church of Christ, and, like Rome, strongly condemns abortion. The Ecumenical Council of Troullo (A.D. 691) decreed (91st Canon): 'As for women who furnish drugs for the purpose of procuring abortion and those who take fetus-killing poisons, they are made subject to the penalty prescribed for murderers.'[12]

But as with Catholic believers in Latin America or Europe, the followers of the Orthodox Church in Yugoslavia, Russia, Greece and other countries resort to abortion frequently.

Islam

Islamic leaders currently set a rather conservative gloss on a basically liberal theology. However, some are beginning to look anew at the ancient problem of abortion.[13] The Grand Mufti of Jordan wrote in 1964: 'The jurists have stated that it is permissible to take medicine for abortion so long as the embryo is still unformed in human shape. The period of this unformed shape is given as 120 days. The jurists think that during this period the embryo or fetus is not yet a human being.'

The Qur'an verses to which the jurists referred describe human embryonic development with words which are poetic, but remain scientifically accurate after a millennium and a half:

> We placed him
> As a drop of seed
> In a safe lodging
> Firmly affixed;
> Then fashioned we
> The drop into a clot
> We developed
> A [*fetus*] lump; then
> We developed out of that lump
> Bones, and clothed the bones
> With flesh;
> Then we produced it
> As another creature.
> So blessed is God
> The Best to Create.

Hindu

Unlike the other great world religions, the Hindu scriptures (the *Vedas*, *c.* 2000–800 B.C.) specifically mention abortion: 'Wipe off, O Pushan, the misdeeds of him that practiseth abortion.'[14]

On the whole, abortion was regarded as a serious crime, to be categorised with incest, murder, or adultery with the wife of your guru.[15] However, exceptions were foreseen and Susruta, an early teacher, advised 'the pregnancy may be terminated to save her life because it is improper to let the pregnant woman die. So the proper step is to induce abortion.'

Clinical

In contrast to the ink spilt over abortion as a subject of ethical controversy, scientifically it has received little analysis. Biologically, medically and epidemiologically it is still an underdeveloped subject. Spontaneous abortion has received less attention than other comparable pathological conditions. The appreciation that it is an important biological mechanism evolved to eliminate developmental defects in the embryo is fairly recent.

The medical literature of abortion was sparse until the 1970s. In the nineteenth century the topic was intellectually untouchable. In the first half of the twentieth century it was highly unpopular. Taussig's book, *Abortion, Spontaneous and Induced: Medical and Social Aspects*, published in 1936, is particularly remarkable for the reason that it is a sturdy plant growing in what is otherwise a largely bibliographic desert. In the post-war world – and even to this day – authors who had useful observations on the medical aspects of abortion could not find journals willing to accept their papers. In the last few years the output of scientific books and papers on abortion has greatly increased. Today it may be commensurate to the available knowledge – although it still does not equal the exuberance of medical literature in other, less significant, fields.

In textbooks of obstetrics and gynaecology, induced abortion has traditionally been mentioned only to be condemned. Very recent editions of the standard works may make a shy mention of new techniques, but nearly all give the impression they want to pass on to the treatment of ectopic pregnancies or prolapses as rapidly as possible.

Pearl, in the *Natural History of Population* (1939),[16] and Glass, in *Population Policies and Movements in Europe* (1940),[17] both commented on the place of abortion in human demography, but they were the exceptions. In many texts on population, abortion remains unmentioned. The topic receives a half-column mention in Bogue's 900-page *Principles of Demography* (1969).[18] Even then assumptions are presented that might be difficult to substantiate, and abortion as a possible factor in family planning programmes is dismissed with the words 'this method of contraception is so highly condemned by Hindu, Moslem and Christian religions that it is not seriously considered as a family planning method.'

Induced abortion is unique amongst medical procedures because it involves two genetically dissimilar individuals – one at the threshold of anatomical development, the other physiologically mature and socially meaningful. It is also unusual amongst medical procedures in that the woman is normally physically and psychologically fit and the indications for operation are usually social and are presented by the 'patient' to her physician, rather than the other way round. The whole problem places doctors in a novel role which many have been reluctant to accept.

During the first three months of pregnancy there are numerous outstanding facts, such as the incidence of embryonic wastage and abnormality, the degree of development of the embryonic nervous system and the emotional impact of the pregnancy on the mother, which point to a qualitative as well as a quantitative difference from later pregnancy.

In this book we deal with epidemiology, and social and technical aspects of induced abortion. We try to face the moral decisions poised by abortion. Professionally we have experience of the disciplines of embryology, gynaecology, sociology and family planning. We have listened, both directly and through the literature, to women who have sought abortions. Private stories of pain, indignity, uncertainty and fright can easily be lost in social surveys and tables of statistics. Therefore, we have chosen seven individual accounts of legal and illegal abortion, from different times and localities.

Subjective and emotional passages, such as those which follow, have more often in the past been published in the anti-abortion literature. On both sides of the debate these illustrate the powerful feelings inextricably bound up with this topic. What ensues in the rest of the volume clearly demonstrates that these experiences can be viewed from an alternative perspective and that early safe abortion, carefully performed with compassion and dignity, is a rational answer to an omnipresent human problem.

An avoidable death

One stifling mid-July day of 1912 I was summoned to a Grand Street tenement. My patient was a small, slight, Russian Jewess, about twenty-eight years old, of the special cast of feature to which suffering lends a madonna-like expression. The cramped three-room apartment was in a sorry state of turmoil. Jake Sachs, a truck driver scarcely older than his wife, had come home to find the three children crying and her unconscious from the effects of a self-induced abortion. He had called the nearest doctor, who in turn had sent for me. Jake's earnings were trifling, and most of them had gone to keep the none-too-strong children clean and properly fed. But his wife's ingenuity had helped them to save a little, and this he was glad to spend on a nurse rather than have her go to a hospital.

Jake was more kind and thoughtful than many of the husbands I had encountered. He loved his children, and had always helped his wife wash and dress them. He had brought water up and carried garbage down before he left in the morning, and did as much as he could for me while he anxiously watched her progress.

At the end of three weeks, as I was preparing to leave the fragile patient to take up her difficult life once more, she finally voiced her fears, 'Another baby will finish me, I suppose?'

'It's too early to talk about that,' I temporized.

But when the doctor came to make his last call, I drew him aside. 'Mrs Sachs is terribly worried about having another baby.'

'She well may be,' replied the doctor, and then he stood before her and said 'Any more such capers, young woman, and there'll be no need to send for me.'

'I know doctor,' she replied timidly, 'but' and she hesitated as though it took all her courage to say it, 'what can I do to prevent it?'

The doctor was a kindly man, and he had worked hard to save her, but such incidents had become so familiar to him that he had long since lost whatever delicacy he might once have had. He laughed good-naturedly. 'You want to have your cake and eat it too, do you? Well, it can't be done.'

Then picking up his hat and bag to depart he said 'Tell Jake to sleep on the roof.'

The telephone rang one evening three months later, and Jake Sachs' agitated voice begged me to come at once: his wife was sick again and from the same cause. I turned into the dingy doorway and climbed the familiar stairs once more. The children were there, young little things.

Mrs Sachs was in a coma and died within ten minutes. I folded her still hands across her breast, remembering how they had pleaded with me, begging so humbly for the knowledge which was her right. Jake was sobbing, running his hands through his hair and pulling it out like an insane person. Over and over again he wailed, 'My God! My God! My God!'

Margaret Sanger (1883–1966)[19]

Career guidance

Not far away from Kobe [Japan] there is a place called Suma, well noted for its scenic beauty, but the place became famous in another sense, because women committed suicide dashing into running trains there almost every week. This tragic practice attracted the attention of a middle-aged social worker,

Mrs Nokubo Joh, a well-known woman of the day. She put up a sign 'Wait a minute' along the railroad track, and reminded the prospective suicider to call on her to talk over personal troubles

A few months later Mrs Joh saw me on the road in the slum. She put her hand on my shoulder, and in a tender voice said, 'Dr Majima, can you imagine how many women came to see me having seen that signboard? All those young girls say that they cannot go on living on account of their pregnancy! I cannot understand why they cannot support themselves with babies, and I can take care of a few of them, but my resources are limited too. So I have been to the Welfare Department of the city for help, and also asked for government support, but all in vain. Can't you do something to help these girls? You could do wonderful work helping these young girls!' I could see her eyes shining with tears, behind her glasses. 'Mrs Joh, do you mean to tell me that I should be an abortionist?'

'Yes, there is no other way out.'

Kan Majima describing an episode in 1917.

A conversion

I was taught obstetrics at The Johns Hopkins Medical School by Dr J. Whitridge Williams, one of the great medical figures of the 1920s. Forceful, confident and didactic, he imparted to us his conviction that induced abortions were either 'therapeutic' or 'criminal'.

I recall the drastic treatment meted out to pregnant women with excessive vomiting: isolation, submammary infusions, rectal clyses and feeding by stomach tube. To resort to therapeutic abortion in these cases was admission of medical failure.

My residency from 1925 to 1929 made me question the wisdom of such restrictive medical policy. In a short period I witnessed three deaths from illegal abortions – a 16-year-old with a multiperforated uterus, a mother of four who died of blood poisoning and a patient in early menopause who fatally misinterpreted cessation of menstruation. A social worker brought me a 12-year-old black child for legal abortion, who had been impregnated by her father. Dr Williams was a court of one to validate abortion requests so I sought his permission. He was sympathetic, but did not believe that continuation of

pregnancy endangered the child's life. When I mentioned the
social injustice of compelling a child to bear her father's
bastard, Dr Williams compromised and said that if I got a letter
from the district attorney, granting special permission, I could
perform the abortion. I failed to get such permission and
delivered the baby seven months later. At about the same time
one of the residents at a neighboring hospital showed me a
child playing with dolls, the daughter of an army colonel, who
had been hysterectomized to eliminate a pregnancy conceived
through 'rape'.

Alan F. Guttmacher (1898–1974)[20]

Social repair

A massive sixteen-year-old girl from a village in the Djurdjura
Mountains wears a blue scarf and a beautiful yellow robe. Her
legs are thick and hairy, and she's never seen a gynaecological
table before. She doesn't know what she's supposed to do on it.
She gets up with her pants on. 'What's this, Madame?' cries
Dr Vasilev. The girl tumbles off the table and looks at us, the
Vasilevs from Bulgaria, me from England, and Fatma who's
running the instruments from the last curettage under the tap.
Fatma confirms: 'Eksesserwell – off with your pants.' Dr
Vasilev sits on the stool, with a sigh and a cigarette, waiting.
The girl reaches up under her robe and pulls down her pants.
They're attached with elastic bands just below her knees. Their
crotch is soaked in blood.

She gets back on to the table and lies there flat, knees tightly
together, and as far from the edge as she can. 'Sob! – Down!'
cries Fatma the cleaner, and the girl consents to shift towards
the end of the table, and even to have her knees separated and
put over the stirrups. But she won't let go of her yellow robe.
She holds it clamped between her legs. Dr Vasilev doesn't
move from his stool. He shakes his cigarette at her: 'Back
home, Madame.'

She relents. She lets Fatma hold her robe back over her
stomach. She clutches my hand. Dr Vasilev's cigarette fizzles
out among the products of the last curettage in the enamel
bowl, and he doesn't bother this time to put on the rubber
apron. The operation takes about three minutes. Towards the
end, the curette is fairly bubbling in the womb. 'It's called "the
song of the curette",' says Dr Vasilev, and he invites me
round to see the pink, frothy blood in the vagina. 'It's the sign

it's nearly finished', he says. An iodine swab and: 'Dayin! – All over!' The girl's eyes are rolling. Her forehead's damp. She's a little shocked. She's been bleeding for two weeks, Fatma tells us. Her husband works in France, and she had to wait for his permission before she could come to hospital.

Ian Young (1964)[21]

A success story

The patient arrives at the Clinic having been counseled by her local clergyman regarding the option of abortion and bearing a note from her local physician stating the date of her last regular menstrual period.

The patient is placed in the lithotomy position on the procedure table. The paracervical block, with use of 1 per cent lignocaine (Xylocaine hydrochloride), is administered in the standard manner. The uterine sound is introduced, followed by careful dilatation with Pratt instruments. The standard appropriate Berkeley curved vacuum curette is introduced, and the procedure is completed.

The patient remains on the procedure table for 10 to 15 minutes after the procedure, while her vital signs are monitored by the counselor. She is then moved to a bed in a resting recovery room, where she is observed for one hour. Her vital signs are recorded every 15 minutes during this period, and she is checked for bleeding. At the end of the hour, if the patient's condition is satisfactory, she is transferred to the lounge recovery areas, where she changes into her clothes and remains two hours for further observation.

Since July 1, 1970, a total of 29,696 appointments have been made for abortion, and 26,000 abortions performed. It should be noted that the Clinic has functioned on the basis of a 16-hour day, seven days a week, and is closed only on legal holidays.

There were no known deaths in this series. The most serious complication of ambulatory abortion is uterine perforation. There were 36 definite perforations, of which 13 required subsequent laparotomy. The perforation in one of these 13 cases was into the right broad ligament, lacerating the uterine venous plexus and the uterine artery and subsequently requiring hysterectomy. The other 12 laparotomies resulted only in suture of the uterine performation, which was bleeding freely.

Bernard M. Nathanson (1972)[22]

A survivor

I found out about this woman through a friend, one of these
friends who are never lacking. She told me you can have an
abortion in such-and-such a place, and I went around in the
street to find the right house. A girl came up to me in the
street and asked who I was looking for. I said 'Look, I'm
looking for such-and-such a person who does such-and-such a
thing.' The girl said, 'My sister does this', and I went to talk
to her. This woman came to my house to do it; I didn't have
to go to hers. She charged something like 50 or 100 escudos,
which in those days (1964) was real money.

She dissolved some pills in lukewarm water in a lavatory,
and then poured the water through the sonda into my womb.
My impression is that this is supposed to dissolve the fetus
inside the mother's womb. I always have had my abortions
between one and two months of pregnancy. Never after that.
After the woman put the tube inside me I almost exploded. A
friend came to my house and said, 'You're shivering with
cold', and I said, 'Throw a blanket over me because I am
dying of cold.' Then my friend said, 'Look, Cristina, I'm
going to take you to the hospital because otherwise you're
going to die here.' I told her, 'Let me stay here because by
now I've had enough of this business, so many kids and so
many problems that I don't know what to do.' So she took me
to the J. J. Aguirre Hospital. My womb was so infected that
the doctors couldn't touch me. One doctor wanted to treat me
and the other didn't. One said to the other, 'If you send her
back home she'll die on the way'. So they operated on me,
scraping my womb clean, almost without anesthesia as a kind
of punishment. They scraped and scraped as if they were
cleaning the inside of a watermelon. Then they asked me who
did this to me and I could tell them nothing. One must not
talk in these situations, and I really wasn't lying because I
didn't know where this woman lived nor did I ever see her
again. This woman had no licence, but I was desperate to find
someone because my pregnancies never have brought me
happiness.

The most beautiful thing in the world is for a woman to have
the number of children that she wants. According to us
Catholics we should have the number of children that God
sends us, but there are times when one cannot anymore
although God keeps sending them. My husband is a hard

worker who doesn't rest day or night. He sells bread from
house to house and works from eight to sixteen hours each day,
and the doctors tell him that he'll end up very sick in the
hospital if he doesn't get some rest. So what do I get from
having seven or eight kids if I can't give them eggs, cheese, or
milk for breakfast.

> Cristina (thirty-one years old,
> four children, seven
> abortions) from Barrio El
> Salto, Conchati, Santiago,
> Chile.

Less eligibility

I am 23 years of age, a teacher, and am also doing part-time
University study. I am living with a man whom I love very
deeply but neither of us feels ready, financially or emotionally,
for marriage and children. My parents do not approve of my
partner.

I was on a low-dosage Pill but, as I was getting repeated
breakthrough bleeding, I had to ask my doctor for a change. I
was off the Pill for two weeks during this time. After I got the
second prescription I began to suspect that all was not normal
and that I might be pregnant, so I went to my doctor. He
arranged for a pregnancy test to be done: it was positive. I did
not want a child at this stage.

My doctor was not very anxious to help me, although he did
agree that it was my own affair, but said that did I realise 'that
if we were later married we would remember that our
first-born had been scraped out of my uterus into a stainless
steel bucket?' – but that it was up to me. He said he would
write a referral letter to the Public Hospital for me.

I was given an appointment for 1.30 pm on a weekday at the
hospital. When I arrived I was interviewed by a clerk at an
open counter which seemed very public.

I was weighed, and I supplied a urine specimen. I was given
a number and then told to wait again. Later I was called, by
number, to a side room and interviewed by a most pleasant
medical student, who recorded answers to various questions.

Next I was told to go to a very small cubicle and strip off. I
then waited for about ten minutes before a nurse called me to
lie on an examination table. It was in another cubicle, with the
curtains drawn, and I could hear the student telling the doctor
about my interview and the doctor disputing what was written

there about dates and times of pregnancy – how could anyone get pregnant in that time? He also made a derogatory remark about the fact that I came from Kalgoorlie.

The doctor then came in with three students. He grabbed my breasts, (which were already sore from the pregnancy) and said, 'Secondary areola', to the students. He did not speak to me nor did he greet me in any way. He then proceeded to handle my breasts very roughly indeed and said, 'Have you ever tried to get milk out of these?'. I said 'Of course not.' He said, 'Well, I'll have a try.' While he was pressing them he said, 'It's really muck stuff – good shaving cream'. He then said to the nice student, 'Well, go on then – get your cancer smear.' He then walked out. The nurse told me to turn on my side and the cancer smear was taken. The student was very kind about this.

The doctor then came back and asked me to spread my legs open. He told the students to examine me internally, after he had done so himself. Then he re-examined me (it was very painful) and told the nice student to do so again. The student said he'd already done so but the doctor insisted and said he'd gone to the trouble of setting up my uterus so that it was intraverted instead of retroverted. He remarked that I was going to have a rotten obstetrical future anyway. He said I was 6–7 weeks pregnant.

I was shocked and appalled and in tears at what was happening to me. The doctor said, 'Are you going to marry the father?' I said, 'No' and he said, 'They're alright for food and bed, but not to marry.' I felt incensed and insulted at the suggestion that the only reason I had for living with M was to get bed and board.

The doctor then said, 'She seems a bit inconsistent but I suppose we'll send her to a psychiatrist.' He then left without saying goodbye. The student apologised for the doctor's behaviour and the nurse told me, 'Never mind, the psychiatrist will simply write a letter.'

I left the hospital and drove home – and I really don't know how I got there. I felt outraged and degraded by the whole experience. My breasts were still terribly sore from his handling them and I feel I can't bear to let a man touch me ever again.

Anonymous (1974)[23]

References

1 Caldwell, T. & Ware, H. (1972). Australian attitudes towards abortion: survey evidence. In Abortion: *Repeal or Reform*, ed. N. Haines, p. 41. Pirie Printers, Fyshwick, Canberra.

2 O'Mahony, J. P. (1974). The beginning of human life. *Month*, **51**, 572.

3 Potts, M. (1975). Natural law and planned parenthood. *Mount Sinai Journal of Medicine*, **42**, 326.

4 Potts, M. (1969). The problem of abortion. In *Biology and Ethics*, ed. F. J. Ebling, p. 73. Academic Press, New York.

5 Noonan, J. T. Jr (1970). An almost absolute value in history. In *Morality of Abortion: Legal and Historical Perspectives*, ed. J. T. Noonan Jr, p. 1. Harvard University Press, Cambridge, Mass.

6 Taussig, F. J. (1936). *Abortion, Spontaneous and Induced: Medical and Social Aspects*. Kimpton, London.

7 Vermeersch, A., *Theologia moralis supra*, nn. 135, 630. Quoted in Noonan (1970); see note 5 above.

8 O'Connell, C. P. (1952). Full-term tubal pregnancy. *American Journal of Obstetrics and Gynecology*, **63**, 1305.

9 Callahan, D. (1970). *Abortion: Law, Choice and Morality*. Macmillan, New York.

10 Fagone, V. (1973). *La Civilta Cattolica*, 16 June and 17 July.

11 Fisher of Lambeth, Lord (1966). *The Times*, 2 November, p. 15.

12 Beric, B. M. (1970). Personal communication.

13 IPPF (1971). *Islam and Family Planning*, vols. I and II. IPPF, Middle East and North Africa Region, Beirut.

14 Hymns of the Athara-Veda (1879–1910), transl. by M. Bloomfield. In *Sacred Books of the East*, ed. F. M. Muller, p. 165. Clarendon Press, Oxford.

15 Chandrasekhar, S. (1974). *Abortion in a Crowded World: Problem of Abortion with Special Reference to India*. Allen & Unwin, London.

16 Pearl, R. (1939). *Natural History of Population*. Oxford University Press, Oxford.

17 Glass, D. V. (1940). *Population Policies and Movements in Europe*. Clarendon Press, Oxford.

18 Bogue, D. J. (1969). *Principles of Demography*. Wiley, New York.

19 Sanger, M. (1938). *An Autobiography*. W. W. Norton, New York.

20 Guttmacher, A. F. (1969). The new law and the abortion problem. In *Therapeutic Abortion*, ed. J. F. Hulka, Carolina Population Center, Chapel Hill, North Carolina. See also Guttmacher, A. F. Abortion: an odyssey of an attitude. *Perspectives in Family Planning*, **4**, 5.

21 Young, I. (1974). *The Private Life of Islam*. Allen Lane, London.

22 Nathanson, B. M. (1972). Ambulatory abortion: experience with 26,000 cases. *New England Journal of Medicine*, **286**, 403.

23 Report by the Abortion Law Repeal Association (1974). 'Report on legal, medical, social and political aspects of abortion relevant to Western Australia', ed. D. White. (Duplicated document.)

1
Definitions, problems and theoretical considerations

Definitions are usually necessary, but often tedious. However, in the case of the extraordinary subject of abortion even the use of the term is revealing of societal attitudes; definitions are confused, slow to change and paradoxical.

The only internationally agreed definitions concern the term 'fetal deaths'* but these are still not widely used. In 1950 the WHO Expert Committee in Health Statistics[1,2] recommended definition of fetal death was adopted by the Organisation, namely 'death prior to the complete expulsion or extraction from its mother of a product of conception, irrespective of the duration of pregnancy'. The same committee also recommended dividing fetal deaths into three categories: early, up to 19 weeks gestation; intermediate, 20–28 weeks; late, over 28 weeks. The last category would be synonymous with the term 'stillbirth' and the early and intermediate with the term 'abortion'. However, not all countries agree to the definition of abortion as loss of the products of conception prior to 28 weeks. Some use a definition of fetal weight (usually 1000 g) rather than age. The intention has usually been to define an abortion as loss of the fetus prior to 'viability' – i.e. it is capable of surviving outside the uterus – but this frontier will retreat rapidly as obstetric technology improves.

In a survey of official definitions in 86 countries it was found that

* To add to the confusion even the spelling of fetus is in dispute. The English and American spellings of 'foetus' and 'fetus' differ. Etymologists and anatomists are agreed that 'fetus' is the correct usage as the word is derived from the Latin *feto* – I bear. However, English clinicians continue to use 'foetus'. The word 'abortion' comes from the Latin *aboriri* – to fail to be born.

38 had no definition whatsoever and the remainder used a variety
of criteria. Some chose to consider an abortion as any delivery before
16 weeks, 28 weeks or sometimes six months, and one even allowed
the term 'abortion' to be used for certain types of term deliveries.
About one country in ten used physiological criteria of viability
rather than a finite time interval; three countries used fetal length;
and one used weight instead of age or viability.

It seems unlikely that the term 'early fetal death' will become
widely used. The word 'abortion' is firmly entrenched in the language even if definition is imprecise. The word 'miscarriage' can
be synonymous with abortion or limited to the description of spontaneous abortions. It is a word favoured by lay writers and is
sometimes used by lawyers. Emotionally, it has fewer of the harsh
overtones of 'abortion' which the lay writer and the jurist sometimes restrict to the description of induced abortions.

Legally, 'abortion' means 'an untimely delivery voluntarily procured with intent to destroy the fetus' although, even in a field where
the use of words is required to be precise, alternative and conflicting
definitions have been given.

The paradox of definitions arises in relation to the Infant Life
Preservation Act of 1929.[3] This piece of English legislation, which
itself had a very long gestation going back to the 1860s, was designed
to deal with cases where the baby was deliberately killed during
delivery. In a sense it was a humane piece of legislation distinguishing between child destruction and murder and, therefore,
avoiding capital punishment. It also included a therapeutic exception for doctors acting in good faith to save the life of the mother.
The wording of the 1929 Act is, 'any wilful act [that] causes a child
to die before it has an existence independent of its mother'. This
definition overlaps with that of abortion. Therefore, until the 1967
Abortion Act an English doctor* could legally destroy a fetus at term
to preserve the life of the mother, but was unable to perform an
abortion for similar reasons when the woman was three months
pregnant.

Fetal loss before the twenty-eighth week of menstrual age can be
disposed of by incineration, or any convenient method, whereas after
this date a stillbirth certificate has to be issued and disposal by
burial or cremation take place, as in the case of an adult.

* For simplicity 'he' is used in the general sense of he or she for doctor,
physician etc. throughout.

The twenty-eighth week of menstrual age accords with the stage of pregnancy when a viable birth may be expected. However, with modern methods for resuscitation at birth and for the maintenance of life of very premature babies, this limit is likely to be lowered.

Methods of estimating the incidence of abortion

Abortion is common but exceedingly difficult to measure. It is difficult to separate induced and spontaneous abortions, as the history of clandestine abortions is often suppressed and the distribution of induced and spontaneous abortions with respect to age and parity is similar. All the evidence on the incidence of illegal abortion must be indirect.

Sometimes clues assist the investigator. Prolonged intervals in the pregnancy history of a cohabiting couple not using contraceptives may point to one or more induced abortions. Conversely, couples who discontinue contraception in order to become pregnant can provide useful information on spontaneous abortion.

Retrospective data

VITAL STATISTICS

In the sixteenth century Henry II of France attempted to make the declaration of pregnancy compulsory, in order to prevent clandestine abortion.[4] The idea miscarried, as it did when attempted 400 years later in Nazi Germany. The next most comprehensive possibility is to make the formal registration of fetal deaths obligatory. Such a requirement is currently in force in New York State but remains as purposeless as the registration of pregnancy.[5]

Registration of legal abortions

The registration of *legal abortion* is a practical and useful possibility in many countries with liberal laws. It is carried out in England, Wales and Scotland, Scandinavia, most Socialist countries, Singapore, Tunisia, India, South Australia and Japan, and in some American states. Data on legal operations provide cross-references to the magnitude of illegal operations in other countries, or at other times, and furnish invaluable evidence about age, parity and socio-economic characteristics of women resorting to abortion; they further permit the evaluation of rare but serious adverse effects of various surgical and medical techniques.

Registration may be the responsibility of the surgeon or of the institution where the operation is carried out. It is an enforceable regulation, giving a reasonable degree of accuracy, but this has the disadvantage that the situation may arise where it is difficult to safeguard the confidential relationship between doctor and patient. Sample surveys of bed usage can be made to estimate the nationwide incidence of hospital abortion cases, if registration is not available.

In Britain registration of numbers is good, although considerable under-reporting may occur among women coming from overseas. Details of age, parity, previous abortions, marital status and home address could be falsified by some women as these data are rarely checked by the surgeon registering the operation. Records are known to be confidential and not open to other government departments, such as the Inland Revenue. Likewise, data from Scandinavia have a high degree of reliability. In New York and other states, registration is usually poor, but some satisfactory comparative studies have been devised by individual centres. In Czechoslovakia, the law is carefully implemented at the district level and the central collection of information is good. In Hungary, all operations are performed in hospital, the system of registration works well and the small size of the nation makes for accurate records. The long series of careful statistics from Hungary and Czechoslovakia are particularly useful, and in the case of the former can be related to the excellent fertility survey conducted in 1966. Less reliance can be placed on the Polish statistics: here private practice persists, and many women wishing to avoid the public atmosphere of a hospital go to private practitioners. Private doctors are required to register the operation, but errors of enumeration are thought to be common. Women from abroad are not itemised separately and may inflate the statistics. Yugoslavia is a federal republic and vital statistics are published for each state. In the underdeveloped areas of the country these may not be as reliable as in the industrialised regions. Compulsory registration of the operation was introduced only in 1960 and the rise in the number of registered abortions that occurred after that date may be spurious. Registration is required in Japan but poorly enforced, and considerable under-reporting seems likely.

One factor is said to be possible tax consequences. In India, a great deal of information is required to be given at the time of registration and the very complexity of the form is probably one of the reasons for poor reporting. In England in April 1971, a prosecution was made involving failure to report legal abortions. Following this event the number of registered operations from several centres jumped, suggesting the repair of some slackness.

Data have been released for only some years from Bulgaria and Romania. No nationwide statistics have ever been issued for the USSR, which is particularly unfortunate because of the fascinating spectrum of economic and ethnic variation represented within that nation and the presumed wide range of birth rates and abortion practice. It is not known what, if any, data are collected nationwide for the People's Republic of China.

As is commonly the case in the registration of vital statistics, the provisional abortion data in certain countries are sometimes amended in the year following their publication, and this has given rise to slight, but important, variations in published data.

Other statistics

Certain other vital statistics, not immediately related to abortion, can be of great value in constructing the total picture of fertility regulation in a country. In nearly all industrialised nations the registration of *births* is satisfactory. On the whole the birth rate follows long-term trends and often remains unchanged in the face of large fluctuations in the number of registered legal abortions, suggesting that transfer in and out of the non-legal sector may be a significant variable.

The numerical registration of *deaths* is very accurate in most developed countries, but the certification of the cause of death is often poor and may be most inaccurate of all in the case of *maternal deaths related to abortion*.

In Britain maternal deaths due to illegal abortion have been used as a measure of the upper limit of the incidence of induced abortion, both by Goodhart[6,7] and James.[8] Two problems arise: namely the accuracy of death certification and the assumed mortality from illegal abortion. Commonsense suggests that death certification among young women who die suddenly in a country well provided with doctors should be satisfactory. However, in practice this is not always the case. A forensic expert[9] reviewing autopsies on cases of sudden death in Britain remarked, in the case of abortion in particular, 'the outstanding impression is one of the unbelievable gullibility and stupidity of doctors asked to examine women found collapsed at home or in the street, sometimes with a previous history of abdominal pain and vomiting'.

In developing countries inaccuracies are even more likely to occur, although a case reported from Mexico City in 1973, where a criminal abortionist fed the bodies of women who died to his dogs and hid the bones under his floorboards, is probably unusual. In some situations death following illegal abortion may be recognised but registered under a misleading cause, either to protect the abortionist or the family. For example, in Italy, registration of a death as due to abortion leads to close and embarrassing questioning of the relatives and a humane doctor usually writes a cause other than abortion on the death certificate.

When illegal abortion can involve several millions of dollars of turnover in a single city and where, as in Australia, the police have been shown to be corruptible, then many things are possible, in either developed or developing countries. Wainer,[10] who knew the illegal abortionists in Melbourne, describes the techniques for disposal of corpses as,

> very similar to those used by the most experienced in the underworld. The best have access to a crematorium after hours; another buried the bodies in a cemetery of a principal town where he had an understanding with the custodian of the cemetery; another knew an undertaker who, for a price, would put the body in the coffin of some old pensioner who had no relatives and there would be a double burial. The most uncouth would put the body in a 44 gallon drum, weight the drum, weld the top onto it, have large holes in it and take it out to the middle of Port Philip Bay to be dumped.

Wainer speculates, 'I wonder how many women on the missing persons files have been accounted for like this?' When the police cannot decide, the epidemiologist may feel justifiably at a disadvantage.

Nevertheless, used critically, deaths ascribed to abortion can sometimes serve as an indirect measure of abortion numbers over time. However, mortality due to abortion tends to decline as standards of medical care rise. Deaths need to be reviewed in parallel with other causes of maternal mortality. The death rate for illegal abortion is most difficult of all to estimate (p. 270).

It would be useful to know the duration of gestation when death due to illegal abortion occurs, and agreement on the details of mortality statistics between different countries would be valuable.

Registration of all abortions

It is possible to demand the certification of all abortion cases – legal, illegal and spontaneous – comparable to the registration of births. It is difficult to distinguish between spontaneous and induced abortions, and at best only those criminal abortions requiring professional medical care will be registered.

Attempts to register all abortions, while not providing the intended information, may reveal trends in the incidence of abortion, although the effects of custom, education and honesty of reporting could also alter the recorded incidence.

Institutional statistics

It can be made obligatory to record institutional statistics on abortion, as in Hungary, or their collection may depend on the enthusiasm of individual workers, as in the USA.

Institutional records are the main basis of morbidity statistics but these are only useful if common definitions are used and both national and international agreement on this topic is needed. Sometimes, however, they do little more than reflect bed availability.

Prosecutions for illegal abortion

In countries where illegal abortion is common, it might be imagined that data on police prosecutions would be useful in following alterations in frequency, but the curious nature of the abortion 'crime' ensures that prosecutions depend more on the attitude of the keepers of the law than on the true incidence of the event, and prosecutions are mainly useful as a qualitative marker of the condition.

PLANNED SURVEYS

Clinical histories

Interested physicians can obtain a useful insight into the epidemiology of abortion. The patient–doctor relationship can assist honesty of reporting, although some cases may have the opposite result. The clinician also has the advantage of being able to look for certain physical signs of interference with the pregnancy, such as infection or vaginal and cervical trauma. Series for study may come from private practice, hospital records or family planning clinics. The incidence of abortion rises with parity, and the probability of the last pregnancy in a fertile lifetime ending in abortion is greater than average. Therefore, data collected from women having deliveries will bias the statistics towards an underestimate of the frequency of abortion, while data collected from hospital admissions for abortion will have the opposite effect. Data collected at the time of any pregnancy event (delivery, abortion or the seeking of contraceptive advice) will omit the infecund and tend to underestimate the subfecund. Again, an opposite bias may manifest itself in clinical histories collected from women seeking advice for gynaecological complaints.

Sample studies

Questions relating to a past history of abortion are becoming increasingly common in KAP (knowledge, attitude and practice) surveys. Pomeroy, continuing the work of Kinsey's group, provided much useful data for the USA[11] and currently KAP surveys have taken place, or are taking place, in many developing countries. Specific surveys on abortion, and not merely as an adjunct to other aspects of fertility control, have begun and, no doubt, will become more common. In some areas, e.g. Latin America, there is an impression that women may respond more honestly to questions on abortion, than to questions on sexual behaviour.

Retrospective surveys present obvious problems of sample selection and material must be carefully presented to allow for the fact that many women will be reporting incomplete fertility histories and, in addition, a changing incidence of induced abortion may affect different age groups unequally. A further complication arises because the factors affecting accuracy of reporting may also vary with time. A greater readiness to report an induced abortion may give rise to a spurious increase in incidence. This latter factor may also interact with a genuine failure, with advancing age, to recall past events in the fertility history.

Randomised responses

One method of investigating the problem of abortion has been developed, which overcomes many of the problems arising from a woman's obvious reluctance to admit to induced abortions. It involves the technique of 'randomised response' reported by Warner[12] and consists of a transparent box containing 35 red balls, 15 blue balls and a window into which a single ball can be shaken. The principle is to attach two statements to the box – one identified by a red ball, the other by a blue ball. The respondent is asked to shake one ball into the window and then comment on the statement which corresponds to the colour of the ball with a simple 'Yes' or 'No'. The box is then reshaken and handed back to the interviewer who thus has no knowledge of which question was answered. Given a large population of respondents, and knowing the ratio of red to blue balls, a meaningful response for the population as a whole can be calculated.

Abernathy and his colleagues at North Carolina University have used this method in abortion studies. In one study the alternative questions in the box were

1. 'I was pregnant at some time during the past 12 months and had an abortion which ended the pregnancy',
2. 'I was born in the month of April'.

Another trial was conducted using the statement, 'At some time in my life I had an abortion which ended the pregnancy'. The procedure was explained to the respondent and a definition of abortion given.[13]

The defect of the procedure is that it can be difficult to convince women that the answers given are truly anonymous and that the apparatus does not conceal some trick.

Prospective studies

INTERVIEWS

A group of women can be interviewed monthly and questioned about their menstrual history. The difference between the number of suspected pregnancies and subsequent deliveries provides a measure of the abortion rate; however, women may give false menstrual data (especially if the nature of the survey is suspected), and genuine physiological and pathological causes of menstrual irregularities cannot be excluded.

PREGNANCY TESTS

In theory one of the most accurate ways of determining abortion rates is to collect urine at monthly intervals for pregnancy tests and correlate the findings with subsequent deliveries. Udry[14] and his co-workers in North Carolina found that only two per cent of women questioned at door-to-door interviews refused to provide urine samples. However, results have been slightly disappointing. The handling of large numbers of specimens proved unpleasant and tiresome and it was difficult to exclude false positives. The woman's own reporting of the pregnancy proved almost as reliable as the test. The group of greatest interest – that is, those women who denied being pregnant but had positive tests – also presented the most problems, as there was no way of dividing cases between false positive tests, unnoticed spontaneous abortions and concealed induced abortions.

Urine can be collected specifically to determine the incidence of abortion, or it may be collected as a part of a project to survey several aspects of community health. In the former case the sample of women willing to co-operate might be biased.

Biological evidence

The rate of spontaneous abortion is high early in gestation and evidence on spontaneous abortion occurring before the first missed period can only be obtained by the systematic study of hysterectomy and post-mortem specimens of uteri. Although difficult to undertake, existing studies in this field require to be repeated and extended and international collaboration should be sought to assemble a meaningful series.

Induced abortion in the total pattern of fertility regulation

Induced abortion is an unexpected and irregular event in the life of any one woman, but in a community it can be a relatively predictable aspect of fertility control. A certain amount is now known about the variables determining human fertility. The fact that the induced abortion rate is frequently the least understood makes it all the more important to review the other factors, as sometimes the abortion rate can be estimated by subtracting the births averted by alternative regulators of fertility from the total theoretical conception rate. By itself, this type of calculation can provide only an imperfect measure of the induced abortion rate, the inaccuracy of which is of the same order of magnitude as, or greater than, that of other methods. However, when used for making comparisons within a community – for example between urban and rural populations, between groups with different socio-economic status or at different points in time – it can be very useful. An overview of all the variables in fertility is also valuable as a check on other methods.

Biological and social variables

The number of conceptions taking place in a population is determined by biological and by social factors.[15,16] Biologically, the number of women at risk for conception is determined by the ages of the menarche and menopause, the prevalence of infertility and by variables immediately related to fertilisation. In many contemporary societies the age of the menarche is falling and that of the menopause rising. The prevalence of primary infertility, that is a man or woman who is sterile from the time of first intercourse, increases with age. Secondary infertility, i.e. failure to conceive after one or more conceptions have occurred, is more common in women than in men and is often related to post-partum or post-abortion infection. Probably three to four per cent of couples who marry in their early 20s suffer from involuntary sterility.

Numerous social variables affect the number of fertile women at risk for conception in the population. One of the most important determinants is the age of marriage. The mean age of marriage in India, 14.5 to 16.0 years, is within a year or two of puberty and may even precede it, although commonly the couple do not live together for some years, until after the *gauna* (or *muklawa*) ceremony.[17] In England and Wales in 1964 it was 22.8 years, but in the early decades of this century it was nearly three years higher. In the USA the age at marriage has fallen even more rapidly than in England.

In general, a low age of marriage is associated with universal marriage, a late age with a significant amount of celibacy. With the passage of time some marital partnerships will be broken by widowhood, divorce or separation. Patterns of migration may be significant in temporarily interrupting marriage relationships.

Social and biological factors often interact. Post-abortion infertility is mostly the result of illegal induced abortion. Social pressures encouraging monogamy, and the tendency to restrict intercourse to marriage partners means that, when fertile women are paired with infertile men, the woman will be barren. On the other hand in those societies where the divorce rate is high, as in contemporary Britain where 'serial monogamy' is becoming a significant demographic feature, the effect of infertility will be mitigated by reassortative mating.

The pregnancy interval

Within a potentially fertile union, a number of possible cycles of reproductive activity can occur. The interval between any two pregnancies will vary, depending on whether regular intercourse leads to (*a*) a conception ending in a live birth followed by breast-feeding, (*b*) a live birth followed by artificial feeding or a stillbirth, (*c*) a spontaneous or induced abortion, and (*d*) whether contraceptives are used to extend the time taken to conceive. In each case the pregnancy interval can be divided into three parts (Fig. 1).

The time taken to conceive is clearly unrelated to the outcome of the conception and is constant in categories (*a*), (*b*) and (*c*). Coital frequency is a variable in the time taken to conceive, but a relatively unimportant one. In one study from the USA, women claiming two coital experiences weekly took 7.0 to 8.5 months to conceive; those with five or more took 4.5 to 5.2 months. Most investigations of the average time taken to conceive (in the absence of contraceptive practices) have not taken into account variations in coital frequency but give results ranging from means of 2.1 to 11.0 months. Potter, in his careful review of the factors affecting the birth interval, accepts five months as the mean period of exposure to intercourse in a woman with normal ovulation prior to conception.[18,19] The

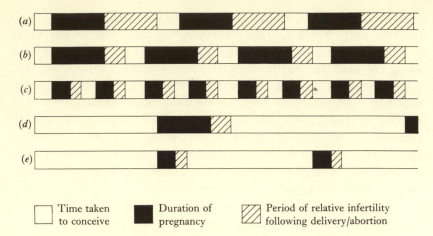

| | Time taken to conceive | | Duration of pregnancy | | Period of relative infertility following delivery/abortion |

Fig. 1. Possible cycles of reproductive activity. (*a*) Term deliveries followed by breastfeeding. (*b*) Term deliveries, or stillbirths, followed by artificial feeding or wet-nursing. (*c*) Spontaneous or induced abortions. (*d*) Term deliveries associated with use of contraceptives. (*e*) Spontaneous or induced abortion associated with use of contraceptives.

range of values arises because of the impossibility of eliminating social variables. The mean conceals an important skew distribution, with many women conceiving rapidly but a few taking well over a year. It is estimated that the average length of time taken to conceive rises by 0.07 per cent per month of the woman's age.

The role of spontaneous embryonic wastage as a possible determinant of the time taken to conceive is interesting (p. 52).[20] In the absence of contraceptive practices, significant variations in the pregnancy interval arise between those pregnancies ending in a birth and those ending in an abortion, because both the length of gestation and the time taken for fertility to return differ. Most induced abortions take place by the twelfth to fourteenth week or earlier. Among any group of wanted pregnancies, or of pregnancies that are not sufficiently unwanted to be interrupted, some will end in spontaneous abortion so that the *mean* duration of gestation will fall short of the textbook figure of 40 weeks. Conversely, spontaneous pregnancy wastage will extend the mean time taken to conceive.

Numerically, the return of fertility after the termination of conception can be the most important variable. The return of fertility after spontaneous or induced abortion is rapid. The return of fertility during lactation is slow:[21] ovulation is delayed and, when it does occur, fertilisation and implantation may be somewhat impaired. In some communities lactation is very prolonged, averaging, for example, 23.5 months in Nigeria 16 months in Bombay. While breastfeeding is an uncertain method of contraception for the individual, mainly because the return of ovulation is unpredictable, in a population it is an important factor. It must also be recalled that some deliveries terminate in stillbirths and, therefore, a more rapid return of post-partum fertility. In fact, stillbirths are often more common in agricultural communities, where lactation is prolonged, than in Western societies.

The Amish and Hutterites – Protestant religious sects that fled from Bern to eastern France and then to the eastern USA – are believed to do little to regulate their fertility.[22] The average number of pregnancies among women of completed fertility in the 1960s was 7.19 and the birth rate 33.3 per 1000. The mean interval from marriage to first delivery (excluding premarital conceptions) is 19.9 months. Subsequent birth intervals average 28.2 months. It is concluded that it takes an average of 10.9 months to conceive and post-partum infecundity lasts 6 to 8 months. Although those who attempt to escape being fruitful and multiplying are supposed to confess their sin before the church congregation, some practice of *coitus interruptus* may occur – and induced abortions are not impossible.

Human data on pregnancy intervals can be illuminated by observations on other primates. Unfortunately, such observations are limited to animals in captivity, a state which may itself alter reproductive performance. The mean 'service interval' between delivery and the next conception is 10.5 months for baboons and 11.8 for the rhesus monkey.[23] Part of the interval is taken up with lactation and, in the baboon, menstruation is re-established at a mean of 7.8 months after delivery, so the mean interval to conception is about 3 months. Following abortion in the first 3 months of pregnancy, menstruation is re-established within 60 days in nearly all animals.

Consideration of the variables determining the pregnancy interval demonstrates that, in the absence of contraception, it will require more than one induced abortion to avert a term delivery and, in the absence of contraception but in the presence of prolonged breastfeeding, it may require two (and could possibly require three) induced abortions to be equivalent to one pregnancy interval ending

Table 1. *Pregnancy intervals*

| | Duration in months | | | | | |
| | No contraception | | | Contraceptive practice[a] | | |
Component	Pro-longed lactation	No lactation	Abortion	Pro-longed lactation	No lactation	Abortion
Post-partum amenorrhea	11	3	1	11	2	1
Anovulating cycles	2	2	0	2	2	0
Ovulating cycles exposed to coitus	5	5	5	50	50	50
Pregnancy	9	9	3	9	9	3
Total	27	19	9	72	63	54

[a] Contraceptive practice assumed to be 90% effective.

in a delivery. If, however, the time taken to conceive is extended even moderately, say from 3–9 months to 12–24, then one induced abortion more nearly averts one live birth.

It must be emphasised that contraceptives are not to be described as taps which turn on or off the fertilising power of sperm, or even traffic lights controlling the release of eggs. They all have measurable failure rates and in biological terms *a contraceptive is an agent which extends the length of time taken to conceive* (see also p. 484).

In short, contraceptive measures alone are inadequate to control human fertility over a fertile lifetime. Induced abortion is an inefficient regulator of fertility, but combined with even a poor use of contraceptives it is a powerful method of reducing achieved family size and of ensuring that any fertility goal can be met.

Maximum conception rate

There is no evidence that human fecundity – the biological capacity for procreation – has varied significantly either from society to society or from one century to another. Although there are wide individual differences in the biological capacity to reproduce, these appear to be fairly constantly distributed amongst human populations and the overall pattern of achieved fertility – the actual number of children produced – is more fundamentally influenced by environmental, social and psychological factors than by any basic physiological variation.

Given a set of social circumstances which were uniformly favourable to maximum fertility, the number of births per married or cohabiting woman might be as high as 20. There is no known society in which such an average has been even remotely approached; at the 1961 Census, there were only 16 women in the whole of England and Wales who had this number of children. The highest recorded average for a whole community is 10 (amongst women living in rural Quebec at the time of the 1941 Census) but in most societies the average is well below six. Of course, six surviving children may be the outcome of a substantially larger number of pregnancies or births and, during the major period of human existence, high birth rates (though never approaching the biological limits) have been offset by high death rates.

This was the situation which prevailed in Europe during the seventeenth and eighteenth centuries and which provided Malthus with the evidence for his thesis that population and food supplies were kept in equilibrium only by the natural checks of war, pestilence and famine. By the late nineteenth century, owing to better diet, improved hygiene and sanitation and advances in medical care, the death rate had fallen dramatically. This new imbalance in the Malthusian equation was reflected in a closing of the gap between numbers of pregnancies and size of completed family, a process which produced a new and unique type of kinship structure. The Victorian era was the first and last period in human history in which the large surviving family was the rule. Nor did it persist for more than a generation; by the late 1870s the birth rate had also started to decline and, during the subsequent 60 years, mortality and fertility fell together to produce a new equilibrium of low birth rates and low death rates.[24,25] The role of induced abortion in this process is examined below (p. 154).

Rates and ratios

Abortion statistics can be expressed in a number of ways. The most useful is as a *rate* per thousand of the population (like a crude birth rate), or as a rate per thousand women aged 15–49 (like an age-specific fertility rate).

A convenient way of portraying abortion statistics, which are often based on hospital or clinic data with a poorly defined denominator, is as a *ratio* of abortions to births. Sometimes this ratio is expressed in relation to all deliveries and sometimes only to live births. It can be a vivid indicator, but it is also a dangerous one. For example, if most women are having six children and three abortions in a lifetime, the ratio is 100:50, but if the mean family size has been reduced to three children and the number of abortions remains three, then the ratio jumps to 100:100. The high abortion ratios in eastern Europe are often quoted in discussions on abortion, but it is commonly forgotten that mean family size is low in these countries, which is a factor inflating the ratios.

When displaying data over long intervals, it can be useful to show abortion rates and birth rates on the same graph and this method has been used frequently in this book.

Indices have been devised to relate abortion statistics to the probability of an individual woman having an abortion in a unit interval of time. Kapor & Beric have suggested an *abortion index*.[26] That is,

$$\frac{\text{number of abortions}}{\text{years of marriage} - \text{one year for each pregnancy}}.$$

An abortion index is restricted to women who have had abortions. It reveals a lot about contraceptive practice and can be used to separate out those women who rely heavily on abortion in the control of fertility, and have an index approximating to one, and those who use abortion to back up contraceptive practices, who have an index of 0.3 or less.

Tietze has created the concept of a *total abortion rate per woman*.[27,28] This is calculated as

the sum of the age-specific abortion rates × 5.

The multiplication by five covers the number of years in each age group, e.g. 15–19. The total abortion rate per woman is related to all women and describes the probability of an individual woman having one or more abortions in a lifetime. It is not difficult to establish that all communities use a combination of abortion and contraception. The society which lowers its birth rate purely by the use of contraceptives or solely by resort to abortion has no basis in reality. As will be seen in Chapter 3, it is likely that the relative use of abortion and contraception varies and that the relationship changes with time.

Some pitfalls
Under-reporting

Accidental under-reporting of spontaneous abortions is likely because the greatest fetal wastage is early in gestation and cases of early abortion can go unrecognised, or be ascribed to menstrual irregularities.

In the case of induced abortion, deliberate suppression of events is common. The topic is culturally difficult to accept for many women in most societies and the criminal status of the operation in some countries greatly reinforces this tendency. In certain cases, only a non-representative minority of induced abortions are admitted. Sometimes induced abortions are totally suppressed and sometimes they are passed off as spontaneous abortions. Most doctors know of the woman who denies interference until she passes a rubber catheter as well as a fetus. Sometimes internal evidence from retrospective surveys suggests the possibility of under-reporting, as when a higher rate of spontaneous abortion is reported among the upper socio-economic classes than among the less privileged, although any biological influence might be expected to act in the opposite direction if at all.

In Hungary a unique situation has arisen where it is possible to measure the degree of under-reporting. In 1966 a fertility survey was carried out on a 0.5 per cent sample of all fertile women. Among the questions asked was one about a past history of induced abortion. Overall, women reported only 55 per cent of the *legal* abortions, which, being registered by the operating surgeon, are known to have taken place.[29] If there is this high degree of under-reporting in a situation where abortion is legally available on request, and where it might be expected to have attained some degree of cultural acceptance, it seems reasonable to predict a greater than 50 per cent suppression of information in the reporting of illegal abortion elsewhere.

Over-reporting

Conscious over-reporting of abortion is very unlikely, but accidental over-reporting is possible. It is known that many more women attempt to induce an abortion than succeed in this goal. Among those who try to induce an abortion using inadequate methods there will be a percentage who miscarry spontaneously, but ascribe the abortion to their own efforts. Since at least ten per cent of all conceptions end in spontaneous abortion it follows that if ten women take sugar lumps as abortifacients one will 'successfully' abort. This statistical possibility is both a pitfall to the medico-sociologist and the basis of a global trade in supposed abortifacient remedies.

Registration of abortion among the unmarried

In several Western communities many, sometimes the majority, of induced abortions occur among the unmarried. However, it is important to remember that in all countries deliveries after marriage are registered as legitimate, whether or not conception occurred before marriage. Premarital conceptions are partitioned between illegitimate births and babies born within nine months of marriage. If termination had not taken place, an unknown number of those pregnancies which might have gone to term would have been legitimate, and, in looking for any possible consequences of abortion in vital statistics of births, attention must not be focused only on those born out of wedlock.

The core of the problem

As has been discussed above, the theoretical maximum conception rate is curtailed by factors limiting cohabitation (such as age of marriage), factors limiting conception (such as contraception), and abortion making its impact after conception.

Sartin, using a high estimate of the maximum conception rate, and Sauvy, taking a lower estimate, both conclude that cohabitation and contraceptive factors are of the same order of magnitude. Fig. 2 shows the number of girls surviving to the next generation.

In attempting to estimate the possible roles of induced abortion and contraception it is most revealing to take a population where the birth rate is declining from a biological maximum to a level characteristic of a contemporary developed country. When the birth (or death) rates alter, the age structure of the population may also change and this in turn will influence the number of fertile couples and the total number of births in the next generation. However, if the fall in the birth rate is relatively slow, these changes are not very large and a community could be envisaged with a constant population and a declining birth rate and, for the sake of the

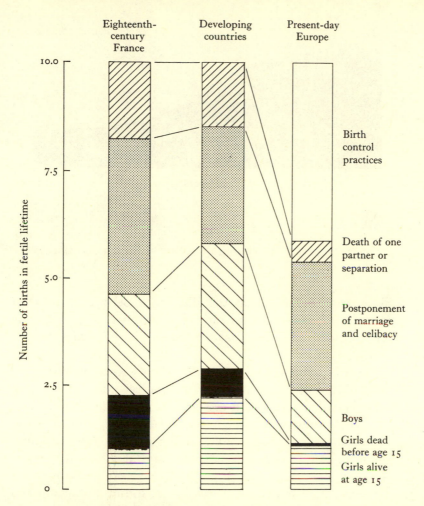

Fig. 2. Total fertility by various factors in three types of population. Assumed potential number of term deliveries = 10.

discussion, a fixed age structure and constant pattern of cohabitation variables. In such a community it is worth considering three hypothetical models.

(i) In theory, a community might lower its birth rate purely by the use of contraception. It might have access to a completely predictable and totally acceptable contraceptive, *or* everyone might be sterilised after having the desired number of children, *or* the unplanned pregnancies which occurred when using less than optimal methods might all be tolerated. In this situation the births prevented

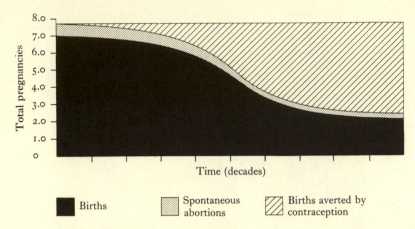

Fig. 3. Hypothetical community using only contraception to control fertility.

by contraception would equal the difference between the initial birth rate and the current birth rate. The number of spontaneous abortions would decline *pari passu* with the number of term deliveries (Fig. 3).

(ii) Conversely, a population might in theory lower its birth rate purely by induced abortion and never use contraceptives. As noted, the total conception rate would rise and the magnitude of the rise would be partly influenced by current breastfeeding practices. As spontaneous abortion is at its maximum prior to the most frequent time for terminating pregnancy, there would also be some rise in the spontaneous abortion rate (Fig. 4).

(iii) A population might use a mixture of induced abortion and contraception, in which case the relationship between the two practices could follow a number of courses. If half the couples use contraceptives and half abortion, the fall in the conception rate experienced by those using contraceptives could be offset by a rise among those resorting to abortion. However, a different pattern will emerge if all the couples use some form of contraception, even if relatively ineffective methods are used, because in these circumstances approximately one induced abortion would avert one birth. The spontaneous abortion rate would remain linked to the total conception rate. In short, when a community uses contraception combined with abortion the total conception rate will fall and the birth rate will fall even lower. An additional complication arises

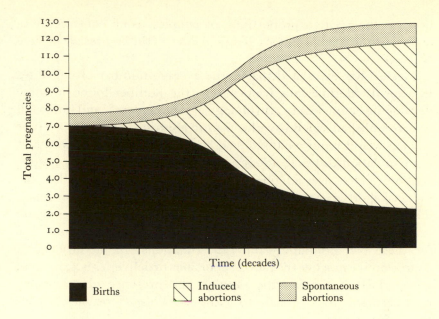

Fig. 4. Hypothetical community using only induced abortion to control fertility.

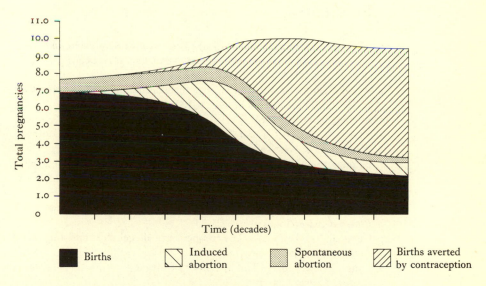

Fig. 5. Model community using contraception and induced abortion to control fertility.

because the relative proportions of couples using contraceptives and resorting to abortion are likely to alter with the passage of time (Fig. 5).

Tietze[28] has calculated that if the average number of deliveries in a fertile lifetime falls from seven (the number found in some developing countries) to 2.2 (biological replacement), and if this fall is accomplished solely by the use of abortion, then the average woman would require 9.6 induced abortions (Fig. 4). However, if the population comes to adopt a reasonable use of effective contraception (Tietze uses a figure of 95 per cent effectiveness) then the induced abortion rate is reduced, by a factor of 14, to 0.7 per woman. The remarkable role of contraception in switching induced abortion rates from high to low is well illustrated by calculating abortion ratios for these two profoundly different situations. In the absence of contraceptive practice the ratio of abortions to deliveries is 436.3 : 100. Using Tietze's figures, the ratio in the presence of reasonable contraceptive practice falls to 31.8 : 100. Potter[30] reaches similar theoretical conclusions.

References

1 World Health Organisation (1969), *Handbook of Resolutions and Decisions of the World Health Assembly and Executive Board*, p. 127 (Resolution WHA 3.6). WHO, Geneva.

2 World Health Organisation (1970). *Spontaneous and Induced Abortion.* WHO Technical Report Series, **461**. WHO, Geneva.

3 20 Geo. V, c. 34 (1929).

4 Sauvy, A. (1969). *General Theory of Population.* Transl. C. Campos. Weidenfeld & Nicolson, London.

5 Baumgartner, Wallace, Lansberg & Pessin (1949). 'The Inadequacy of Routine Reporting of Fetal Deaths.' Quoted in U.N. ST/SOA/Series A/B/12–28.

6 Goodhart, C. B. (1969). Estimation of illegal abortions. *Journal of Biosocial Science*, **1**, 235.

7 Goodhart, C. B. (1964). The frequency of illegal abortion. *Eugenics Review*, **55**, 197.

8 James, W. H. (1971). The incidence of illegal abortion. *Population Studies, London*, **25**, 327.

9 Johnson, H. R. M. (1969). The incidence of unnatural deaths which have been presumed to be natural in coroners' autopsies. *Medicine, Science and Law*, **9**, 102.

10 Wainer, B. (1972). *It Isn't Nice*. Alpha Books, Sydney.
11 Gebhard, P. H., Pomeroy, W. B., Martin, C. E. & Christenson, C. V. (1959). *Pregnancy, Birth and Abortion*. Heinemann, London.
12 Warner, S. L. (1965). Randomized response: a survey technique for eliminating answer bias. *Journal of the American Statistical Association*, **60**, 63.
13 Abernathy, J. R., Greenberg, B. G. & Horvitz, D. G. (1970). Estimates of induced abortion in urban North Carolina. *Demography*, **7**, 19.
14 Udry, J. R., Srisomany Keovicht, Burnright, R., Cowgill D. O., Morris, N. H., & Yamarat, C. (1971). Pregnancy testing as a fertility measurement technique: a preliminary report on field results. *American Journal of Public Health*, **61**, 344.
15 Potts, D. M. (1972). Limiting human reproductive potential. In *Reproduction in Mammals*: vol. 5, *Artificial Control of Reproduction*, ed. C. R. Austin & R. V. Short, p. 32. Cambridge University Press, London.
16 Guttmacher, A. F. (1952). Fertility of man. *Fertility and Sterility*, **3**, 281.
17 Baxi, P. G. (1957). A natural history of childbearing in the hospital class of women in Bombay. *Journal of Obstetrics and Gynaecology of India*, **8**, 26.
18 Potter, R. G. (1963). Birth intervals: structure and change. *Population Studies, London*, **17**, 162.
19 Potter, R. G., Wyon, J. B., Parker, M. & Gordon, J. E. (1965). A case study of birth interval dynamics. *Population Studies, London*, **19**, 81.
20 Sheps, M. C. (1964). Pregnancy wastage as a factor in the analysis of fertility data. *Demography*, **1**, 111.
21 Chen, L. C., Ahmed, S., Gesche, M. & Mosley, W. M. (1974). A prospective study of birth interval dynamics in rural Bangladesh. *Population Studies, London*, **28**, 227.
22 Sheps, M. C. (1966). Analysis of reproductive patterns in a demographic isolate. *Population Studies, London*, **19**, 65.
23 Asanov, S. S. (1972). Comparative features of the reproductive biology of hamadryas baboons (*Papio hamadryas*), grivet monkey (*Cercopithecus aethiops*) and the rhesus monkey (*Macaca mulatta*). In *The Use of Non-Human Primates in Research on Human Reproduction*, ed. E. Diczfalusy & C. C. Stanley, p. 472. WHO and Karolinska Institute, Stockholm.
24 Banks, J. A. (1954). *Prosperity and Parenthood*. Routledge & Kegan Paul, London.
25 Potts, M. (1972). Models for progress: United Kingdom (1919–1939) and China People's Republic (1957–1971). In *New Concepts in Contraception*, ed. M. Potts & C. Wood, p. 213. Medical & Technical Press, Lancaster & Oxford.

26 Kapor, M. & Beric, B. M. (1972). Personal communication.
27 Tietze, C. & Dawson, D. A. (1973). Induced abortion: a factbook. *Reports on Population/Family Planning*, **14**, 1.
28 Tietze, C. & Bongaats, J. (1975). Fertility rates and abortion rates, simulations of family limitations. *Studies in Family Planning*, **6**, 114.
29 Klinger, A. (1969). The Hungarian fertility and family planning survey. In *Family Planning and National Development*, Proceedings of the Conference of the Southeast Asia and Oceania Region of the IPPF, Bandung 1969, p. 68. IPPF, London.
30 Potter, R. G. (1972). Additional births averted when abortion is added to contraception. *Studies in Family Planning*, **3**, 53.

2
Spontaneous abortion

At conception everyone of us receives an equal contribution of genetic material from each parent. Every sperm and each egg carry a unique assortment of parental genes and every fertilised egg is an unprecedented and unrepeatable object. However, reproduction and embryonic development are imperfect processes, associated with what appears to be great biological wastefulness.

Nearly all laymen, and many doctors, think of human reproduction as the coming together of a perfect sperm and egg which go on to produce an embryo, which in turn slowly enlarges into a lovely baby. They recognise that occasionally mild developmental anomalies will occur, and, very rarely, serious abnormalities, but little more. Nature is not like that. Misunderstandings about the nature of conception and illusions about the 'miracle' of development are a misleading starting point for dealing with the clinical and ethical problems presented by abortion.[1]

The complexity of the vertebrate organism does not require emphasis. Faced with the need to transform the coded genetic information found in the chromosomes into the reality of another generation, systems appear to have evolved in which there is an excessive production of gametes (eggs and sperm), a generous number of which become fertilised, but only some of which will develop to term. At several stages in the reproductive process, screening mechanisms exist which eliminate abnormal products. It is as if a car production line was run with a labour force only partially capable of interpreting the complex blueprints set before it. Instead of attempting to make a perfect vehicle each time, the assembly line is frequently inspected and defective products destroyed.

For every egg that is fertilised and develops, many hundreds are wasted. For every sperm that fertilises, hundred of millions are lost. even though each individual gamete is unique. The detection and elimination of reproductive errors is a natural process, as essential in life as the body's ability to deal with infective organisms, or the property of the mammalian nervous system to store past information. Spontaneous abortion is one such process of detection and elimination. Clinically, it can be messy, but it is as natural as the healing of a wound or recovery from tonsilitis.

Spontaneous abortion
Clinical

Excluding ectopic pregnancies, where the embryo has implanted in a site other than the uterine cavity, any separation of the placenta from the uterine wall results in uterine haemorrhage. Clinically this appears as vaginal bleeding, which is usually the first sign that an abortion is taking place.

In some cases – those of threatened abortions – the bleeding is slight and, particularly if the woman rests, may stop completely and the pregnancy continue unaffected. More commonly, bleeding is followed by rhythmical contractions of the uterus felt as 'labour pains'. The bleeding increases and the contents of the uterus are partially or wholly expelled. The contractions and retractions of the uterine muscle clamp down upon, and constrict, the blood vessels that previously supplied the conceptus and, as soon as the uterus is empty, bleeding virtually stops. If it continues it is usually because material remains in the uterus or cervix when surgical removal is necessary.

Causes

MATERNAL

Severe generalised diseases and virulent infections, especially those causing high body temperature (e.g. malaria), can cause spontaneous abortions, but this is rare. More usually, the maternal factors that give rise to abortion involve local physical or physiological changes in the genital tract.

Certain congenital abnormalities of uterine development predispose to abortion without preventing conception. Another common cause of abortion, particularly in older women and certain racial groups, is the presence of uterine fibroids – benign tumours which develop within the uterine wall and distort both the uterus and the uterine cavity. Their presence interferes with effective implantation, with the development of the placenta, and is thought to predispose to an abnormally irritable uterus. In both these cases abortion tends to be recurrent, but the cause can often be successfully treated. A third local cause is incompetence of the uterine cervix, usually resulting from a previous incident where the cervix has been suddenly overstretched. It may follow normal delivery but is more likely to be a consequence of a previous dilatation of the cervix for uterine curettage or therapeutic abortion (p. 219).

The role of hormone deficiencies in spontaneous abortion is controversial. That progesterone deficiency can be responsible for abortion is unquestionable. However, the administration of hormones to a woman who has previously had an abortion, without first establishing that hormone deficiency was the cause, though it is commonly performed both in Great Britain and in the United States, is both illogical and potentially damaging. (The administration of diethylstilboestrol to pregnant women with a previous history of abortion is thought to have been responsible for cases of vaginal cancer in girls of the next generation.)[2,3]

When pregnancy occurs in the presence of an intrauterine device (IUD) the probability of spontaneous abortion is increased. Among 722 pregnancies in the Cooperative Statistical Program for the Evaluation of Intrauterine Devices, between 40 and 50 per cent are thought to have aborted spontaneously. In the case of an IUD with a tail, the abortion rate was reduced by removing the device, whereas, in the case of a tailless device, probing and manipulation increased the possibility of abortion to 80 per cent of the cases.[4] Unfortunately in these data, as in so many other studies of abortion, it is difficult to separate the iatrogenic from the biological; while a foreign body appears to increase the probability of abortion *per se*, the woman who is practising contraception by the use of an IUD is also highly motivated to terminate the pregnancy and, as Lewit says, the possibility must be borne in mind that women with a tailed IUD in place may 'manoeuvre the device after the pregnancy has been diagnosed and thus induce abortion'. A few of the pregnancies which occur with an IUD *in situ*, and persist beyond the first trimester of pregnancy, appear to be at risk to develop intrauterine infections, leading to fetal death and abortion and sometimes to severe maternal disease which may also culminate in maternal death.

All obstetricians can recall instances where spontaneous abortions have followed a strong emotional shock. Sudden news of death or injury to a loved one in war, or road traffic accidents, may be followed within hours by the onset of abortion. Sudden disclosure of marital infidelity may produce the same result. The mechanisms by which such psychological factors work upon the pregnant uterus are of great theoretical interest.

FETAL

In clinical practice no adequate cause is found for the majority of spontaneous abortions. Numerically, fetal causes are probably more important than maternal.

Specimens for anatomical investigation can be collected in one of three ways. The first is to examine the products of what are believed to be spontaneous abortions, although inevitably cases considered to be spontaneous will include some induced abortions. The second is to collect material from induced abortions. Here study is limited because certain intervals that are of interest to the embryologist are not yet routinely interrupted surgically and because both vacuum aspiration and dilatation and curettage damage specimens. The third is to investigate every uterus removed in a series of hysterectomy specimens. There will always be some women who were pregnant without being aware of it, although the number will be small, and it requires great skill and patience to recover fertilised ova or the early embryo when it has first implanted and is only a millimetre in diameter.[5]

Abnormalities of development can be assessed by anatomical and histological inspection of spontaneous abortions and/or by the study of fetal chromosomes. Both methods have their limitations. Many spontaneous abortions have been dead for some time, and the products of conception may be so damaged during the miscarriage that proper examination is impossible. In the case of chromosomal investigations, it is necessary to culture the cells for a while and, if (as quite frequently happens) growth does not occur, it is difficult to determine whether this was because of lethal abnormalities in the material, damage during abortion, or because the fetus had died so long before the abortion occurred. Overshadowing these difficulties are the obvious problems of collecting material.

Table 2. *Spontaneous abortion and abnormal development*

	Number abortions	Per cent abnormal
Kuwait (1968–70)	209	50.0
USA (1936–41)	1000	61.7

The first method of collecting material, mentioned above, is also historically the oldest. In the 1880s, the continental anatomists W. His and C. Giacomini called attention to the high incidence of abnormalities among embryos aborted in the first 10 or 12 weeks of pregnancy. By 1908 F. P. Mall[6] had assembled material from 434 cases of assumed spontaneous abortions and found that 37.5 per cent showed abnormalities. The great American embryologist, A. T. Hertig, in the 1940s and 50s carried on the study of early human developments with great thoroughness.[7-10] Work from contemporary Kuwait, where the criminal abortion rate is thought to be low and where there are important social and nutritional differences compared with the USA, makes an interesting comparison (Table 2).[11] Recently, it has been found that up to one-third of the pregnancies that terminate spontaneously have chromosomally abnormal fetuses. Many of these affected embryos would also be anatomically abnormal and some of those, classified as normal by histologists such as Hertig, might in fact have shown chromosomal anomalies had they been so investigated.

Human chromosomes consist of 23 pairs, of which 22 are identical and one pair is either XY or XX, viz. the sex chromosome. An abnormality often analysed is the occurrence of three chromosomes (trisomy) instead of the two normally found. Mongolism is one such abnormality. Trisomonies (other than those of the sex chromosomes) are found in 10 per cent of spontaneous abortions, but in only 0.2 per cent of the general population.

The largest series of chromosomal studies on human material comes from the work of Carr and his colleagues in Canada.[12,13] In a series of 227 spontaneous abortions, where it was possible to culture the cells, abnormalities were found in 22 per cent. Trisomonies were the most common type of abnormality.

TERATOLOGY

Teratology, the study of embryonic abnormalities and the factors that cause them, is a difficult science. Even gross associations – as in the relationship between thalidomide and limb deformities – have not always been recognised immediately. Experimental findings in one species do not always apply to another. An agent that damages the embryo at one stage of pregnancy may be without danger at another, may require a different concentration or duration of exposure, or yet again may have a deleterious action on a different organ system. Changes at the biochemical and molecular level that give rise to teratological damage are numerous and include genetic mutations, chromosome aberrations, altered nucleic acid function, enzyme inhibition, altered energy sources, lack of biochemical precursors, changed membrane characteristics and osmolar imbalance.

Most teratological agents cause a rise in the abortion rate or in the congenital abnormality rate at birth, depending upon the dose and the time in pregnancy when they acted. The range of potentially dangerous agents grows yearly and includes virus diseases, drugs, and ionising radiation. Cigarette smoking increases fetal loss and the prematurity rate at delivery.[14] It is not intended here that we review this large and important problem, except to consider one theme which relates sociology to physiology.

COITAL BEHAVIOUR

Once an egg has been released from the ovary, or the sperm deposited in the female reproductive tract, they undergo an ageing process. In experimental animals such ageing is associated with abnormal embryonic development.[15-19] Recent work suggests that over-ripe gametes are associated with an above-average incidence of human embryonic abnormalities. In 15 cases of congenital abnormality, Cohen[20] obtained temperature charts (which indicate the time of ovulation) and records of coitus for the cycle of conception. In five cases, ovulation and the fertilising intercourse were separated by 48 hours, in three there was a four-day delay and in one case, which gave rise to a trisomy, there was a five-day delay. In one, small, case-control retrospective study of mentally deficient children in the Netherlands, Jongbloet[21] found the greatest number of abnormal children had been born as a result of accidental conceptions to parents using the rhythm method, when, if fertilisation occurs,

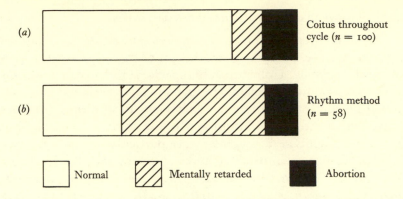

Fig. 6. Coital patterns and pregnancy outcome. Pregnancies among 35 couples with at least one mentally retarded child divided into (*a*) those conceived as planned pregnancies with coitus taking place throughout the menstrual cycle, and (*b*) those conceived as accidental pregnancies whilst the rhythm method was being used.

it is likely to be associated with the disjunction of coitus and ovulation (Fig. 6). There was no measurable change in the spontaneous abortion rate in this group, but Guerrero[22,23] found that 30 per cent of conceptions ended in abortion if coitus was delayed for three days after ovulation. He also showed that the sex ratio appears to alter as the time of ovulation and coitus become separated. If the fertilising coitus takes place eight or more days prior to ovulation, two-thirds of the progeny are male. It is not clear if this effect is the result of differential survival of male and female sperm, or differential loss of male and female embryos after fertilisation.[23]

It has also been suggested that use of the rhythm method of contraception is correlated with certain abnormalities of implantation, such as ectopic pregnancy and placenta praevia (the placenta implanted partly or totally over the cervix).[24–26]

Thibault[27] believes that 'human fertilisation should no longer be dependent on the chance of coitus', but when conception is desired coitus should be planned to coincide as closely as possible with ovulation.

LABORATORY AND DOMESTIC ANIMALS

Something is known about fetal and maternal causes of abortion in domestic animals and there is a large literature involving laboratory animals. Unfortunately, species differences are so significant in reproductive physiology that animal experiments give only limited insight into reproductive behaviour in women. Differences in the role of the corpus lutum and in the puzzling process of the maternal recognition of pregnancy are particularly striking. Nutritional deficiencies will produce abortion in animals, but have to be very severe. Certain types of maternal stress predispose to spontaneous abortion, e.g. mares mated soon after foaling miscarry four times as frequently as those mated later. Serious overcrowding in mice communities raises the incidence of prenatal wastage.

Estimates of early fetal loss in cattle, horse, sheep and swine vary from 10 to 60 per cent.[28,29] Similar findings have come from studies on prenatal wastage in rodents and on a population of wild rabbits.[30] In monkey colonies the probability of spontaneous abortion is partly related to the length of time that has elapsed since the last delivery. If conception occurs within one month, over one-quarter of conceptions will abort; if two to three months, one-fifth, but when the interval is over four months the rate of detectable abortions falls to seven per cent of all pregnancies.[31] The same variable may also be relevant in cases of human abortion.

Epidemiology of spontaneous abortion

Incidence

In the large majority of cases it is impossible to distinguish clinically between induced and spontaneous abortion, other than by relying on the history given by the woman herself. For example, in the early 1960s in one hospital on the outskirts of London, about 375–400 cases of abortion were admitted annually out of a total of under 1500 gynaecological admissions.[32] At that time only 6–12 therapeutic abortions were performed yearly. By 'superficial' history and findings, evidence of induced abortions was recorded for about 50 cases, but in 1963 all abortion admissions were interviewed by one person and, after their confidence had been gained, the women were more ready to admit interference. Nevertheless, one severely ill woman with renal failure maintained, right up to the time when the last rites were administered by her priest, that her abortion was spontaneous. When the fetus was passed, and she began to recover, a rubber catheter appeared with it.

Because of these difficulties only a handful of authors have conducted credible surveys of spontaneous abortion, assembling a reasonably representative cross-section of fertile women, taking care to exclude induced abortion as far as possible and setting out their results using *life-table* techniques.

'Life-table' methods were devised to aid the study of mortality statistics. It is possible to calculate the proportion of a population of individuals at a given age (x) who will survive for a unit time $(x+1)$, and the age-specific mortality rate for that interval $(Mx+1)$. The technique is very appropriate for the study of fetal death. In dealing with adult deaths this unit interval is commonly a year. In the case of fetal wastage, one- or four-week intervals are more appropriate. Owing to the uncertainty concerning the magnitude of fetal loss prior to the first missed period, an arbitrary starting point in pregnancy must be selected as the point of entry for the individual case in the population under study.

Although few reliable studies have been completed, they come from geographically varied countries. In 1953, French & Bierman[33] carried out both retrospective and prospective studies of pregnancy loss in the Hawaiian Island of Kauai, which has a population of 30000. In the prospective study, which gives a higher incidence of fetal loss than the retrospective one, women were encouraged to report their pregnancies to the study team soon after missing a period. Three thousand pregnancy histories were collected over three years. Twenty-four per cent of all pregnancies recognised at the end of the first lunar month of pregnancy ended in abortion. No attempt was made to partition spontaneous and induced abortion, but the induced rate was assumed to be low in the outer Hawaiian islands population – a supposition which has been partly confirmed since the repeal of the abortion law.[34]

Similar studies have been conducted in India and Pakistan, but here the women were visited in their homes, instead of being asked to report to the study team. In India, as part of the Khanna Study of family planning which focuses attention on many aspects of fertility in a group of Punjabi villages, Potter, Wyon, Gordon and New[35, 36] collected 1765 pregnancy histories which had been reported at monthly home-interviews. Some 105 pregnancies per 1000 ended in abortion. Despite the effort put into the study, Potter and his collaborators were wary of their own result and pointed out that there was circumstantial evidence of inaccuracies. In 20 per cent of term deliveries cyclical bleeding has been *reported* for more than 56 days after the last menstrual period, possibly because many women postponed admitting their pregnancies. By inference, another group probably never reported a pregnancy and sought an illegal abortion, or else had a spontaneous abortion that was never recorded. It is interesting that retrospective studies collected in the same area only revealed one-fifth of the fetal loss detected in the prospective studies.

Across the border in Lahore, Pakistan, Awan[37] conducted similar studies between 1963 and 1965. The area concerned was 8 km from Lahore and contained a population of 30000, mostly with an income *per capita* of less than 50 rupees ($6.8) a month. All married women were visited monthly and 1147 pregnancies were registered. As in Hawaii, the induced abortion rate was thought to be low, but in addition a careful effort was made to distinguish induced from spontaneous abortion. Some women admitted interference, others had clinical signs such as sepsis and yet others were known to have expressed regret at conceiving the pregnancy, or to have sought an artificial interruption (see also Table 9, p. 99).

In the USA between 1958 and 1960, Shapiro, and his co-workers,[38] (1962 and 1971) collected approximately 12000 cases of pregnancy from the records of the Health Insurance Plan of Greater New York. This plan covers antenatal care, delivery and postnatal services. It covers a cross-section of the population, although incomes are higher than in the general population and few unmarried girls use the Plan. Women usually seek advice early (75 per cent of women by 12 weeks) and induced abortions were thought to be few, although this last assumption may well be questioned in view of experience gained since the repeal of the abortion law. Shapiro and his colleagues analyse their data in two ways: first, as specific death rates for selected stages of gestation against the cumulative total of women who sought antenatal care at any time during pregnancy (any abortions that had occurred); and secondly, per 1000 pregnancies registered by the specified stage of pregnancy. The curves are widely different early in pregnancy, because most women only registered for antenatal care after the seventh week. However, the few women

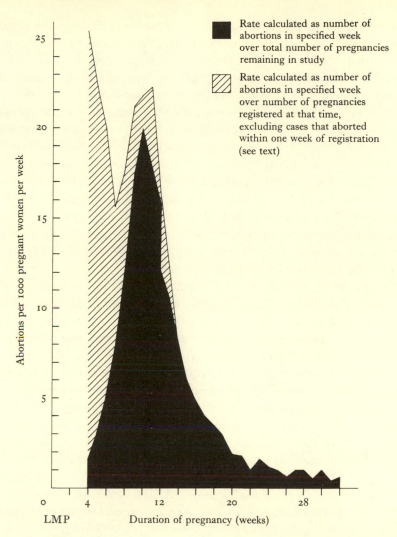

Rate calculated as number of abortions in specified week over total number of pregnancies remaining in study

Rate calculated as number of abortions in specified week over number of pregnancies registered at that time, excluding cases that aborted within one week of registration (see text)

Abortions per 1000 pregnant women per week

LMP   Duration of pregnancy (weeks)

Fig. 7. Spontaneous abortions by duration of pregnancy. LMP = last menstrual period.

who seek help early may do so for the very reason that they are about to abort. In order to reduce this possible bias, women who aborted in the first week after they sought antenatal care were excluded from the life-table calculations. Therefore, the rates shown in Fig. 7 may represent a low estimate of fetal loss.

Tietze, Guttmacher & Rubin[39] and Pettersson[40] have used populations of women in which the exclusion of induced abortion should have been particularly easy. In the first case, 1497 pregnancies were followed up in women who had discontinued the use of contraceptives in order to have a baby. Seven per cent aborted. In the second case, Pettersson followed a group of 463 women who had applied for legal abortion in Sweden. As the decision-making machinery in Sweden is very time consuming, sufficient spontaneous abortions occurred, whilst awaiting approval or refusal, to permit life-tables to be constructed. Twelve per cent aborted after the seventh week of pregnancy. It seems unlikely that many women resorted to induced abortion whilst actually awaiting a decision on their request. (In this particular series there were only two applications refused – although the refusal rate is higher in many other groups.) The discrepancy between the two studies is interesting; perhaps Tietze and his co-workers were dealing with women of less than average fertility, or they missed many early abortions.

A trial, using pregnancy tests, conducted in the area north of Bangkok, Thailand, provides an ingenious attempt to determine the spontaneous abortion rate.[41] About 1000 women were involved. The women were told they were being tested for diabetes and urine was collected at six-weekly intervals. Approximately 12.5 per cent of women were found to be pregnant on each test occasion. Nearly 39 per cent of the 15–19 year age group, but only about 7 per cent of the over 35 age group had positive tests. On questioning, only one per cent of women with positive pregnancy tests denied pregnancy. This is within the limits of error in pregnancy testing, but it is important to note that this small group contained half the women who were subsequently thought to have abortions. Of the women who were tested in the initial round and then again six weeks later, 21 had aborted; amongst those tested in the second round six weeks later, another five had aborted. In seven cases the pregnancy test ceased to be positive, but the women denied being pregnant on either occasion. If all the pregnancies that gave positive tests but were not followed by delivery are assumed to have aborted, and false positives are believed to be unlikely, then the maximum fetal wastage was 16 per cent of the total conceptions. However, the margin of error of the pregnancy tests overlaps the magnitude of the very variable the trial was set up to measure, and the results, while useful, may not be any more accurate than those from technically less sophisticated tests.

The several studies quoted can be supplemented with the relatively larger literature relating to retrospective clinical case histories,[42] such as that of Pearl,[43] who analysed 38000 pregnancy histories, and Crew,[44] who reviewed the then existing literature, for the 1927 World Population Conference, and found the unweighted mean of 20 different studies to be nine spontaneous abortions per 100 pregnancies, with a range from 5.1 to 12.9.[45] Two UK studies are worth mentioning. In 1949 Lewis-Faning[46] found a rate of 9.4 per 100 pregnancies (excluding induced abortion) in a study of over 8000 pregnancies. Maximum loss occurred in the second and third months of gestation. In 1958 Stevenson, Dudgeon & McClure[47] published a detailed study of pregnancy outcome from women resident in Belfast: 1127 abortions were identified among 1110 women and represented 11.8 per cent of total recognised pregnancies. The authors regarded this as a minimum estimate and in a study based on past obstetric history they found 15.8 per cent of pregnancies ended in abortion. Illegal abortion was assumed to be rare in the group under consideration, but this may well have been an unwarranted assumption.

The effect of age, parity and other factors

Several of the characteristics of women having spontaneous abortions can be determined more closely than the absolute rate. Results are qualitatively similar in most studies. In general, spontaneous abortion is most common among the very young, in women over 30 and of higher parity (Figs. 8 and 9). Ethnic, nutritional and other differences between groups are more difficult to unravel, as the differences being sought are of the same order of magnitude as the degree of inaccuracy present in nearly all surveys.

The findings of Shapiro and his colleagues[38] that abortion is more frequent in non-white women may reflect racial or environmental differences, but the possibility of concealed illegal abortion accounting for the difference seems more likely in view of the evidence available on New York women, who now have free access to legal abortion. In the absence of additional evidence to the contrary, it is reasonable to assume that the spontaneous abortion rate is similar in all communities and at all times.

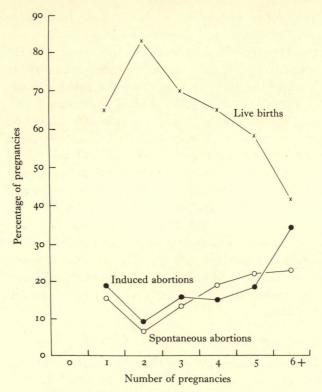

Fig. 8. Outcome of pregnancy by parity.

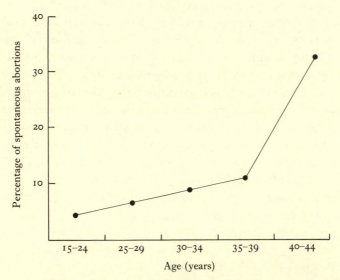

Fig. 9. Percentage of spontaneous abortions in different age groups in a number of planned pregnancies.

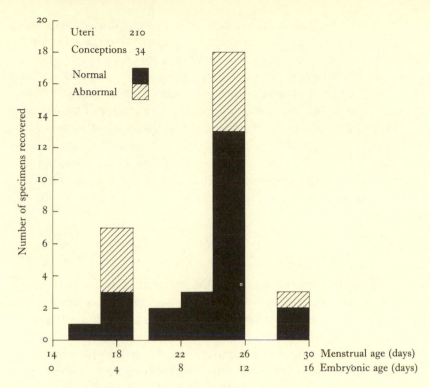

Fig. 10. Embryonic abnormalities (thought to be incompatible with continuation of the pregnancy) detected prior to and shortly after the first missed period.

Early embryonic mortality

Fetal wastage before the clinical or immunological diagnosis of pregnancy is possible is the most difficult of all to measure, but is of some importance as the limited evidence that is available suggests that the rate of loss is then at its maximum. On the basis of observations on hysterectomy specimens, Hertig & Rock estimated that 90 per cent of human fertilised eggs remained viable at the late blastocyst stage, 58 per cent proceeded to implantation, but only 42 per cent survived to the twelfth day of pregnancy.[8,9] (Fig. 10). The incidence of clinically silent, spontaneous fetal wastage prior to menstruation[48] has been measured by Bonachera & Botella-Llusia, who found evidence of products of conception in 2.4 per cent of a series of 1000 women having routine investigations for primary infertility.[49]

Unfortunately, the available data on very early human pregnancy are limited to small groups, or come from unusual or biased samples. The use of 'menstrual regulation' techniques and the recent emergence of immunological pregnancy tests, which depend on very sensitive radioactive tracer techniques and which are reliable before the first missed period, may soon provide a new wave of knowledge.

James[50] has analysed Hertig's series, together with other biological and clinical data, and concluded that one fertilised ovum in three perishes before pregnancy is recognised and one in four or five is lost after the diagnosis of pregnancy has been established. In total he estimated that one fertilised ovum in two is aborted spontaneously.

Conclusion

In summary, embryonic development is an inaccurate and unreliable process. It appears that a machinery has evolved for identifying, and eliminating by spontaneous abortion, the great majority of embryonic mistakes. Congenitally abnormal babies can be regarded as errors of development that for some reason were not detected and aborted during development. Mongolism, for example, probably survives because it is the result of a relatively *minor* defect in the separation of one of the smallest chromosomal pairs in the human cell. Other, potentially more damaging, trisomies are known mainly from specimens of early pregnancy, since they are virtually always aborted. At present approximately 1 in 50 babies has some degree of congenital abnormality, mostly of a mild order. If spontaneous abortion did not occur, perhaps one in ten, or even one in five, of all babies would be abnormal and most of the defects would be much more severe than those found in the present spectrum of congenital disease. A number of moral considerations flow from the proper understanding of the messy, but healing, process of spontaneous abortions.[51]

On the one hand, it is illuminating to consider that in the present state of medical knowledge not more than ten per cent of spontaneous abortions are the result of causes that are amenable to medical treatment. On the other, it is necessary to reflect on the implications of treatments that new technologies may facilitate. Already some gynaecologists perform routine amniocentesis on women over 35 and offer therapeutic abortion in cases of fetal chromosomal abnormalities. In contrast, supposing a drug could be discovered, as is biologically possible, which might prevent spontaneous abortion – how should it be used?

The most vociferous resistance to induced abortion has come, and continues to come, from Catholic thinkers, whose teaching in relation to reproduction derives from *natural law* not revealed religion. As biologists now read the statutes of natural law, they commend spontaneous abortion as an exceptionally common and inescapably necessary process. A final poignancy is added by the fact that the one method of contraception recommended by Catholic thinkers may well be associated with an increase in some of the very abnormalities which abortion attempts to eliminate. For millions of people the quality of life is diminished by this double misreading of nature's ordinances.

References

1 Potts, M. (1969). The problem of abortion. In *Biology and Ethics*, ed. F. J. Ebling, p. 73. Academic Press, New York.
2 Herbst, A., Ulfelder, H. & Poskanzer, D. C. (1971). Adenocarcinoma of the vagina. *New England Journal of Medicine*, **285**, 390.
3 Greenwald, P., Barlow, J. J., Nasca, P. C. & Burnett, W. S. (1971). Vaginal cancer after maternal treatment with synthetic estrogen. *New England Journal of Medicine*, **285**, 390.
4 Lewit, S. (1971). Outcome of pregnancy with intrauterine devices. *Contraception*, **2**, 47.
5 Hertig, A. T. & Rock, J. (1973). Searching for early fertilised ova. *Gynaecologic Investigation*, **4**, 121.
6 Mall, F. P. (1908). A study of the causes underlying the origin of human monsters. *Journal of Morphology*, **19**, 1.
7 Rock, J. & Hertig, A. T. (1948). The human conceptus during the first two weeks of gestation. *American Journal of Obstetrics and Gynecology*, **55**, 6.
8 Hertig, A. T. & Rock, J. (1959). A series of potentially abortive ova recovered from fertile women prior to the first missed menstrual period. *American Journal of Obstetrics and Gynecology*, **58**, 968.
9 Hertig, A. T., Rock, J., Adams, E. C. & Menkin, M. C. (1959). Thirty-four fertilized human ova, good, bad and indifferent, recovered from 210 women of known fertility. *Pediatrics, Springfield*, **23**, 202.
10 Hertig, A. T. & Edmonds, A. W. (1940). *Archives of Pathology*, **30**, 260.
11 Hathout, H. (1972). Looking at abortion material. In *Induced Abortion: A Hazard to Public Health?* ed. I. R. Nazer, p. 216. IPPF, Beirut.

12 Carr, D. H. (1967). Chromosome anomalies as a cause of spontaneous abortion. *American Journal of Obstetrics and Gynecology*, **97**, 283.

13 Carr, D. H. (1972). Chromosomal anomalies in human fetuses. *Research in Reproduction*, **4**(2), 3.

14 Mulcahy, R. & Knaggs, J. F. (1968). Effect of age, parity and cigarette smoking on the outcome of pregnancy. *American Journal of Obstetrics and Gynecology*, **101**, 844.

15 Blandau, R. J. & Jordan, E. S. (1941). The effect of delayed fertilization on the development of the rat ovum. *American Journal of Anatomy*, **66**, 275.

16 Witschi, E. & Laguens, R. (1963). Chromosome aberrations in embryos from overripe eggs. *Developmental Biology*, **7**, 605.

17 Witschi, E. (1968). Natural control of fertility. *Fertility and Sterility*, **19**, 1.

18 Shauer, E. L. & Carr, D. M. (1967). Chromosome abnormalities in rabbit blastocysts following delayed fertilization. *Journal of Reproduction and Fertility*, **14**, 415.

19 Butcher, R. L. & Fugo, N. W. (1967). Delayed ovulation and chromosome anomalies. *Fertility and Sterility*, **18**, 297.

20 Cohen, J. (1972). Personal communication.

21 Jongbloet, P. H. (1971). *Mental and Physical Handicaps in Connection with Overripeness Ovopathy*. Stenfert Kroese, Leyden.

22 Guerrero, R. (1973). Possible effects of the periodic abstinence method. In *Proceedings of a Research Conference on Natural Family Planning*, ed. W. A. Uricchio & M. K. Williams, p. 96. Human Life Foundation, Washington D.C.

23 Guerrero, R. (1974). Association of the type and time of insemination within the menstrual cycle with the human sex ratio at birth. *New England Journal of Medicine*, **291**, 1056.

24 Iffy, C. (1961). Contribution to the aetiology of ectopic pregnancy. *Journal of Obstetrics and Gynaecology of the British Commonwealth*, **68**, 441.

25 Iffy, C. & Wingate, M. B. (1970). Risks of rhythm method of birth control. *Journal of Reproductive Medicine*, **5**, 96.

26 Iffy, C., Wingate, M. B. & Takobovits, A. (1972). Post-conception 'menstrual' bleeding. *International Journal of Gynaecology and Obstetrics*, **10**, 41.

27 Thibault, C. (1970). Normal and abnormal fertilisation in mammals. *Advances in the Biosciences*, **6**, 63.

28 Corner, G. W. (1923). The problem of embryonic pathology in mammals with observations upon intrauterine mortality in the pig. *American Journal of Anatomy*, **31**, 53.

29 Perry, J. (1954). Fecundity and embryonic mortality in pigs. *Journal of Embryology and Experimental Morphology*, **2**, 308.

30 Frazer, J. F. D. (1955). Fetal death in the rat. *Journal of Embryology and Experimental Morphology*, **3**, 13.

31 Asanov, S. S. (1972). Comparative features of the reproductive biology of hamadryas baboons (*Papio hamadryas*), grivet monkey

(*Cercopithecus aethiops*) and the rhesus monkey (*Macaca mulatta*). In *The Use of Non-Human Primates in Research on Human Reproduction*, ed. E. Diczfalusy & C. C. Stanley, p. 472. WHO and Karolinska Institute, Stockholm.

32 Diggory, P. (1966). A gynaecologist's experience. In *Abortion in Britain*, Proceedings of a Conference held by the Family Planning Association, ed. T. Fox, p. 88. Pitman Medical, London.

33 French, F. & Bierman, J. M. (1962). Probabilities of fetal mortality. *Public Health Reports*, **77**, 835.

34 Smith, R. G., Steinhoff, P. G., Diamond, M. & Brown, H. (1971). Abortion in Hawaii: the first 124 days. *American Journal of Public Health*, **61**, 530.

35 Potter, R. G., Wyon, J. B., New, M. & Gordon, J. E. (1965). Fetal wastage in eleven Punjab villages. *Human Biology*, **37**, 262.

36 Wyon, J. B. & Gordon, J. E. (1971). *Khanna Study: Population Problems in the Rural Punjab*. Harvard University Press, Cambridge, Mass.

37 Awan, A. K. (1969). *Provoked Abortion Amongst 1447 Married Women*. Maternal and Child Health Association of Pakistan, Lahore.

38 Shapiro, S., Levine, H. S. & Abramowicz, M. (1971). Factors associated with early and late fetal loss. *Advances in Planned Parenthood*, **6**, 45.

39 Tietze, C., Guttmacher, A. F. & Rubin, S. (1959). Unintentional abortion in 1,497 planned pregnancies. *Journal of the American Medical Association*, **142**, 1348.

40 Pettersson, F. (1968). *Epidemiology of Early Pregnancy Wastage*. Scenska Bokforlaget Norsteds, Stockholm.

41 Udry, J. R., Srisomany, Keovicht, Burnright, R., Cowgill, D. O., Morris, N. H. & Yamarat, C. (1971). Pregnancy testing as a fertility measurement technique: a preliminary report on field results. *American Journal of Public Health*, **61**, 344.

42 Wiehl, D. G. (1938). A summary of data on reported incidence of abortion. *Milbank Memorial Fund, Quarterly*, **16**, 88.

43 Pearl, R. (1939). *Natural History of Population*. Oxford University Press, Oxford.

44 Crew, F. A. E. (1927). Concerning fertility and sterility in relation to population. In *Proceedings of a World Population Conference*, ed. M. Sanger, p. 214. Edward Arnold, London.

45 Tietze, C. (1953). Introduction to the statistics of abortion. In *Pregnancy Wastage*, ed. E. T. Engle. C. Thomas, Springfield, Ill.

46 Lewis-Faning, E. (1949). Family limitation and its influence on human fertility during the past fifty years. *Papers of the Royal Commission on Population*, vol. **1**, HMSO, London.

47 Stevenson, A. C., Dudgeon, M. Y. & McClure, H. I. (1958). Observations on the result of pregnancies in women resident in Belfast. II. Abortions, hydatidiform moles and ectopic pregnancies. *Annals of Human Genetics*, **23**, 395.

48 de Moraes-Ruehsen, M. D., Jones, G. S., Burnett, C. S. & Baramki,

T. A. (1969). The aluteal cycle. *American Journal of Obstetrics and Gynecology*, **103**, 1059.

49 Bonachera, E. M. & Botella-Llusia, J. (1956). The unknown abortion as a cause of apparent primary sterility in women. *Annali di ostetricia e ginecologia*, **78**, 34.

50 James, W. H. (1970). The incidence of spontaneous abortion. *Population Studies, London*, **24**, 241.

51 Potts, M. (1975). Natural law and planned parenthood. *Mount Sinai Journal of Medicine*, **42**, 326.

3
Epidemiology of induced abortion

The world literature on the incidence of induced abortion is difficult to survey because of the irregular quality of much of the data. The limitations of various types of source, reviewed in Chapter 2, should always be borne in mind. Additional analyses of some national records are presented in Chapter 13, where the relationship between contraceptive practice and abortion is discussed.

Records of legal abortions are considered before illegal, and the available material is broken down geographically. An attempt is made to relate abortion statistics to the general demographic development of the country concerned. For a number of countries, the abortion rate and the birth rate per 1000 of the population are illustrated. Abortion laws are only mentioned in so far as is necessary to explain abortion statistics and the main review of legislation is reserved for Chapters 11 and 12. Material related to the UK and the USA is further expanded in Chapters 9 and 10, respectively.

Incidence of legal abortion
The USSR

The USSR was the first country in the world to permit legal abortion on an extensive scale. In 1920, three years after Lenin came to power, the Soviet government decreed that any pregnant woman could be aborted on request. This first and only pre-war experiment in legal abortion lasted until 1936 when a restrictive law was reintroduced.

It is unlikely that accurate statistics relating to the years 1920–36 will ever be available. It is thought that 18–20 pregnancies in every 100 ended in legal abortion. In cities the percentage was higher: in

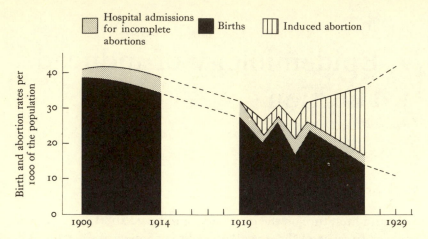

Fig. 11. Number of births, incomplete and induced abortions
registered in Moscow (1909–29). No records are available for
the years 1914–18. After 1927 the incomplete and induced
abortions were not registered separately. The law was made
liberal in 1920.

Leningrad in 1929 there were 39058 births and 53512 legal
abortions,[1] whilst in Moscow in 1934 there were 57000 births and
154854 abortions.[2] In the country as a whole, for the year 1934, one
report estimated 700000 legal abortions and three million births. The
Danish Abortion Commission Report of 1929, after taking evidence
from the USSR, accepted a rate of 8.1 abortions per 1000 of the
population, which approximates to the current rate found in Japan
and Czechoslovakia. Over 85 per cent of legal abortions were
performed in the first eight weeks of pregnancy and only one in 200
after 12 weeks.[3] However, the great economic and ethnic variation
in the country rendered nationwide data, even if they were accurate,
less useful than in other countries. Taussig,[4] who had visited Russia,
says abortion was rare among Kalmucks, Kirgis and Burjat people
– Moslem peoples of Asiatic Russia.

Gens[3] provides some interesting statistics for 14 cities. There is
no significant difference between Moscow (Fig. 11) and the other
cities. The sudden changes in 1922 and 1924 probably result from
irregularities of registration. It is also known that some women
came from outside Moscow to seek legal abortion. (In Gens' original
tables, the figures of 3809 and 3810 admissions for incomplete
abortion appear three years running, suggesting errors of tran-

scription, as well as of collation.) Nevertheless, within these limitations, a striking rise in abortion rates can be seen, associated with
a comparatively small decline in the birth rate. This pattern is
probably characteristic of a community which has a moderate or a
poor use of contraceptives (see p. 471).

In November 1955, shortly after the end of the Stalin era, all
restrictions on legal abortion were removed for a second time.
Regrettably, nationwide statistics on this second experience of legal
abortions are almost as poor as in the first.[5]

Demographic and economic diversity still persist in the USSR.
The country can be broadly divided into a series of 'European'
Republics with birth rates of 14 to 17 per 1000 of the population and
still falling, and a series of 'Asian' Republics with birth rates of 30
or more, which are steady or even rising. In the Baltic Republics
only one in 100 families has four or more children, while in Kazakhstan the corresponding figure is one in four. One-third of the
mothers with 10 or more children come from Moslem areas of the
USSR, which make up only 11 per cent of the total population.[6,7]

No doubt legal abortion rates also vary greatly. David[8,9] has
summarised the available information, which has been painstakingly
gleaned from a number of sources. The Russian publication, *Socio-
Hygienic Aspects of Regulation of Family Size* by Sadvokasova,[10]
quotes a four-fold rise in legal abortions between 1954 and 1966.
Berent[11] computed 7.5 million abortions annually in the USSR –
there are less than five million births. Sadvokasova maintains that
in the urban areas abortions exceed births, and Mehlan quotes
annual rates from her publications of 165 abortions and 61 live births
per 1000 fertile women. In the countryside the trend is reversed with
92 births per 1000 fertile women and 63 abortions. David[12] gives data
from a Moscow State University thesis by Katkova, for which she
studied abortion in a sample of married women over the age of 20
and living in an urban area. Between 1960 and 1965, 95 per cent
became pregnant at least once, 28 per cent had one abortion, 32 per
cent two abortions, and 14 per cent more than two abortions. These
high figures are confirmed by Sokolova,[13] who carefully avoids
providing absolute figures, but quotes the percentage of pregnancies
ending in abortion in Leningrad in the 1960s (Table 3).

Local nationalism persists in the USSR. Currently, the most
restless republics, Estonia, Latvia, Lithuania and the Ukraine, have
high abortion rates and low birth rates. In Latvia 93 out of every

Table 3. *Pregnancy outcome in the Leningrad district (1961–67)*

| Year | Pregnancy outcome (% of total live births and abortions) | |
	Live births	Abortions
1961	29.2	69.8[a]
1962	24.6	73.8
1963	22.9	75.5
1964	20.7	77.7
1965	19.7	78.7
1966	19.4	79.0
1967	18.3	79.9

[a] The remaining pregnancies ended in stillbirths or ectopic conceptions.

100 married women over 20 years of age report at least one abortion.[14] The politically less active central Asian Republics of Kazakhstan, Turkmenistan, Uzbekistan, Kirgizia and Tadzhikistan, contain 20 million people, have low abortion rates and high birth rates and are doubling in population in the course of a generation. In the long run, their claims are likely to become more insistent and more important.

Some of the factors leading to high induced-abortion rates in the Soviet Union are the non-availability of contraceptive services (oral contraceptives, for example, are not used) combined with an inadequate distribution of poor-quality, aesthetically unacceptable condoms. There is a high degree of urbanisation, limited living accommodation and a very high incidence of women employed outside the home.

Japan

Between 1638, when Shogun Ivemitsu closed Japan to outside intercourse, until 1853, when Commodore Perry forcibly ended the period of Seclusion, the population of Japan is thought to have remained constant at around 30 million. In the latter half of the nineteenth century, it grew to 45 million. During this period Japan

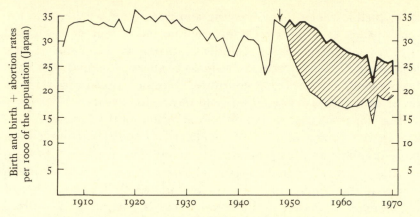

Fig. 12. Registered live birth and legal abortion rates per 1000 of the population in Japan (1906–70). In 1966 tradition held that it was unlucky to have a girl child (the Year of the Fiery Horse) and there was a decrease in the total births and probably some falsification of the birth certificates for girls born late in the year. (Arrow indicates year of legal change. Heavy line denotes birth+abortion rate; shaded area shows abortion rates.)

underwent very rapid industrialisation. By the standards of many countries attempting to undergo industrialisation in the second part of the twentieth century, the rate of population growth was relatively slow at about 0.6 per cent per annum, while the gross national product grew at 4 per cent per annum during 1880–90. In the 1920s the population passed the 60 million mark, was densely packed in relatively small islands and became one of the motives for the acquisition of an overseas empire.

When the Pacific War ended in September 1945 that empire was lost. The country had to accommodate three million civilian repatriates, as well as a similar number of soldiers. The income *per capita* had been halved since pre-war days and on top of her other hardships the country, like other post-war industrial nations, experienced a 'baby boom' as families were reunited. The illegal abortion rate rose and in 1948 a liberal abortion law was enacted (see p. 412). The new law was not seen as a measure to curb birth rates, although it provided the backcloth against which the birth rate fell. It was a liberal law, liberally interpreted. Registration is required but is incomplete. Reported abortions climbed from a quarter of a million in 1949 to well over a million in 1959, or two abortions for every three births. Since that time, the abortion rate has fallen and the relationship to improving contraceptive usage will be discussed later (p. 465). The degree of under-reporting has been analysed by Muramatsu[15,16] and the decline in legal abortions appears to have been a genuine one. It has continued into the 1970s: in 1973, 30000 fewer abortions were reported than in previous years.

The impact of contraception and abortion on the Japanese birth rate is well known (Fig. 12). The effect on family structure is even more dramatic and the Japanese household now averages 3.53 (3.29 urban; 4.17 rural) members. Households with four family members comprise the largest single group (21.5 per cent).[17] The number of big families with five or more members is declining and only 8 per cent of the non-farming households have more than three children. Nuclear families account for over half (55.4 per cent) of the total, this amount rising to two-thirds among wage-earners. The change from extended to nuclear families is one of the most profound that can occur and no doubt the resort to abortion in Japan has been an engine of social change during this transition.

Eastern and Central Europe

The socialist countries of eastern and central Europe changed their abortion legislation in the decade and a half following World War II (p. 404).[18,19] Beginning in 1947 with the German Democratic Republic, there was then a burst of legislation in Bulgaria, Czechoslovakia, Hungary, Poland and Romania in 1956 and 1957. Liberalisation sometimes occurred in stages, as in Yugoslavia where abortion became legal for medical reasons in 1951 and on social grounds in 1961. Always there are practical or legal restrictions on abortion to be performed after 12 weeks. The alteration of the laws occurred at a time of falling birth rates, amongst a generation who perceived life as one of economic hardship, when many women worked outside the home and when housing was in very short supply.

The registration of legal abortions is moderately good to exceptionally accurate (Figs. 13 and 14).[8,20-23] The demographic changes which have taken place have been unusually rapid, but they appear to be of the same type as those found in western European societies. When it comes to the socio-economic variable which controls fertility, the Iron Curtain appears to be particularly transparent. Berent[11] has demonstrated that the socio-economic variables affect-

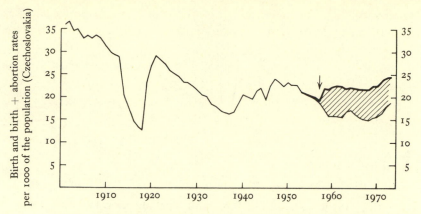

Fig. 13. Registered live birth and legal abortion rates per 1000 of
the population in Czechoslovakia (1901–73). Note the low birth
rates during World War I and the Depression, although
abortion was illegal. (Arrow indicates year of legal change.
Heavy line denotes birth+abortion rate; shaded area shows
abortion rates.)

ing fertility – such as urban/rural residence, education, housing
and female employment – are outstandingly similar to those well
known in western Europe and North America. For example, in
Hungary (1955), 20.7 per cent of rural births were fourth order or
higher, while the figure for the towns was 13.1. In 1967 the
percentages had fallen to 12.2 and 5.9, respectively, but the differential persisted. In Bulgaria 2 per cent of births to non-manual
workers were of fourth order or higher orders, and 13 per cent among
manual workers and 15 to 30 per cent among agricultural workers
were fourth order or higher. By income, those with one child were
on average twice as rich as those with six. With respect to education
the range was widest of all: 0.1 per cent births to families with higher
education being fourth order or higher, against 60.8 per cent of those
born to illiterates. Twenty-seven percent of women of fertile age in
Sofia are said to have had *two* or more abortions in a 12-month period
during 1967–68.[24]

The significant thing about eastern Europe appears to have been
the rate and magnitude of change in important variables. Before
World War II, approximately three-quarters of the population were
agricultural; today over half are urban. The most rapid change, and
probably the most telling from the point of view of fertility, has been

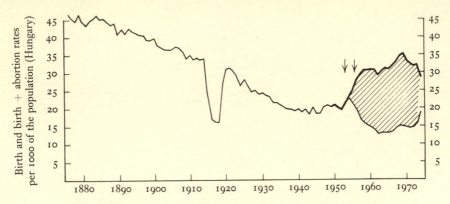

Fig. 14. Registered live birth and legal abortion rates per 1000 of the population in Hungary (1876–1974). (Arrow indicates years of legal change. Heavy line denotes birth+abortion rate; shaded area shows abortion rates.)

the increasing employment of women, and today in the USSR, German Democratic Republic and Czechoslovakia between two-thirds and three-quarters of all married women are at work. The effect of employment can be illustrated from the Protestant, industrialised, Czechoslovakian regions of Bohemia and Moravia where working women have on average 1.87 children each, whilst those who stay at home have 2.2.[25]

Scandinavia

For a long time the Nordic countries, especially Sweden, appeared in the eyes of the remainder of western Europe and of the USA to be places where legal abortion was common. The reality was somewhat different.[26–28] Legal abortion in Scandinavia is now over 30 years old, but came at a time of low birth rates and when the countries concerned had already reached the end of the demographic transition. Until recently the number of abortions performed was low (Figs. 15 and 16) and of more interest to the psychiatrist, so often involved in the decision-making, than to the demographer or social scientist attempting to review the variables in the control of human fertility. The small number of registered abortions shows that a law, by itself, is not the only factor determining the incidence of hospital operations.

Sweden and Denmark both went through two distinct phases. In the first, which lasted until the late 1960s, not very liberal laws were

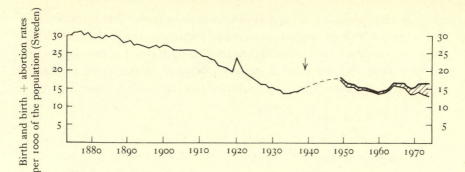

Fig. 15. Registered live birth and legal abortion rates per 1000 of the population in Sweden (1874–1974). (Arrows indicate years of legal change. Heavy line denotes birth+abortion rate; shaded area shows abortion rate.)

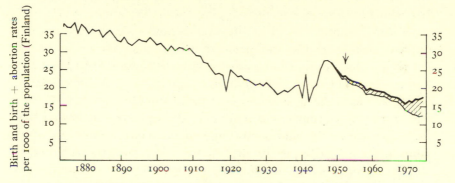

Fig. 16. Registered live birth and legal abortion rates per 1000 of the population in Finland (1874–1973). Note how the law was liberalised later than in Sweden, but medical practice is as liberal. (Arrows indicate years of legal changes. Heavy line denotes birth+abortion rate; shaded area shows abortion rate.)

cautiously interpreted; in the second, very recent, phase there was some widening of legislation combined with a significant relaxation of codes of medical practice. In Sweden for the first five years after the 1939 law less than 1000 operations a year were performed (a rate of under 0.1 per 1000 of the population). By 1950 the rate had risen to nearly 1 per 1000 but then it fell back to a new low of 0.37 per 1000 in 1960. In 1967 the rate again passed the 1 per 1000 mark and has continued to rise. During the same period the rate in eastern Europe and Japan was four to ten times as great. Within three years of altering the British law the abortion rate reached that found after 30 years of legal abortion in Sweden and Denmark. The same rate occurred within three *months* of the repeal of the New York law. In many ways, Britain and Scandinavia arrived at the same stage in the evolution of legal abortion practices at the same moment, despite the different times at which they crossed the starting line.

Switzerland

Article 120 of the Swiss Penal Code, in force since 1942, permits abortion if 'serious harm' would follow the pregnancy. It is open to a divergency of interpretations, and the incidence of legal abortion varies greatly between different cantons. In some Protestant cantons there is approximately one abortion to two births, in some of the Catholic cantons less than one abortion to 200 births and some cantons report no legal abortions at all. In the country as a whole in 1966 there were 21 839 legal abortions and 110 738 births.

Stamm[29, 30] estimates 50 000 illegal abortions a year in the country and suggests that the incidence of illegal abortion 'is lower in countries where women have ready access to the advice of a physician and to therapeutic abortion' than in countries, such as Switzerland, where access to legal abortion is very unequally distributed. The use of oral contraceptives in Switzerland is approximately half that found in the USA and *coitus interruptus* (and *coitus interruptus* combined with the use of the rhythm method) accounts for over half the contraceptive practice of the country. The pattern of contraceptive use and the birth rate are much like those of neighbouring northern Italy, Austria, the northern provinces of Yugoslavia and East Germany, where there are considerable data on the incidence of induced abortion, and Stamm's estimate of the number of illegal operations seems reasonable.

United Kingdom

The impact of the 1967 legislation on the number of abortion operations taking place in the UK is fully discussed in Chapter 8. It is noted there that the number of hospital abortion operations rose in response to the public debate preceding the 1967 legislation. Statistics for this period are available from sample surveys of bed occupancy carried out in National Health Service (NHS) hospitals and the number of private operations has been estimated.[31]

Registration of abortions since the Abortion Act are published for England and Wales and for Scotland. The Act does not apply to

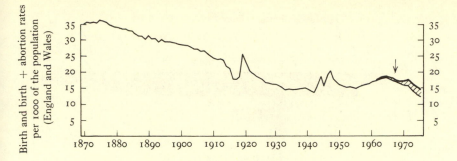

Fig. 17. Registered live birth and legal abortion rates per 1000 of the population in England and Wales (1870–1975). (Arrow indicates year of legal change. Heavy line denotes birth+abortion rate; shaded area shows abortion rate.)

Northern Ireland. In 1970 nearly 11 per cent of terminations were on women from overseas. A number of these women were probably resident in the UK at the time of conception, but many more visited the country to obtain the operation (see also Chapter 9 on the working of the 1967 Abortion Act). However, between 1974 and 1976 the number of women coming from foreign countries declined by 52 per cent. Abortions to residents of England and Wales fell by 8400 or 7.7 per cent.

United States

From 1967 to 1973 a variety of abortion reform and repeal laws were passed in over 20 states. A dramatic increase in numbers of legal abortions occurred from 1970 onwards. In 1973 the Supreme Court declared the remaining restrictive laws, and most reformed laws, unconstitutional (see Fig. 18 and also Chapter 10).

There is no nationwide system of abortion registration in the USA. However, in 1970 the Center for Disease Control in the USA Department of Health, Education and Welfare assembled statistics covering part or all of a selection of 17 states that then had repeal, reformed or restrictive legislation.[32] The material covered an aggregate of 1 213 919 live births and 177 113 legal abortions in 1970, giving a ratio of legal abortions to live births of 14.6:100. Considerable under-reporting of legal abortions is known to occur, and the true ratio in these states was probably nearer 25:100. When the ratio of reported legal abortions to live births was calculated for state residents (including out-of-state operations), the ratio was highest

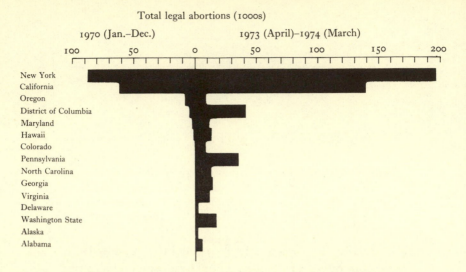

Total legal abortions (1000s)

1970 (Jan.–Dec.)   1973 (April)–1974 (March)

100   50   0   50   100   150   200

New York
California
Oregon
District of Columbia
Maryland
Hawaii
Colorado
Pennsylvania
North Carolina
Georgia
Virginia
Delaware
Washington State
Alaska
Alabama

Fig. 18. Total number of legal abortions in selected states of the USA in 1970 and 1973–74. (i.e. before and after the Supreme Court ruling).

in the Atlantic states of New York, New Jersey and Pennsylvania (17.4:100) and the Pacific states of Washington, Oregon, California, Alaska and Hawaii (16.4:100), and lowest in the west, south and central states of Arkansas, Louisiana, Oklahoma and Texas (0.4:100).

The experience of New York State was influencial throughout the country. Women from every other state of the Union, as well as from a number of foreign countries, had terminations in New York. In 1970, in 20 states in the eastern USA, the ratio of legal abortions to deliveries was 10:100 or over, largely as a result of terminations obtained by residents of those states who travelled to New York. In another eight states the ratio exceeded 5:100. The fertility rate per 1000 women aged 15–44 years for the USA as a whole was 77.5 in July 1971 and had fallen four per cent in six months. The relation between live births, legal abortions and illegal abortions for New York residents is considered on p. 138.

In all states where monthly records were available, the number of abortions doubled in 1970, both where the ratio of abortions to deliveries was high (as in Oregon, which had repealed its law) and where it was low (as in Georgia, which then had a reformed law cautiously interpreted and limited to accredited hospitals). By 1970,

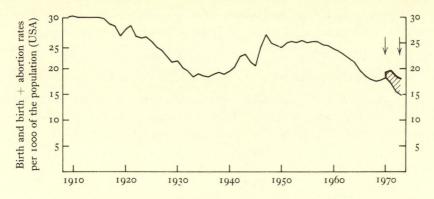

Fig. 19. Registered live births and calculated legal abortion rate per 1000 of the population in the USA (1909–73). (Arrows indicate New York and Supreme Court rulings. Heavy line denotes birth+abortion rate; shaded area shows abortion rate.)

in those states where data are available, the abortion rate per 1000 fertile women was higher than that of the UK or Scandinavia, but lower than that of eastern or central Europe or Japan.

Nationwide experience since 1973 has been reviewed by the Guttmacher Institute[33] and the American National Academy of Sciences.[34] The abortion rate in all states is illustrated on p. 349.

People's Republic of China

China contains a fifth to a quarter of the world's population – 750 to 1000 million in 1970. Abortion became legally obtainable in 1957 (p. 414) but national statistics on the operation have never been made available. China is unique in including abortion as part of a national family planning campaign. The population growth rate of the country is said to have fallen below two per cent per annum for the first time in 1966, which is a remarkable achievement equalled by no other country in a similar state of development.

Some small insight into the incidence of induced abortion is available from isolated statistics quoted by visitors to the country. A visitor to a hospital in 1963 reported 7292 deliveries, 1000 terminations and 2000 contraceptive clients in the year. In 1964 one 650-bed hospital in Peking had 28 beds reserved for abortion and performed approximately 20 abortions a day.

The family planning programme was revitalised after the Cultural

Revolution and all methods of fertility regulation are now freely available. Vacuum aspiration equipment is found in most of the 70000 commune hospitals.[35]

Other countries

A number of countries have liberalised their abortion laws recently and it not yet certain if the rate of legal terminations has stabilised or is still rising. In some cases, official statistics have yet to be published and assessments must be based on the experience of individual centres.

SINGAPORE

The number of legal abortions performed in Singapore grew from 1886 in 1970 to 6600 in 1974. At the same time, the number of hospital admissions for spontaneous and induced abortion has fallen. In 1964 there were 4295 and in 1973 there were 1243. There were 14.9 legal abortions per 100 live births in 1974. Singapore, like Britain or Scandinavia, changed her abortion law in the context of a society with a good use of contraception.[36]

In the Republic of Singapore, the overwhelming majority of deliveries are performed in Kandang Kerbau Hospital. (It is this hospital which appeared in the *Guinness Book of Records* as having the world record number of deliveries annually – although, since the family planning campaign began in Singapore, this dubious distinction has passed to a hospital in Caracas.) The Kandang Kerbau Hospital is also the main hospital for terminations in the State and the ratio of deliveries to abortions reflects island-wide experience: in 1970 there were 1410 legal abortions to 29379 deliveries; and in 1971 approximately 4500 terminations; one surgical team performed 4386 vaginal terminations, 44 hysterectomies and 30 saline inductions. Termination has been closely linked with contraceptive advice and the opportunity for sterilisation. In 1970 three women had repeat operations. A 'menstrual regulation clinic' was opened in 1973 and by 1974–75 was dealing with 18 to 20 patients a day.[37]

CANADA

In many areas of Canada, as in England, there was a marked rise in the abortion rate while legislation was under discussion. In London, Ontario, for example, there were four hospital abortions in 1962, 42 in 1968 and 119 in 1969. Throughout the country, in the first 12 months after abortion law reform (September 1969 to August 1970), there were 4375 legal abortions and 364300 live births: a ratio of one abortion to 83 deliveries or approximately one-tenth of the corresponding ratio in England and Wales during the first year of operation of the 1967 Act. The number of legal abortions rose to 11152 in 1970, to 30949 in 1971 (8.3 per 100 deliveries) and 43200 in 1973 (12.9 per 100 deliveries). However, the average conceals wide variations. In British Columbia in 1971–72 there were 23.7 abortions to 100 live births, but Newfoundland and Prince Edward Island only 2.0. Within states, there was also variation between hospitals. Some hospitals set arbitrary limits to the number of abortions they would perform each month, and many excluded non-residents. There was very little crossing of provincial boundaries. For example, of the 5568 operations performed in Ontario in 1970, only 54 were on residents of other provinces.[38]

The magnitude of the change that has overtaken the country can be judged by the statistics of British Columbia. In 1965, before the law was changed, there were 98 legal abortions for approximately two million people. By the 1970s there were 8200 abortions. As in many places, changes in attitudes towards abortion have been accompanied by liberalisation of all attitudes towards fertility regulation. In Vancouver General Hospital in 1965 there were 20 legal abortions and 25 sterilisations. By 1972 there were approximately 3000 legal abortions and approximately 1000 women received tubal ligation. The number of vasectomies also rose in the Province. Whereas throughout Canada, before the law was changed, abortion caused approximately 10 per cent of all maternal deaths, by 1972 there was only one abortion death amongst the 54 women who died as a result of pregnancy and delivery.

The Canadian health system will meet the costs of medical treatment undertaken outside the country and many Canadian women from conservative states travel to the USA. About 5500 Canadian residents had abortions in New York State in 1973.

AUSTRALIA

The law in South Australia was liberalised in 1969. In 1970, 1330 terminations were performed; in 1971, 2519; and the 1972 figure appears as if it will be at the same level. The distribution of unmarried women (over 50 per cent) and age groupings are much as in Britain. When illegitimate deliveries, pregnancies conceived before marriage, and abortions on single women are combined, the total extra-nuptial conception rate accounts for 77 per cent of known conceptions in the 15–19 age group, 21 per cent in the 20–24 age group and only 9 per cent in the 25–29-year-olds.[39] The problem of the young unmarried pregnant girl in Western society and the effect of liberal abortion legislation is further discussed on p. 110.

TUNISIA

Tunisia changed its abortion laws in 1965. By 1968, after an administrative initiative had been taken to make sure the law was implemented, there were 2200 terminations annually (1.2 abortions to every 100 deliveries). In 1969 the number rose slightly to 2862,[40] but by 1974 it had rocketed to 12400, or between six and seven legal abortions per 100 live births[41] (Fig. 20).

INDIA

The implementation of a reformed Indian abortion law began in the first half of 1972. In spirit, the law is a slightly more liberal modification of the 1967 British Act. In practice, the initial regulations concerning supervision and reporting of the operation were complex and unrealistic. While the Indian parliament had spoken of one to two million illegal abortions in the country annually, it seems that only 24000 legal abortions were registered in the first year (1972–73).[42,43] Probably many surgeons preferred to do the next operation, rather than complete the paperwork on the previous procedure, and other doctors will have avoided reporting any cases at all because they will have chosen not to register their institutions, as registration could be both difficult and time consuming. A desire for too much detailed information about legal operations aborted the possibility of gathering useful data and led to bureaucratic infertility in the field of statistics. In 1974–75, 90700 abortions were registered. In 1975, the regulations concerning registration and the administration of licensed places were revised, and both the total number of operations and the accuracy of registration may be expected to improve.

CUBA

Culturally, and from the point of view of religion, Cuba is part of Latin America. It is Catholic, poor, has a high birth rate and a low death rate. Since the late 1960s, *de facto* abortion on demand has been available. The number of operations has climbed steadily from a ratio of 11.7 to 100 live births in 1968 to 66 in 1974.[44] This latter figure (corresponding to 131 500 abortions nationwide) is at a level characteristic of many eastern European countries when they first reformed their abortion laws and is typical of a community beginning to control its fertility (Fig. 20). The Cuban statistics add verisimilitude to the estimates of illegal abortions from other Latin American countries.

Countries with restrictive abortion laws

Therapeutic abortion is occasionally performed in countries with strict anti-abortion laws. In Belgium all abortions are illegal, even when the life of the mother is to be saved, but Hubinont reports one abortion in 174 deliveries in his department at the Saint-Pierre University Hospital, Brussels, in 1958–61, and one in 128 over the years 1963–66.[45] In France the national therapeutic abortion ratio prior to the 1975 reform was believed to be 0.05 to 0.5 operations to 1000 deliveries.[46]

Although it is generally felt that the problem of illegal abortion is becoming more serious in many developing countries, therapeutic abortion often remains uncommon. For example, in the Caribbean few therapeutic abortions are performed, usually at a ratio of approximately one to 500 deliveries. In 1971 in Jamaica there were 20 therapeutic abortions, 19 in Trinidad, 10 in Guyana but 65 in Barbados. Curaçao, the former Dutch colony, is an exception following the unwritten precedent of its mother country in that the number of hospital abortions has risen rapidly in the early 1970s. In Curaçao there were approximately 500 hospital abortions in the year 1971–72.[47]

Israel is another country which has inherited the British law of Queen Victoria, this time through the years of the British Mandate prior to 1948. Nevertheless, since a 1952 District Court case in Haifa, the attorney general has not prosecuted doctors performing abortions, except in extreme circumstances. The law is not enforced and doctor-performed abortions are readily available, at least to the more prosperous social groups. In 1966, 1967 and 1968 there were approximately 47000 live births annually and an estimated 26000 abortions each year – 1200 in hospitals and 25000 performed in private clinics. Only one death due to induced abortion was recorded during three years. The proportion of women having at least one abortion is highest (51.8 per cent) for immigrants from Europe and

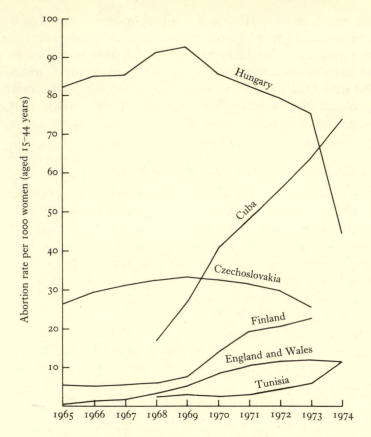

Fig. 20. Legal abortions per 1000 women aged 15–44 for selected countries (1965–74).

the USA and lowest for women born in Asia and Africa. Thirty per cent of Israel-born women report at least one induced abortion. Only 1.3 per cent of all Arab women report having an induced abortion.[48, 49]

Bickers estimated that there was one therapeutic abortion to 1000 deliveries in the American University of Beirut[50] and Hathout reported nine legal abortions among 32 000 deliveries in the late 1960s in Kuwait. (There were 8000 admissions for spontaneous and illegal abortion over the same interval.)[51]

As already noted, hospital abortion rates are a useful indicator of national opinion on abortion, rates often rising *before* legal changes. The USA is a good example of this trend. A survey of legal abortions made between 1963 and 1968, covering a sample of hospitals with three million deliveries a year, showed a rise in legal abortion ratios from 1.27–5.19:1000 deliveries.[52] In Melbourne (Victoria, Australia) there were about 20 terminations annually at the Woman's Hospital in the 1960s. In 1972 an estimated 500 were carried out and the rate in the state (where the law is restrictive) approximated to that in South Australia (where the law has been reformed).

Figs. 11 to 17 and Fig. 19 illustrate the role of legal abortion against the background of the demographic transition in selected developed countries. Fig. 20 illustrates abortion rates per 1000 fertile women and shows some of the trends that can be discerned in recent years. Cuba and Tunisia are the only developing countries for which comparable statistics are available.

Incidence of illegal abortions

Developed countries in the twentieth century

With few exceptions, data on induced abortion prior to 1900 are mainly qualitative in type (see Chapter 5). For the greater part of the twentieth century, induced abortion has been illegal in most developed nations, but some attempts have been made to estimate the magnitude of the problem. While the epidemiological work that has taken place has not been commensurate with the health and demographic implications of the problem, the universality of induced abortion in nations undergoing the demographic transition ensures that some data are available for nearly all countries. Summed, these data tell a consistent story, even though in isolation one nation's observations may appear a doubtful foundation for any conclusions. Additionally, the pattern of illegal abortions partially uncovered may be checked against the experience of those countries that, at varying stages of the demographic transition, have come to permit legal abortion on social as well as medical grounds.

BRITISH ISLES (1900–67)

The iceberg of induced abortion may not have risen any higher from the water as the nineteenth century gave way to the twentieth in Britain, or have grown any bigger, but perhaps the fog that had previously surrounded it grew a little thinner. Detailed studies of the factors controlling the birth rate began to be made.[53]

Table 4. *UK: incidence of abortion (spontaneous and induced) in hospital and birth control clinic records*

Year	Locality	Number Women	Number Pregnancies	Percentage of pregnancies ending in abortion
1845	Manchester	2000	8681	14.1
1897–98	Oxley	898	3964	15.7
1903	Birmingham	6000	14430	16.0
1909–13	Birmingham	3009	11430	17.7
1924–28	Birmingham	1000	3228	18.4
1925–29	Sheffield	6444	20260	17.4
1920s–30s	Society for the Provision of Birth Control Clinics	10000	34959	9.7
1936	London	17931	22559	6.8
1937	London	635	—	20.8

Perhaps the best was Elderton's careful study of the factors leading to a decline in the birth rate in northern England in the years immediately prior to World War I.[54] It emphasised the role of abortion and its relatively ready availability, but did not attempt to assign to it any numerical value as a factor in the decline.

From the second decade of the century onwards, several authors published data based on clinical records and hospital admissions (Table 4). A British Medical Association Committee attempted to review the topic of abortion in 1936 but added little new material.[55] One year later, a Ministry of Health, *Report of an Investigation into Maternal Mortality* cautiously declined to separate induced from spontaneous abortions but concluded 'From statements made in the areas visited . . . the impression has been gained that the practice of artificially-induced abortion (a) is frequent and appears to be increasing; (b) is more prevalent in some districts than others; (c) is not restricted to any one class.'[56]

Much of the early twentieth-century evidence was summarised in the *Report of the Inter-Departmental Committee* in abortion,[57] and Glass, writing in 1940, gave some additional information culled from papers presented to that committee, but otherwise unpublished.[58] The Committee estimated a total of 110000–150000 abortions a year and suggested 40 per cent of these were illegal. There were approximately 600000 deliveries annually.

T. N. Parish set a new standard of academic and clinical excellence in the analysis of abortion material when he published a paper entitled, 'A thousand cases of abortion' in the *Journal of Obstetrics and Gynaecology of the British Empire* in 1935.[59] His study was based on cases of abortion admitted to St Giles Hospital in Camberwell. At that time, admissions for abortion constituted two per cent of all hospital admissions in the London area[60] and the total death rate from abortion for England and Wales stood at over 450 per annum, of which more than 250 were notified as being septic. In Camberwell the admissions rose from 147 in 1924 to 293 in 1934, and in the same period the birth rate for the borough declined from 18.2 to 13.2 per 1000. Another investigator, Pierce,[61] used ectopic pregnancy as an ingenious measure of the conception rate in the area and noted that between 1923 and 1928 there was a 50 per cent increase in hospital admissions for abortion relative to admissions for ectopics. In Parish's series, criminal interference was admitted in 486 of the 1000 cases, in 246 there was no evidence of interference and in the remainder it was impossible to comment on the etiology of the condition. Self-induced abortion appeared to be reported more readily than the activities of the criminal abortionist. Women with sepsis would be more likely to enter hospital than those who had more successful operations. In contemporary Chile it is thought that one-third of all criminal abortions find their way to hospital (p. 442), but whether this sort of proportion existed in the days before antibiotics is difficult to say.

Imperfection of statistics on illegal abortion has always led to genuine differences of interpretation. In 1937 the *Medical Press and Circular* (a British medical periodical which ran for over a century) published a series of papers on 'Declining fertility'. Possibly they were inspired by the Prime Minister's Budget speech for that year in which he looked forward with apprehension to the time 'when the countries of the British Empire will be crying out for more citizens of the right breed, and when we in this country will not be able to supply the demand'. In one article Professor Young,[62] a member of the Population Investigation Committee, reviewed 'The part played by contraception and abortion'. He disagreed with the view that induced abortion had increased in the preceding decade. At the same time, he noted that, while maternal deaths from childbearing were declining, abortion deaths remained constant, and, as a ratio of total maternal deaths, abortion deaths rose from

Table 5. *Five hundred consecutive cases of abortion, Camberwell, London (1962–64)*

	Total number of abortions	Number of illegally induced abortions	Percentage induced abortions
	500	300	60
Religion			
Protestant	334	200	60
Roman Catholic	105	63	60
Jewish	1	—	—
Race			
White	340	238	70
Black	100	38	38
Cypriot	60	24	40

10.5 in 1930 to 18.2 to 100 deaths in 1935. Young attempted to escape from this paradox by invoking arguments about 'innate fertility' and in emphasising the effect of nutrition on reproduction.

A handful of studies on abortion preceded[63] and succeeded World War II. Obeng also studied abortion cases admitted in the Camberwell area, London.[64] Between 1956 and 1966, admissions for abortion rose from 210 to 340 per annum. Obeng made a careful study of 500 consecutive cases of abortion admitted between 1962 and 1964 (Table 5). It is one of the few relatively fixed points in the socio-medical history of abortion in the years prior to the 1967 Act. Each case was interviewed on admission. Eighty-four per cent of the women were married, most had one or more children, belonged to social classes IV or V and were between 21 and 30 years old. There was no correlation between religion and the probability of abortion. Two hundred and fifteen admitted interference with the pregnancy and in another 85 there was trauma to the genital tract or infection diagnostic of induced abortion so that, overall, 300 cases (60 per cent) were induced abortions. In half of the remainder, a firm diagnosis of spontaneous abortion was made and the remaining 20 per cent were classified as doubtful. Certain collateral evidence confirmed the overall picture: for example, 12 per cent of the women had been booked for antenatal care and this subgroup tended to be admitted relatively later than the other women, suggesting that mainly they had spontaneous abortions.

Among the pressures in favour of abortion was one that may have been underestimated elsewhere, namely unpleasant experiences at previous term deliveries. Eighteen women confessed to inducing abortion to avoid 'going through another pregnancy and labour like that again' and in two cases the women had a history of heart disease but had been refused sterilisation.

A national opinion poll carried out in 1966 on a random sample of 3500 women showed that of the 2000 women who completed the questionnaire, 91 were women who had had at least one abortion. By extrapolation, it was estimated that a minimum 30000 women resort to backstreet abortionists. Women are more likely to conceal abortions than to invent them, and there is evidence that confidential surveys such as this underestimate the incidence of abortions.

Since the reform of the abortion law in the UK, a significant number of women have come from the Republic of Ireland to seek abortion in Britain (see Chapter 9). Undoubtedly induced abortions have always happened in Eire, although there has not been the intellectual climate to attempt to measure their incidence. In an Irish pastoral letter of 1931, the Most Rev. Dr Fogarty of Killaloe referred to:

> illegitimate intercourse between the sexes. This sin is surely bad enough in itself, but when it is followed by wicked mothers or their friends bordering the savagery of King Herod and murdering newborn infants to hide their shame or to save trouble, you have a crime of shocking depravity...the administration of the law is entirely too indulgent with this inhuman and disgusting criminality.[65]

UNITED STATES

In the USA, as in the UK, clinical observation provides some witness to the scale of illegally induced abortion.[66-69] From one in ten to one in four of pregnancies usually ended in abortion. Findley provided one clinical judgement in 1922 of the proportion thought to be illegal: '...abortions in the United States have become so common that, instead of being regarded as a crime, it is a laudable and justifiable means of limiting the size of families'.[70]

A few observers designed special surveys of pregnancy

Table 6. *Illegal abortions: USA married white women*
(*1925–50*)

Decade analysed[a]	Induced abortions	Spontaneous abortions	Total abortions	(*n*)[b]
1925	23.6	14.5	37.9	(827)
1930	24.3	13.3	37.6	(1074)
1935	18.3	16.9	35.2	(1282)
1940	13.5	18.4	31.9	(1372)
1945	12.3	18.1	30.4	(1070)
1950	10.4	19.4	29.8	(423)

[a] The data were broken down to give averages for overlapping ten-year intervals.
[b] *n* = Total number of pregnancies reported.

wastage.[71–73] Stix[72] found in 1935 that among 3106 conceptions, 23.3 per cent were reported to end in induced abortion, and 1.3 per cent in stillbirths. The data are much like that already noted for Britain. Pearl brought a good deal of academic insight to the problem of abortion.[74] In studies in New York and Chicago, he found a pregnancy wastage of 13.3 and 11.9 per cent, respectively, although only 2.8 and 1.6 pregnancies in 100 admitted illegal interference. In his *Natural History of Population*, he reviewed more extensive data and discerned certain important socio-economic correlates of induced abortion.[75]

The archives of Kinsey's Institute for Sex Research include retrospective data on pregnancy and abortion extending back to the 1920s and collected between 1938 and 1955.[76] Unfortunately, the pioneer nature of the group's work made it impossible to use a random sample of the population. Instead the sample is biased towards upper socio-economic groups, while the southern and western states are under-represented. Nevertheless, within the sample, the data are more satisfactory than others that are available. They are particularly interesting in showing a high illegal abortion rate among married women in the 1920s and early 1930s and a relatively low one in the 1950s (Table 6). Among married black women, the induced-abortion rate was lower than among white women. Since the Gebhard study, this relationship appears to have been reversed. In 1970, in the last study in the USA before the widespread availability of legal abortion, Abernathy and his co-workers found a high rate of illegal abortion throughout the population.[77] The survey used the randomised response method described previously (p. 28), applied to a probability sample of 1300 women aged 18 to 44 in urban North Carolina. On the basis of their findings, the authors estimated the total number of abortions in the USA as 700000 per annum – a number approximating to the legal rate reported five years later.

A straightforward device for investigating illegal abortion is to question illegal abortionists directly.[78, 79] Whittemore interviewed five illegal abortionists and a number of patients in a city with a population 'between 100000 and 300000'. Assuming the groups interviewed represented the total professional skill available to the community in this field and discounting self-induced abortions but allowing for the known rate of legal terminations, Whittemore estimated 390000–860000 abortions annually in the USA – a figure also consistent with those of Abernathy and with later experience.

The experience of legal abortion among New York residents, when linked to birth rate statistics, indicates a high illegal abortion rate prior to repeal (p. 138). Records of 2857 women with septic abortions in New York shortly before the law was changed showed 52 per cent were unmarried, 43 per cent white and 40 per cent Roman Catholic. Seventy-two per cent were admitted before 13 weeks.[80]

OTHER DEVELOPED COUNTRIES

All European countries have made some attempt to investigate induced abortion. There is a considerable literature from France, Italy, Germany, the Low Countries, and Greece. None of it is inconsistent with the available data from Britain prior to 1967, though it suffers from the same inevitable limitations.

Numerically the largest survey of abortion comes from the compulsory registration of the event in Germany during the National Socialist period of government. Problems associated with abortion registration have already been discussed (p. 22), but the very magnitude of the German exercise commands attention.[81] Taussig quotes authors who believed there was one illegal abortion for every live birth in Hamburg in the 1930s.[4] Peller interviewed many women in Vienna in the interval 1920–24.[82] The birth rate had fallen 70 per cent in 30 years to a low of 12 per 1000. By 1928 the average couple was having 1.2 births. Peller estimated that the abortion rate was 20–21 per 1000 women of reproductive age and judged that the falling birth rate was quarter to a third the result of women having abortion and two-thirds to three-quarters the result of contraceptive practice (which would have been largely *coitus interruptus*). Illegal abortion has also remained a problem in West Germany and Austria since World War II.[83] Stamm has reviewed illegal, as well as legal, abortions taking place in Switzerland.[84]

Scandinavia in the 1930s seems to have had some of the characteristics of contemporary eastern Europe: a gross reproduction rate of 0.8 to 0.9, 60 per cent of the population using *coitus interruptus*[85] and a high induced-abortion rate.[86] In 1930 there were 10 445 abortion admissions against 94 220 live births[87] and informed observers such as Ottensen-Jenson put the total number of induced abortions at approximately 50 000 a year.[28] In Oslo municipal hospital abortion admissions rose from 1121 in 1920 to 2331 in 1933. In the mid-1930s an official committee estimated 3500 to 5400 induced abortions for 46 000 deliveries but estimates, based on patient histories from an Oslo family planning clinic, found abortion ratios (spontaneous and induced) of 28.2–34.3:100 births,[88] although the legal abortion rate was low until recently.[89] In Denmark the birth rate was slightly higher and the estimates of abortion somewhat lower – 1000–6000 against 66 000 births.[58]

Among the nations of pre-industrial and early industrial Europe, France always had an exceptionally low birth rate. It must be assumed that *coitus interruptus* and induced abortion have long been common. In the twentieth century these traditional methods were supplemented by the commercial distribution of condoms, but medically based contraceptive services remain poorly developed. In 1965 the previously restrictive anti-contraceptive legislation was partially amended. In 1975 the abortion law was liberalised.

At the end of the nineteenth century, at a time when there were about 850 000 deliveries in the country (approximately equal to that in the UK in the 1960s), the number of induced abortions was variously estimated at 100 000 to 500 000 annually.[90] By the 1930s observers seem to favour the higher figure and Glass quoted the President of the Superior Commission for the Birthrate as saying of abortions in 1937, 'It is estimated that the figures range between 300,000 and 500,000 per year . . . and I believe the latter figure is closer to the truth.' In the towns it was thought at this time that there were more abortions than live births and in Paris Dalsace put the ratio at 125 abortions to 100 births. The same high figures have been suggested for the decades after World War II with ratios of between one abortion for three deliveries and one and a half abortions for one delivery, some commentators putting the number of induced abortions as high as 1 200 000 annually.[91–93] In 1967 The National Institute for the Study of Demography estimated 250 000 to 300 000 criminal abortions a year.[94]

Belgium, urban and industrialised, has a record of abortions that may be even higher than that for France or Britain.[95–97] Theoretically the law will not permit abortions even to save a woman's life. Professor Keiffer, of the University of Brussels, in a memorandum to the Ministry of Health in the mid-1930s, estimated that 750 000 induced abortions took place in Belgium between January 1919 and December 1923 (over the same period there were 749 470 births).[58] Other observers also believed the abortion : birth ratio approached unity. Today the birth rate is low (13.8 per 1000 in 1972) the desired family size is 2.5 and, when contraceptive usage has been studied, *coitus interruptus* is found to be the commonest method (used by over 40 per cent), calendar rhythm next (used by a quarter of the couples). The use of appliance methods, IUDs and Pills is low. When questioning pregnant women, it has been found that at least one-third are 'displeased' with their being pregnant and over half claimed they became pregnant while using a contraceptive method. One author concludes, 'Considering the incidence of ineffective contraceptive practices, it may be wondered how these data can be reconciled with the demographic reality of the low mean family size. The main explanation must be sought in the corrective effect of abortion, of which even the lowest estimates lead to quite impressive figures.'[98]

In a survey of obstetricians' opinions in the 1960s, 73 per cent believed the Belgian law to be too restrictive.

In Holland, in a six-year study on one Amsterdam hospital, involving 400 inpatients and 3000 outpatients treated for abortion, one-quarter admitted induced abortion. Allowing for spontaneous abortion it was estimated that one in seven of all pregnancies was terminated by illegal abortion.[99] Other estimates have put the level higher. Married women who already had children predominated in these studies, although changes in the behaviour of the young unmarried have probably been important recently. No firm relationship has been demonstrated in Holland between a woman's social class and the likelihood of a criminal abortion, although there appears to be a positive correlation with the ineffective use of contraceptives and perhaps also marital discord.[100-102]

The estimates for illegal abortion rates in Italy prior to World War II are lower than those for her more industrialised neighbours. Nevertheless, the role of induced abortion as a major factor in the declining birth rate was appreciated and one Italian gynaecologist believed a three- to four-fold increase in abortions took place between 1908 and 1928.[58] An investigation at the Institute of Pediatrics of the University of Turin at the time of World War I found 12 per cent of pregnancies ended in abortion. Only 3.5 per cent of this total admitted illegal interference. The residual figure of spontaneous abortions would be compatible with the natural incidence of the condition but an element of under-reporting seems likely in view of the religio-cultural strictures against abortion. In 1935 Allaria estimated one abortion to 10 deliveries. In Sicily the post-war abortion rate has been estimated at 23.9 per 1000 of the population.[103] The relatively low abortion rate between the wars was accompanied by a high birth rate of 30 per 1000. By 1968 the birth rate had fallen to 17.6, the same as that of England and Wales two years earlier. In the towns it was thought that there were more abortions than live births.

Italy is a country where it is useful to try to estimate the induced abortion rate by a process of exclusion, using factual data on fertility and on the known variables of cohabitation and contraceptive practice. In its fertility, as in the degree of industrialisation and economic progress, Italy is really two nations. In the wealthy north, the birth rate is very low, e.g. in Piedmont, the area centred on Turin, it was 13.4 per 1000 in 1965. In the poor south the birth rate is high, for example, in Calabria, in the 'toe' of Italy, in 1965 the birth rate was 24.1 per 1000, or 30 per cent above the national average. In the mid-1960s the age of marriage was very similar to that in the UK and 50 per cent of girls did not marry until after the age of 25. All forms of contraception were illegal in Italy until 1971, when the Constitutional Court struck down Fascist laws dating from 1931. The anti-contraceptive laws had been unequally applied, but it seems reasonable to assume that contraceptives were less readily available than in, say, neighbouring Slovenia, where there is government-supported family planning. Yet with a birth rate of

19.2 in 1965 (higher than the corresponding Italian level) Slovenia had more abortions than live births. In Hungary in 1965 the birth rate was 13.1, or almost equal to that in Piedmont. Again a good deal was known about contraceptive practices, which were as good in Hungary as in Italy; Italian men are unlikely to accept the suggestion that they are less virile or more sexually perverted than their neighbours, so it is difficult to avoid the conclusion that illegal abortions in northern Italy are as numerous, or more numerous, than legal abortions in Hungary (see p. 401).[104–106]

The ratio of septic abortions to deliveries for hospital admissions can run as high as one in three in many northern Italian urban areas[107] and is compatible with the inferred high abortion rate. There is evidence of a serious under-registration of maternal deaths due to illegal abortion, because doctors are reluctant to enter a cause of death that they know will expose the family to harrowing investigations by the police. Only 150 cases of illegal abortion came to the courts between 1955 and 1965.

There are few data on illegal abortion from the USSR prior to the World War I. The birth rate in Moscow in 1909 was 35.4 per 1000 and the rate per 1000 of the population for admission to hospital for incomplete abortions was 1.3. By 1914 the birth rate had fallen to 31.0 and the abortion admission rate risen to 3.2.[4] The country was then in the situation found in many developing countries today.

Australia, Canada and New Zealand behave demographically like Europe and North America.[108,109] Recent studies, based on the activities of a sample of doctors carrying out illegal abortions, suggest a total of 45 000–90 000 criminal abortions yearly in Australia. There are only 11.5 million people in Australia and there is one of the highest consumptions *per capita* of oral contraceptives, so the rate, if correct, is suprisingly high. However, the birth rate is falling and a quarter of the population is Roman Catholic and may have below average contraceptive practices.

A survey, based on a random probability sample of 2400 New Zealanders found 1.2 per cent of the women aged 15–44 years reported an illegal abortion in 1971. Extrapolated to the whole population, this would suggest 7000 illegal abortions annually (approximately 10:100 live births).[110] The nature of the study probably provides a minimum estimate only. Interestingly, twice as many women confessed to attempting an abortion as to succeeding. Illegi-

Table 7. *Ratio of abortions to 100 pregnancies by ethnic group and religion. Hospital admissions, Israel (1968)*

Jews (Country of origin)							
Israel	Asia	North Africa	Europe & USA	Subtotal	Moslems	Christians	Overall total
22.4	26.6	26.9	35.7	27.1	8.7	14.0	23.3

timacy and premarital conceptions (13077 of 25245 first conceptions were premarital in 1970) are an even more serious social problem in New Zealand than in the UK.[111] Contraceptives are less readily available and abortion is illegal, suggesting these two variables are not the determinants of patterns of premarital behaviour. Perhaps opportunities for sexual congress are greater than in the UK: a high proportion of teenagers own cars (the legal age of driving is 15), the beaches are deserted and the weather not inclement.

In Israel, abortion is easily available, although illegal, and the variety of ethnic and religious groups make a sociologically interesting situation (Table 7).[112-114] Overall, it is thought a third of all women have had abortions.

In Greece, as in Hungary, a 0.5 per cent sample of married women under age 50 was surveyed in the late 1960s. The women each reported one abortion for every two births, the rate was four times as high in the towns as in the villages and rose with parity. Semiliterate women had three times as many abortions as university educated women. The national total of illegal abortions is estimated to be 60000 to 100000 annually.[115-119]

Contemporary developing countries

Evidence concerning the incidence of induced abortion in societies which currently have high birth rates is fragmentary. There is, of course, strong negative evidence of a relatively low abortion rate. When the birth rate is 40 or more per 1000 it is approaching the maximum that the unrestrained human reproductive system can achieve and there is little room for a large number of artificial terminations.

Abortion is known, and occasionally resorted to, in every peasant rural society in every developing country, but it is usually at a low rate. In urban communities it is sometimes common.

Table 8. *Induced abortion in Latin America*

Country	Year of study	Induced-abortion rate per 100 pregnancies	Birth rate per 1000 of the population (1967)	Annual rate of increase in population	Income *per capita* in 1966 (US $)
Argentina	1964	25.3	22.3	1.5	705
Bolivia	1969	1.2–8.5	44	2.6	118
Brazil	1964	18.2[a]	38	3.0	252
Chile	1964 & 1966	16.6–23.2	28.4	2.4	474
Colombia	1965–66	13.6	34.9	3.2	285
Costa Rica	1962–64	11.1	39.2	3.4	362
Ecuador	1967	11.1[a]	40.4	3.4	188
El Salvador	1958–63	20.0 (17.0)	44.4	3.7	240
Guatamala	1964	14–15 (7–7.5)[b]	43.0	3.1	255
Honduras	1962–63	17.5	44.2	3.4	199
Mexico	—	13.9	43.4	3.5	446
Panama	—	30.0[a]	38.2	3.3	451
Paraguay	1961–65	19.0	45	3.2	175
Peru	1960	3.8–7.2	31.9	3.1	320
Uruguay	1968	32.6	21	1.2	570
Venezuela	1968	19.6[a]	43.5	3.5	744

No estimates of abortion rates are available for Nicaragua or Surinam.
[a] Only available studies include spontaneous as well as induced abortions.
[b] Main entry based on survey of spontaneous as well as induced abortions, but percentage illegal also estimated.

LATIN AMERICA

The first useful study of induced abortion in Latin America was made as recently as 1962. Armijo and Monreal startled the Seventh Pan American Congress on Social Medicine by demonstrating a very high rate of induced abortion in Chile.[120, 121] In 10 years these workers, and a number of others, have published a series of papers which have resulted in clearer understanding of the pattern and dynamics of induced abortion in Latin America than in most other continents (Table 8). Many of the studies have been carried out under the auspices of CELADE (Centre Latinoamericano de Demografía – the population research bureau of the United Nations, located in Santiago). Part of this review is based on a document prepared by the Western Hemisphere Region of the International Planned Parenthood Federation from the source materials at their disposal.[122]

The original Chilean studies remain amongst the most detailed and now have an added importance, as changes in abortion rates, resulting from family planning programmes, can be monitored (p. 442). Some 3800 interviews were carried out on a sample of households (women aged 20–50 years) in the three cities of Santiago, Concepción and Antofagasta. A quarter of the women admitted at least one induced abortion and a quarter of this quarter had had three or more abortions.[123] In Santiago alone, it is suggested that there are 50000 illegal abortions a year – that is almost half the total number of legal abortions occurring in England and Wales, for a single city with one quarter the population of London.

For a brief interval during the Allende regime in Chile, abortion was approved as a hospital procedure in one selected area of Santiago. Using money available for research purposes from a large international health organisation, Chilean physicians performed 3250 hospital abortions in the Barrof Luco area of the capital. The results were carefully analysed. Without publicity, the number of hospital abortions rose rapidly until a ratio of one abortion to every two births was reached. This transfer of abortions from the back street to medical facilities caused a measurable decline in admissions for complicated abortions and it is estimated that the US $30000 which the pilot scheme cost saved approximately US $200000 in clinical care of incomplete abortions. The birth rate and infant mortality in the area also fell. For political reasons these findings are unlikely to be published in the near future. They are buried in international archives under the heading *Acute Pelvic Inflamatory Disease in Santiago, Chile*.

Studies from other Latin American countries give similar results.[124–129] Over a quarter of all pregnancies from a sample of hospital patients in Buenos Aires ended in illegal abortion,[130, 131] and in Uruguay three-quarters.[132] In Colombia the Ministry for Public Health, section for Materno-child Welfare, estimated (1968) that in urban areas a quarter of all pregnancies end in abortion, but they did not attempt to distinguish between spontaneous and illegal events. Additional material is summarised in Table 8 although it would be misleading to extrapolate to the whole of a nation data from many of the samples quoted. Socio-economic characteristics of women resorting to abortion and the relationship between the probability of induced abortion and contraceptive practice are discussed elsewhere (p. 454).

The burden of human suffering caused by criminal abortion in Latin America is huge and grows daily. The cost of treating an abortion patient is estimated at ×4.5 the cost of a Caesarean operation and ×9 the cost of a normal birth. Stycos[133] has written:

> In the early 1960s studies by Chilean public health physicians showed that four out of every ten admissions to Santiago's emergency services were abortion complications, that one out of every five maternal deaths was due to abortion...
> Distinguished physicians, such as University del Valle's dean of medicine, could begin to insist that women 'are earnestly looking to our profession for help. It is not a Catholic problem nor a moral problem, nor a political problem, it is a health problem. Our people are asking the doctors for an answer.'

The answer they were given in most, but not all, countries of Latin America was the provision of contraceptive services, through a variety of non-governmental routes. It was not exactly giving vinegar to those crucified in the control of their own fertility, but it was a small measure handed over in a leaky vessel.

CARIBBEAN

Illegal abortion is a familiar and an apparently worsening problem on all the islands of the West Indies. Community-based surveys have not been attempted, but observations by individual obstetricians on hospital records provide some data. Hoyte[134] analysed admissions to the General Hospital, Port of Spain, Trinidad. Overall, 34.6 per cent of pregnancies ended in abortion, the incidence as a percentage of conceptions being at a maximum in the 45–49 years age group. The number of annual admissions rose from 1200 in 1956 to 2000 in 1963. Most women were admitted at less than 12 weeks of gestation. The cost of illegal abortion is considerable: 1234 women spent 4409 days in hospital and nearly half required antibiotics or blood transfusion. By 1971 Port of Spain Hospital was handling over 8000 deliveries a year and had 2803 abortion admissions. The level of unavoidable admissions, amongst which abortions are a significant part, was so great that for eight months in 1971 no routine gynaecological operations whatsoever were performed.[135] The Victoria Jubilee Hospital in Kingston, Jamaica, has similar problems.[136] It is the largest in the country and handled 14000 deliveries and 2586 abortion admissions (one to five deliveries) in 1971. There is a 12-bed abortion ward and two women must frequently share the same bed. In the public hospital in Guyana there are over 7000 deliveries a year and in 1971 there were 1962 abortion admissions. Barbados is a small island of about 300000 inhabitants, with a moderate birth rate (21.9 per 1000 in 1971). In 1971 in five hospitals throughout the island there were 800 abortion admissions against 5000 institutionalised deliveries.

Criminal abortion is the largest single cause of maternal deaths in many Caribbean countries. Five women died in the Jubilee Hospital in 1971, and over the five years 1964–68 abortion deaths accounted for 19 out of a total of 82 maternal deaths in Jamaica. In Guyana in 1971 eight women[137] died, and in Barbados one. It is generally felt that the problem of induced abortion is becoming more serious, especially accelerating in the later years of the 1960s.

ISLAMIC NATIONS

The nations of Islam, from Morocco to Indonesia, encompass over 10 per cent of the world's population. They are countries of moderate to very high birth rates (Egypt 39, Turkey 43, Kuwait 60, per 1000) and they are at varying stages of economic development. Only Tunisia permits induced legal abortion on other grounds than to save the mother's life, although changes of practice *de facto* are occurring in Bangladesh, Malaysia and Indonesia and a change *de jure* in Iran is likely to be implemented shortly.

Some of the most reliable data on illegal abortion come from the prospective study organised by Awan in Pakistan and already referred to in relation to spontaneous abortion.[138] The rapport established between the interviewers and the women in the study area during the two years of the project, and the close questioning of those whose pregnancies ended prematurely, are thought to have given unusually reliable answers about deliberate interference (Table 9).

Retrospective surveys are available from several Islamic countries. Yaukey surveyed fertility control in the Lebanon.[139] Among a sample of Moslem villagers it was reported that 0.2 pregnancies in 100 ended in illegal abortion. Christian villagers admitted no induced abortion at all. However, in the urban counterparts of these communities 8–14 pregnancies in 100 were reported to have been terminated deliberately. Bickers estimated that 2000 illegal abortions occurred annually in the Lebanon in the late 1960s. However, only 70 of 300 abortion cases admitted to the American University Hospital in Beirut conceded illegal interference.[140]

The evaluation of family planning efforts in Turkey has been frank

Table 9. *Illegal abortions: Lahore, Pakistan (1963–65)*

	Observed
Population of area studied	29490
Women 14–50 years	4582
No pregnancies (2-year period)	1447
Total fetal loss	156
Admitted illegal abortions	28
Diagnosed illegal abortions	12
Total induced abortions	40 (27 per cent of total fetal loss)
	Calculated (life-table techniques)
Total fetal loss per 100 conceptions	18.85
Induced abortions per 100 conceptions	5.73
Induced abortions per 100 live births	7.06

and relatively detailed.[141] The government has included family planning in health services since 1965. Early surveys of family planning practice show a high incidence of abortion[142] and a survey carried out by the Hacettepe Institute of Population Studies in 1968 included questions on several aspects of abortion.[143] A sample of over 3000 women was taken from urban and rural areas spread over the country. The hostility of some women who refused to answer questions on abortion, combined with variations in the reported rate of spontaneous abortions, suggests that there may have been irregular reporting of induced abortions. Nevertheless, the raw data give a high rate of induced abortion. For example, nearly half the urban women report one or more abortions in a lifetime and the induced abortion ratio was 38 to 100 live births. Over the country as a whole there were an estimated 168000 abortions a year or 16 to 100 live births.

Studies based on hospital or family planning clinic experience are becoming more common. Alavi-Naini[144] carried out a particularly interesting analysis in Teheran (1967–70) when she followed up 452 pregnancies, within an upper- and middle-class community who had

had positive pregnancy tests. It might be argued that those who feared pregnancy would be over-represented in such a sample, but the practice of confirming a pregnancy in this way is widespread among urban Iranians. Two of the pregnancies (0.5 per cent) ended in hydatidiform moles, 241 (68.3 per cent) in deliveries, 51 (14.4 per cent) were reported to have ended in spontaneous abortions and 59 (16.7 per cent) in induced abortions. Some of the spontaneous abortions may have been misreported and induced abortions may well have been relatively frequent among the 99 women lost to follow-up. Daneshbod and his colleagues[145] used a different route for surveying illegal abortion when they analysed maternal deaths coming for autopsy (1963–69) at the Saadi Hospital, Shiraz, Iran. Six out of 44 deaths were the result of septic abortions and there was one suicide, a girl of 20, 12 weeks pregnant. Of course, there is no way of telling if women dying of abortions were more or less likely to reach hospital than those dying at or after delivery.

Larsen[146] has approached the problem of measuring induced abortion in Iran through an ingenious demographic analysis. He compared age-specific marital fertility rates for rural and metropolitan women. In the 20–24 year age group they are exactly comparable (360 per 1000), but after age 25 the rates diverge, the rates for Teheran being only 40 to 67 per cent of the rural rates. A physiological basis for the differences seems out of the question. Therefore the differences must be caused by variations in contraceptive and abortion practices. In 1968 only 33 per cent of women in Teheran claimed to have ever used contraception (half of this number used *coitus interruptus* and the other two quarters each used condoms and oral contraceptives). Assuming an overall contraceptive use-effectiveness of 60 per cent and a ratio of abortions to births averted of 1.4:1, Larsen calculated the role of induced abortion for different hypothetical levels of contraceptive use within the community. The results can only be approximations, but the logic of the calculations gives the magnitude of the answer some weight (Table 10).

In Basra University Maternal Hospital, Iraq, there are approximately 300 deliveries a month. The number of admissions for incomplete abortion is even greater and may reach 14 a day. The female population is mainly engaged in agricultural work. Ten pregnancies in a lifetime, of which half may end in abortion, is not an uncommon occurrence in this part of Iraq. The sexual demands on the woman

Table 10. *Estimate of induced abortion in Teheran, Iran*

Age (years)	15–19	20–24	25–29	30–34	35–39	40–44	Total
Marital fertility rate							
rural	316	360	359	295	227	150	—
urban	330	360	240	170	150	60	—
Births averted in urban population[a]	—	—	9600	10800	5500	5000	30900
Births averted by contraception[b]	—	—	8200	7200	4600	2400	22400
Calculated number of abortions[c]	—	—	2000	5000	1300	3600	11900

[a] Calculation based on 1966 urban population
[b] Calculation based on 33 per cent of women using contraceptives (1966 knowledge attitude and practice study estimated real usage 30 per cent). Assumed contraceptive efficacy 0.6.
[c] Calculation based on 1.4 induced abortions for each birth averted.

can be extreme; intercourse during labour or within a day of delivery has been reported. It is usual for several girls to be admitted each week – usually on Thursdays and Fridays as these are the preferred days for marriage – with vaginal haemorrhage consequent on a violent first intercourse.

Egypt has a higher degree of urbanisation than most other Moslem countries. There is clinical evidence of a relatively high induced-abortion rate. In many urban hospitals there are half as many abortion admissions as deliveries. Foda[147] investigated induced abortions among hospital patients, a sample of urban women and a sample of rural women. He found the rural women reported one induced abortion for 75 living children, the town-dwellers one for 35 and the private patients one for three. Kamal[148] and his co-workers, in a study of 800 women coming into hospital with abortions or for delivery, found 35.5 per cent of cases had had induced abortions (these cases consumed 50 per cent of the hospital budget). Toppozada[149] found a slightly lower percentage reported by private patients in Alexandria, but, allowing for inaccuracies of reporting, the total of 185000 abortions annually in Egypt estimated by Foda seems not unreasonable.

Ethnically, Malaysia is half Moslem Malay and half Chinese and Indian. The main information on abortion comes from surveys of hospital admissions for abortion at the General Hospital, Kuala

Lumpur. In the first, 1961–62, 239 out of a sample of 1000 admissions were classified as septic. In 1968–69 only 3.6 per 1000 were classified as septic. However, over three-quarter were 'incomplete/complete'. Possibly, diagnostic criteria rather than admission rates had altered although the authors noted that more private, medically supervised, abortion clinics had opened in the decade and possibly the family planning programme was having an impact. A survey of University Hospital patients in 1973–74 recorded 3.9 per cent induced, and 18.4 per cent spontaneous, abortions among 3921 reported pregnancies.[150, 151]

At a single hospital in Amman, Jordan in 1969, there were 734 deliveries and 397 abortion admissions.[152] However, as 90 per cent of deliveries are at home and hospitals deal mainly with complicated cases, these statistics probably do not reflect the true picture. Jordan has a gross reproductive rate of 3.4 and induced abortion is likely to be less common there than in some neighbouring countries.

INDIA

India contains one-seventh of the world's population. For more than 20 years the government has been engaged in an increasingly massive family planning programme, but during the same period the *annual* increase in the population has risen from five million to 13 million. Where small successes have been obtained they are probably partly the result of illegal abortion. In urban hospitals the ratio of abortion admissions to deliveries is as high as 30–40:100.[153–159] The ratio appears to be rising (p. 421). In Gandhigram the ratio of total fetal loss (abortions of all types and stillbirths) rose from 13.5:100 pregnancies in 1964 to 21.2 in 1967, while the marital fertility rate fell from 22.1 to 21.4 per 1000 women aged 15–44.[160] In 1972 the Indian abortion law was liberalised (p. 421).

KOREA, TAIWAN, PHILIPPINES AND THAILAND

Korea and Taiwan have more than usually vigorous family planning programmes, and abortion, although illegal, is widely practised. A moderate change in the Korean law occurred in 1973, but it is too early to evaluate its effect. Good retrospective surveys of induced abortion, based on adequate samples, have been completed giving data on frequency, socio-economic correlates, relationship with contraceptive practice and changing incidence with time.

Hong[161,162] has conducted two careful retrospective surveys on probability samples of married women aged 20–44 years in 1963 (3204 women) and 1968–69 (2228 women) from Seoul Special City. Unlike Western countries, less than 0.5 per cent of births take place to girls under 20, the illegitimacy rate is of the order of two per cent and terminations to unmarried girls account for only five or six per cent of all induced abortions, so that the parameters chosen do not exclude a numerically significant number of women resorting to abortion. The induced-abortion ratio rose from 17:100 pregnancies in 1961 to 31 in 1963 and to 40 in 1969. By 1970 there was one induced abortion for every 1.3 deliveries – an estimated 100000–120000 a year for the metropolis; that is, there were as many illegal abortions in this one city as legal abortions in Britain in the same year. Hong concludes that the ratio of abortions to births exceeded unity in 1972.

Part of the rise in the abortion ratio has been the result of a fall in the number of births, itself a result of improved contraceptive practice. In 1963 a married woman in Seoul could expect to have, on average, 5.8 births and 3.2 abortions by age 45. By 1968 she could expect 4.6 births but still 3.2 abortions. The ratio of births to abortions changed because the total number of conceptions declined as a result of improved contraceptive practice.

However, the picture is further complicated by changing age-specific rates, a rise in abortions in younger age groups accounting for a real increase in the total number of induced abortions in Seoul. This important pattern of changes will be explored more fully in Chapter 13.

Hong traced 510 deaths to women aged 15–50 years in Seoul, Korea. Maternal deaths composed the second largest group of deaths (13.3 per cent) during the reproductive years and 22 of 58 deaths in this category were caused by the complications of induced abortion. Hong estimated deaths due to abortion to be 3.7 per 10000 abortions (maternal mortality 9.1 per 10000 deliveries). The most frequent cause of death was suicide (25.9 per cent), and probably some part of this component related to the control of human fertility.[163]

Taiwan, like Korea, has a relatively effective family planning programme, which is mainly based on the intrauterine device (IUD).[164,165] The scale and change in abortion rates also appear to be similar to those in Korea, rising from 9 per cent of pregnancies in 1964 to 10 per cent in 1965; 12.3 per cent in 1967; and 20 per cent in 1968. (See also p. 474.) Chow & Liu used the random response test (p. 28) in a sample of 1100 women: 28.2 per cent admitted one or more abortions, compared with 12.7 per cent in a control group in a normal interview situation. Even in the former case, under-estimates are likely; in a group known to have had abortions, only 40 per cent responded positively in the random response test.[166]

The Philippines are economically poorer than either Taiwan or Korea. Government-sponsored family planning predictably came late in a country that is 86 per cent Roman Catholic and where the importation of any contraceptive was illegal until 1969. The birth rate is still in the mid-40s per 1000 and the annual growth rate one of the most rapid in the world. Induced abortion is a particular problem in urban areas. One hospital in Manila, for example, has 80–85 deliveries a day and 10–15 abortion admissions. In the urban area of the city, the birth rate fell from 46 in 1962 to 32.9 per 1000 in 1968. Although *coitus interruptus* is well known and there had been an illicit supply of condoms, together with some medical use of IUDs and Pills (before importation became legal), it is interesting to speculate how much of the decline must have been due to induced abortion. The problem of abortion in the Philippines seems destined to worsen.

Thailand is at least partially representative of the nations of Southeast Asia. It has a high birth rate (over 40 per 1000) but an acceptance and openness about family planning not found in the neighbouring Indian subcontinent. Although land inheritance can be through the female, the nuclear family structure ensures that decision-making rests with the fertile couple. One unpublished survey based on a random sample of the population has been conducted and suggests a relatively low incidence of induced abortion. But a very high incidence of induced abortion is found among the massage parlour girls. In a sample of 180 young women from this profession 92 per cent has had induced abortions – which were usually obtained from physicians and cost about 3000 bhat ($30). The girls earn about 10000 bhat ($200) a month.[167]

More representative information is available from hospital statistics. There were 14442 deliveries at the Chulalongkorn Hospital in Bangkok in 1969, and 1299 abortion admissions, about one in five of which had clinical signs of sepsis and, no doubt, an unknown additional proportion had been induced but without undue complications.[168]

AFRICA

Much of Africa has relatively low densities of human settlement. The birth rate is the highest for any continent (estimated 47 per 1000 of the population). Until the 1970s all the nations of sub-Saharan Africa had restrictive abortion laws, mainly dating from the time of colonial rule, or (as in the case of the Portuguese territories) as a consequence of persisting rule from Europe, but in 1972 Zambia reformed its law along the lines of the British 1967 Act. West Africa has particularly strong traditions of high fertility but in urban areas there is, as in all other developing countries, an accelerating problem of induced abortion.

At the Korle Bu Hospital in Accra, Ghana, over half the beds in the Department of Obstetrics and Gynaecology are used for abortion admissions, which averaged 2890 annually against 9277 deliveries, for 1967–69. The abortions make up 60–80 per cent of all minor surgery, use some 50 per cent of the blood supplied for transfusion in the hospital and put a considerable strain on the hospital resources. One in 300 women admitted with an abortion dies and there is a significant morbidity. For example, one 24-year-old mother of two children had had her uterus and bowel perforated by the illegal abortionist and required a hysterectomy and resection of a gangrenous bowel. Thirty per cent were nulliparous and the commonest single age group was 20–24. The majority were married but often had only been married for a short interval.[169] In Lagos in 1972, there were 1990 abortion admissions and 19322 deliveries at the Island Maternity Hospital.[170]

Kinshasa, capital of Zaïre, is one of the most rapidly growing capital cities in the world, having doubled its population (now 1.7 million) since the country was created after the Congolese civil war. The Mama Yemo hospital is the only hospital obliged to admit patients in need of care. There is a 120 per cent daily occupancy of the beds in the hospital as a whole and 44000 women were delivered in the 390 obstetric beds in 1972 (maximum 163 deliveries a day). Abortion admissions account for 60 per cent of all the gynaecological cases (3182 out of 5985 in 1972). The ratio of abortions to deliveries was 7.2:100, which is low by the experience of many other 'jumbo' maternity hospitals in the developing world. On the strict criterion of either patient history or clinical evidence of trauma, only 19 abortion admissions were *proven* illegal abortions. Nevertheless, sepsis among abortions is common (40 per cent of cases are infected) and the mortality high (11 deaths in 1972 or 341 per 100000, cf. maternal mortality, 140 per 100000). Among the 11 deaths, four were proven illegal abortions.[171]

It should be noted, however, that sepsis *post partum* is common and some genuinely spontaneous abortions may become infected because of the low standard of hygiene and quack (or self) treatment.

The same pattern of low-to-moderate induced abortion is found elsewhere, in sub-Saharan black Africa.[172] Rapid growth in urban areas, combined with some slight rise in the number of beds available, may be expected to lead to an increase in the number of admissions for incomplete abortion, but many statistics also suggest a genuine rise in the number of illegal abortions. At the Mulago Hospital, Kampala, admissions for incomplete abortion rose from 881 to 1518 per annum in the five-year period 1963–67.[173]

A survey of medical perceptions of illegal abortion was conducted in Nigeria by asking physicians to make guesses about certain aspects of abortion and then, for a subsample, to refine their views in the light of their colleagues' opinions – the so-called Delphi technique. It was concluded that induced abortion was more common than any other operation, that most were performed by medically qualified personnel (although this may be an artifact of the methodology), that dilatation and curettage was most frequent and that the typical woman seeking an abortion was married, educated and desperate.[174]

The mortality among those women reaching hospital after an illegal abortion is often high. In 1972 there were 17 deaths in 3275 abortion admissions in Korelbu, Accra; 3 in 229 in Lagos Teaching Hospital; 11 in 751 in Victoria Hospital, Mauritius; 6 in 244 in West Sierra Leone; and 11 in the Mama Yemo Hospital, Zaïre, out of 3182. Young girls, especially students, in many parts of Africa are particularly vulnerable to unwanted pregnancies. In 1972, 18 pregnant teenagers were admitted not to the obstetric wards but to the burns unit of the Mama Yemo Hospital, after self-immolation with kerosene. They had 50–90 per cent body burns.[171]

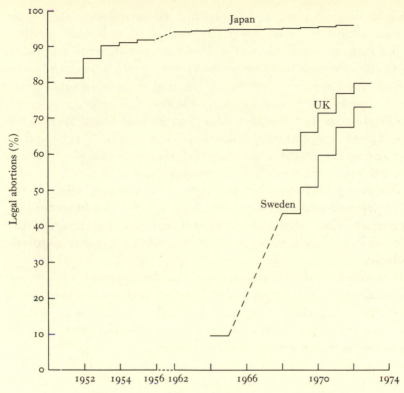

Fig. 21. Percentage of legal abortions performed in the first 12 weeks of pregnancy by country and year.

Duration of gestation

Many legal abortion statistics record the duration of gestation at the time of operation. It is a most important variable and the physical, economic and emotional costs of the operation rise rapidly after the first 12 weeks (see also Chapter 6). Many people would argue that the ethical problems also multiply as pregnancy progresses.

Nearly all women seek advice before the twelfth week of pregnancy and delay is almost invariably provider induced. Mild degrees of legal reform, a cautious medical profession and, in particular, decision-making committees are associated with a high proportion of operations spilling over into the second trimester. Sweden is the most forceful example of a country where the provision of services has led to undue delay (Fig. 21). In Japan, by contrast, readily available services and a straightforward law permit more than 95 per cent of women to obtain abortions at 12 weeks or less; in Uruguay 92 per cent of abortions were before the twelfth week and 64 per cent before the eighth. There seems no reason why a similar situation should not be reached in the USA in the near future. Britain unfortunately has tended to follow the Swedish error.

The fragmentary available data suggest that illegal abortionists have a good record of early operation. Moore-Čavar[173] reviewed the literature of several different countries and found that 78–96 per cent of operations were completed in the first 12 weeks.

The young unmarried are an exception to the generalisation that delay depends upon the provider. They can be slow in recognising pregnancy. They often delay telling their parents, or seeking other help, and in this aspect, as in many others, present particular problems.

It would be rational to advertise the need to seek advice early where abortion is legal for social reasons, just as immunisation or family planning advice have been advertised. Britain is an example of a country where the climate of opinion does not yet permit this necessary aspect of public health education.

Age and parity

Age and parity of abortees are the simplest characteristics to gather and considerable data are available. Statistics from the experience of legal abortion in England and Wales is reflective of the situation in many countries, both where abortion is legal and where it is illegal (Fig. 22). Deaths reveal something of the structure of the population resorting to abortion where it is illegal. For example 64 per cent of 223 women dying of abortion in California (1957–65) were married, and 58 per cent had four or more children, and most of these deaths were probably due to criminal abortion. On the other hand, a higher death rate for abortion for black (7.15 per 10000) than white (0.8 per 10000) Americans may have reflected more difficult access to safe operators for the black community.[175]

Induced abortion is common when pregnancy is common. Numerically, women in their 20s have the bulk of abortions. However, the social and economic pressures to restrict family size are maximum at the extremes of fertile life. A significant number of

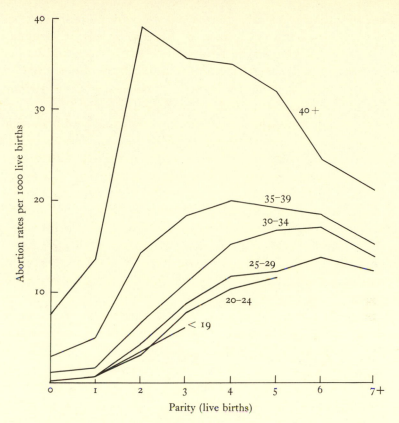

Fig. 22. Abortion ratios by age and parity (married women, England and Wales, 1969).

pregnancies in the young are conceived outside marriage. This effect is most marked in industrialised nations, but is also emerging in the urban areas of some developing countries (see below). For older women, all over the world, economic and to some extent emotional pressures to limit family size rise with age and parity – each variable being significant by itself and both also acting in concert. Therefore, although the total number of abortions contributed by teenagers and women over 35 is always a minority part of the abortion total, the ratio of abortions to live births rises in these age groups (Fig. 23).

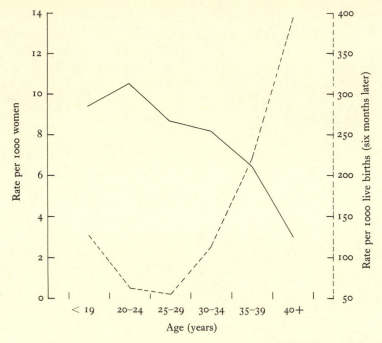

Fig. 23. Legal abortion rates by age (England and Wales, 1970).

Marital status

All societies penalise childbearing among the unmarried, although the degree of restraint varies. In some countries, such as Britain, America, the socialist countries of the USSR and eastern Europe, and Scandinavia, the unmarried mother can expect certain elements of protection and assistance from society. Nevertheless, the task of bringing up a bastard remains formidable. In some other countries, e.g. the remainder of continental Europe or Australia, the difficulties will be somewhat greater. Elsewhere, e.g. in the Lebanon and many Moslem countries, a premarital pregnancy may lead to a girl being murdered by her own family. In some hospitals when a pregnancy is diagnosed in an unmarried girl, she is passed into police protection. In general terms the more powerful the deterrent the fewer the pregnancies among the unmarried, but the greater the incentive for abortion when they do occur.

The unmarried woman's ability to obtain an abortion varies.

Where abortion is legal and widely known to be relatively easy to obtain, as in Britain or America, many girls will find their own way to services. Where abortion is illegal and unmarried girls lead cloistered lives, as in the Lebanon, it is correspondingly more difficult to find access to an abortion directly. In both situations efforts are likely to be made to bypass the parents. A case is known from Washington of an unmarried girl who flew to a New York outpatient clinic for a termination, telling her mother she had gone to the Metropolitan Museum of Art. It finds its parallel in the equally genuine case of a girl in Iran, whose uncle brought her to a medically qualified abortionist for a saline infusion, so timed that she could go home for the night and hopefully deliver the next afternoon. It was a deception maintained at horrendous emotional and physical cost to the girl. While pressures vary, overall patterns are rather similar, and in the USA the younger the girl the later she comes to abortion, presumably largely because of delay in telling her parents, perhaps partly mixed with an initial denial of the reality of pregnancy.

The mean age at which women marry influences the abortion rate amongst the unmarried ones. In much of the developing world, marriage is early, the parents making the choice of marriage partner and taking the young bride into the extended family. Therefore the interval of risk for premarital pregnancy is brief, as marriage follows soon after puberty. In many industrialised nations, the mean age of marriage is often in the early or middle 20s, so that women are exposed to the risk of premarital pregnancy over a number of years at a time when biological fertility is high but they are relatively inexperienced in contraceptive practice. In pre-industrial Europe the peasantry sometimes had a mean age of marriage as high as the late 20s, but the amount of premarital intercourse, as measured by the illegitimacy rate, was low – although the premarital conception rate, later legitimised by marriage, was moderate in extent.[176] In industrialised nations since World War II, there may have been some increase in the extent, and a decline in the age of initiation, of premarital sexual activity.

When abortion is legal and registered the publication of statistics on the unmarried often arouses controversy. However, it seems unlikely that the state of the law determines the basic pattern of resort to abortion in the community. The variation in the proportion of unmarried women obtaining legal abortions in different countries

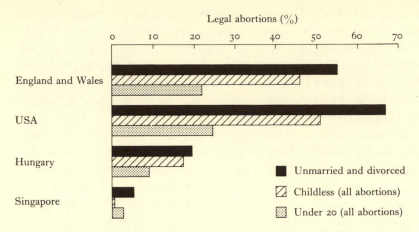

Fig. 24. Percentage distribution of legal abortions by marital
status, prior births and age for selected countries (1973).

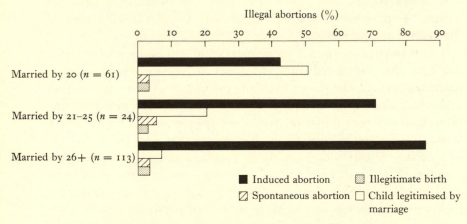

Fig. 25. Illegal abortion (USA, 1940–49). Outcome of
premarital conceptions.

(Fig. 24) appears to reflect deep cultural differences that are unaffected by the availability or non-availability of legal abortion. Gebhard and his co-workers[76] found high termination rates for
premaritally conceived pregnancies in the USA, a generation before
abortion was legally available for social reasons (Fig. 25). By contrast, in Singapore, which has a liberal law, only five per cent of
abortion applicants are unmarried.

However, the number of unmarried women having legal abortions is a major variable determining the proportion of all legal abortions that occur to young and to childless women (Fig. 24). Unfortunately, for the young nulliparous abortion presents more technical, as well as more emotional, problems than it does for the older parous woman (see also Chapter 6).

The urban areas of some developing countries seem likely to begin to follow the Western pattern in the foreseeable future. For example, in one large centre in Bombay the proportion of unmarried girls seeking legal abortions rose from two per cent in 1972 to eight per cent in 1973, and at the Wadia Hospital in Bombay 35 per cent of those having legal abortions were unmarried.[177] The change is probably not as rapid as the bald statistics suggest. It is probable that, initially, some of the unmarried faked married names, and the transfer from illegal to legal abortions may be occurring at different rates among the married and unmarried. Roman Catholic girls in Bombay are over-represented among the unmarried seeking termination. Some Moslems are seeking abortions for the first pregnancy, because they were married when very young and are then divorced as soon as they become pregnant. Although categorised in statistics as married, they are analogous to the unmarried girl in a Western community who is abandoned by her boyfriend when pregnancy occurs. In Allahabad, Uttar Pradesh, three to eight per cent of urban women, and 9.2 per cent of rural women, having abortions are unmarried.[178]

Socio-economic status

Abortion rates and ratios amongst different socio-economic groups are determined by the combination of varying pressures to control fertility and differing degrees of contraceptive success. Income, education or social class, as defined by various indicators, have all been used as criteria in the analysis of both legal and illegal abortion rates. At first glance it seems difficult to distinguish any universal pattern, as the most privileged groups have sometimes the highest rates and sometimes the lowest. However, early in the demographic transition, as in India, there is a strong correlation between education level and abortion rates: illiterate women report three per cent of conceptions ending in abortion, those who reached middle grade education nine per cent, and high school 11 per cent.[178,179] Possibly some levelling off in abortion rates is apparent amongst couples with university education for in this group 12 per cent of conceptions end in abortion. Where the demographic transition is more established, as in Rio de Janeiro, the relationship can be the reverse – the higher socio-economic groups report an abortion rate one-tenth of that of the lowest groups.[127] In this situation, contraceptive practices are probably overtaking abortion practices amongst the socially privileged.

The relationship between contraceptive practice and abortion in different social groups is reviewed separately in Chapter 13.

Urban/rural differentials reflect socio-economic differences and in many developing countries the variation is gross – the variables separating the villager from the town dweller may be more significant than those separating comparable urban classes in developed and developing societies. The largest migration in human history is currently taking place as millions of people leave traditional village societies and move into the exploding cities of the Third World. The demographic experience of the historical shift towards urbanisation in Europe and North America differs from that of current trends in Asia and Africa, although there may be certain parallels in Latin America. European urbanisation was accompanied by a rise in death rates, especially in infant mortality.[180-182] The expectation of life in England and Wales in 1841 was 40 years, but in London only 35 and in Liverpool and Manchester 25. Modern, mass preventive medicine is so efficient that the killing diseases of nineteenth-century cities are at least partially controlled, and adverse urban/rural differentials in infant mortality have been reduced or reversed. High ratios of fertility in many Asian and African urban areas have not yet shown the beginning of a decline.

Probably nineteenth-century cities, like twentieth-century ones, had higher abortion rates than rural areas. In the Ukraine, during the interval when abortion was legal between the two world wars, Peller found the highest abortion rates were in towns and cities (Fig. 26). The village emigrant takes some time to adopt the new patterns. In Santiago in the early 1960s women who had lived in the city for less than 10 years had 13.3 induced abortions per 100 pregnancies, while those who had lived there for over 10 years had 26.0.[120] Urban residence may mean something very different for the unmarried than the married. In Thailand half the serious cases of criminal abortion, in one series in Bangkok, had come from the provinces and lived alone in flats or hostels.[183]

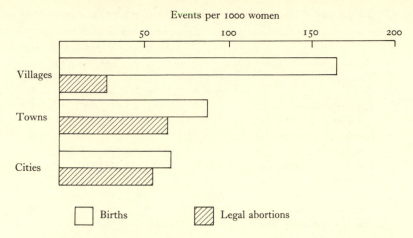

Fig. 26. Outcome of pregnancy among Russian women aged 15–49 (Ukraine, 1927).

Research surveys from the Hacettepe Institute, Ankara, Turkey, cover a wide cross-section of the nation. As usual, it is difficult to separate induced from spontaneous abortion, but the average fetal wastage reported across the country is 24 abortions per 100 deliveries. It is reasonable to assume that over half this loss is provoked, but it is the variation in rates that is revealing. In the rural areas, 13 pregnancies in 100 are reported to end in abortion. In Ankara, Istanbul and Izmir, the figure is 97 in 100, with other urban areas falling in between. Amongst urban Turkish women with no schooling, the ratio is reported as 18 abortions to 100 deliveries, but for the wives of business and professional men the ratio is 109:100.[184]

Yugoslavia presents a particularly fascinating comparison; it is a test-tube of demographic change, containing within its borders a number of diverse semi-autonomous states all exposed to liberal abortion laws.[185] The central and southern parts of the country have little industry, religious beliefs run deep and the majority of the population is engaged in agriculture based on village settlement. Near the Italian border, in Slovenia and Vojvodina, the country is industrial and well developed. There has been considerable migration towards the industrialised areas in recent years and this is particularly marked in the case of the province of Vojvodina where Slav-speaking people have been encouraged to settle near the Hungarian border. There is a three-fold variation in birth rates between

Table 11. *Socio-economic aspects of abortion in Yugoslavia*

		Kosovo	Vojvodina	Slovenia
Birth rate per 1000	1954–54	43.5	23.3	22.8
	1970	36.0	12.6	16.4
Illiteracy among women over 10 years old (%)	(1971)	43.5	13.1	2.5
Employed persons who are female (%)	(1971)	17.0	31.0	42.1
Income *per capita*: dinars	(1960)	52000	147000	279000
Infant mortality per 100 live births	1950–54	154.6	120.2	70.6
	1970	93.9	34.2	23.3
Number of examinations for contraception per 1000 fertile women	1968	17	269	266
Number of women per gynaecologist		27600	9000	6300
Number of abortions per 1000 live births	1960–64	—	504–1321	535
	1965	—	—	523
	1966	—	1431	481
	1967	636	1824	485
	1968	—	1531	—
	1970	—	1609	450

industrialised areas such as Vojvodina and Slovenia and poor areas such as Kosovo, Bosnia and Herzegovina. There is a two-fold variation in the percentage of working women in the labour force and in other parameters such as literacy, income and even expectation of life and infant mortality (Table 11).

Vojvodina had a particular social history which created a strong tradition of abortion, long before liberalisation of the law. Traditionally, on the father's death, farms were divided between all the sons in the family. A similar tradition applied in Ireland, where in the late eighteenth and early nineteenth century, as the population grew, the farms were subdivided so that when the potato harvests failed in the mid-1840s the tiny plots could not support the families who depended upon them. One and a half million died and nearly one million emigrated. In Vojvodina the people adopted the alternative solution of strict family limitation, using a combination of *coitus interruptus* and illegal abortion. As in Ireland the demographic imperative extracted a cruel tribute while the death and mutilation consequent on induced abortions in Serbia became known as the

Table 12. *Socio-economic advance and abortion*

Completed family size

	Women living in		
Women born in	Vojvodina	Herzegovina	Bosnia
Vojvodina	2.60	—	—
Herzegovina	2.68	3.20	—
Bosnia	2.80	—	5.10

Pregnancies, deliveries and abortions per woman

	Deliveries	Induced abortions	Spontaneous abortion	Total pregnancies
Women born in and resident in Vojvodina	2.6	3.2	0.3	6.1
Women born elsewhere and living in Vojvodina	2.9	1.9	0.1	4.9

White Plague.[186] Today the old traditions persist, the birth rate is very low (14.4 per 1000) and the net reproduction rate is below replacement (0.85). There is an expanding, but by no means universal, use of contraception and a liberal abortion law has brought an old problem into the open. In 1969 there were 41 000 legal abortions in Vojvodina and 4500 hospital admissions for spontaneous and criminal abortion among a total population of two million people.

In all republics except Slovenia the number of legal abortions is still increasing. But in Slovenia, a decline began in 1965 that has not yet come to an end. In 1965 there were 523, and in 1970 450, abortions per 1000 live-born children.[187] Yugoslavia demonstrates, between different states of the same country, the pattern of abortion in relation to birth rate which has been described during the historical process of the demographic transition for a single homogeneous nation such as Britian, or between different social classes at a single instant of time, as in Chile (Fig. 51, p. 470).

The effect of migration across socio-economic frontiers has also

Table 13. *Family size by generation*

	Total deliveries		
	Per women in study	Per maternal grandmother	Per maternal great-grandmother
Women born in and resident in Vojvodina	2.6	5.3	5.6
Women born elsewhere and living in Vojvodina	2.9	5.9	7.6

been studied in Yugoslavia. Beric[188] surveyed 2000 families, comparing women born and still living in Vojvodina, women born and resident in Herzegovina and the families of the sisters of immigrants who remained in Herzegovina. The total number of conceptions in the three groups is comparable (Table 12), but the average family size is smaller in the economically advanced areas. Abortion plays a major role in this adjustment. Beric has also accumulated data allowing a comparison between generations and it can be surmised that the differences in abortion rates mediated by socio-economic factors in different parts of the country in the 1960s had their parallel in historical terms in a single locality (Tables 12 and 13).

Some sociological variables have been little investigated but may be of interest. For example, in Melbourne, Australia, 72 per cent of women having abortions were eldest, second born or only children and only 3 per cent were youngest children in a family. However, the sex of the older siblings was not correlated with the likelihood of resort to abortion.[189]

In the context of abortion research, socio-economic factors are usually regarded as determinants of abortion rates. But in sociological terms, abortion must be seen as a prime factor in socio-economic change. The differences in income *per capita*, education, literacy and female employment that characterise socio-economic advance are dependent on a reduction in achieved family size. No society has made such an adjustment without significant recourse to abortion – whether legal or illegal. Induced abortion has been and is an intrinsic element in social progress.

Religion

In contrast to the influence exerted by socio-economic pressure, urbanisation and the need (or freedom) of women to work, religious influences are slight.

Explicit statements by a religious group on abortion appear to be poor predictors of behaviour within that group. In some developing countries, such as Brazil or Iran, the culture is relatively homogeneous for one religion and, with the possible exception of urban élites, beliefs are ingrained, but in Europe and North America genuine religious belief is declining rapidly and statistics can mislead unless they include measures of religiosity. When certain religious groups adopt forceful attitudes towards abortion, their propagandists may tend to sidestep the problem of the frequency of induced abortions within the group, while their opponents may be unduly eager to emphasise the point. A woman seeking abortion may conceal her allegiance to a religion opposed to its use, because she may feel her religion might bias the gynaecologist against acceding to her request. A more obvious distortion could arise in retrospective studies, if women of certain religious faiths conceal past abortions more than others.

Among 7600 couples studied by Weill-Halle in France, 742 reported an aggregate of 1704 induced abortions.[190] Broadly, the distribution of religious belief was similar in the abortion group and in the total sample. One of the main effects of religion was not to stop abortion, but to create problems of conscience. The ratio of those who said they had such problems to those who said they had not, was six to one among practising Catholics, two to one or less among non-practising Catholics, and equally divided among Jews and non-believers. Practising Catholics and Protestants had slightly fewer abortions than non-practising Catholics, non-believers or Jews. Practising Catholics also wanted additional children six times as frequently as non-practising couples. Among a sample of Hawaiian women whose decision to have a baby or an abortion was analysed, unmarried Catholics resorted to abortion less often than Protestants or agnostics.[191]

In Latin America, the great majority of women are Catholic and, as has been pointed out, abortion is common. Hutchinson[127] in Brazil found some differences in incidence according to religion and religious practice. Among practising Catholics, 3.2 per cent had had at least one abortion, against 9.2 per cent in the total sample of 1734

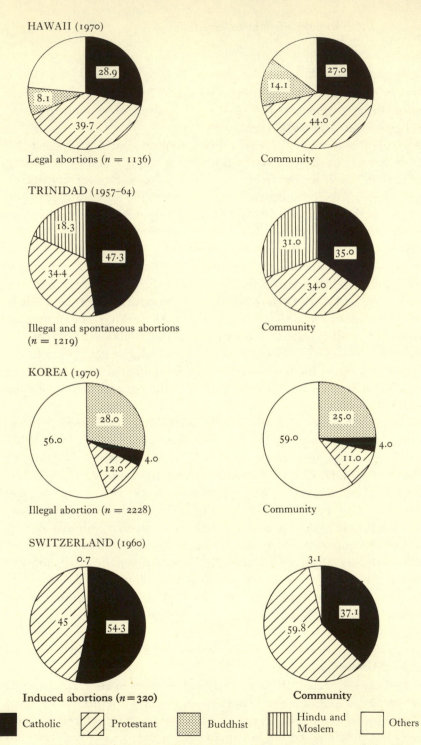

HAWAII (1970)

28.9

8.1

39.7

Legal abortions (n = 1136)

27.0

14.1

44.0

Community

TRINIDAD (1957–64)

18.3

47.3

34.4

Illegal and spontaneous abortions
(n = 1219)

31.0

35.0

34.0

Community

KOREA (1970)

28.0

56.0

12.0

4.0

Illegal abortion (n = 2228)

25.0

59.0

11.0

4.0

Community

SWITZERLAND (1960)

0.7

45

54.3

Induced abortions (n = 320)

3.1

59.8

37.1

Community

Catholic   Protestant   Buddhist   Hindu and Moslem   Others

Fig. 27. Distribution of religion by place and by women having
induced abortions.

women. However, non-practising Catholics had a slightly above-average resort to abortion (9.8 per cent claiming one or more artificial terminations) and were at a level above the Protestants (8.7 per cent), although the exact significance of these variations is difficult to analyse. Interestingly, in parts of Latin America, Miro & Rath found a *positive* association between church attendance and contraceptive practice.[192] Among the small number of Jews in the sample, 14.3 per cent claimed one or more abortions and this characteristic association is probably significant.

It is more common, however, to find induced-abortion rates unrelated to religious observance, and sometimes religious beliefs act paradoxically. Data are available from areas as far apart as Trinidad, USA, UK,[193] India and Switzerland demonstrating an over-representation of Catholics among women seeking and having abortions (Fig. 27). Approximately two per cent of the population of the city of Bombay are Roman Catholic, but Catholic women make up about 12 per cent of those having abortions. The impression of local observers is that the Catholics are not more wealthy than other women seeking abortions, but rules of chaperonage are less strict among Catholics than Hindus.[194]

In the UK, religious affiliation is not recorded in the registration of legal abortions. Sample surveys (Fig. 27) are available and the Lane Committee commented, 'Despite the opposition of the Catholic Church to abortion the proportion of Catholics among women having abortions does not seem to be much lower than that among fertile women in general. As with contraception, many women may be rejecting their Church's teaching in this field.' Possibly Catholics are inhibited from using effective contraceptive methods by religious constraints and are burdened with a higher rate of unplanned conceptions than other groups. In broader terms, it may be useful to regard them as a subgroup at an earlier stage in the evolution of birth control practices than the rest of the community, and therefore characterised by the use of a combination of contraceptive and abortion practices that is biased towards the latter. Thus the finding would seem to support the hypothesis that couples set themselves well-defined goals of family size and, although they use differing combinations of abortion and contraception to achieve these, in the last analysis no system of beliefs effectively deflects them.

At a political level it is possible that the froth created in public discussions of abortion policies is at a maximum where the conflict between intellectual belief and emotional response is greatest.

It can be stated that the role of religion in determining societal standards concerning the legality of abortion is out of all proportion to its impact on the individual's decision to seek or not to seek an abortion.

References

Four sources have been used particularly frequently in reviewing the epidemiology of abortion and are the origin of much of the numerical data:
David, H. P., Kalis, M. G. & Tietze, C. (ed.) (1973). *Selected Abortion Statistics: An International Summary.* Transnational Family Research Institute, Washington DC.
Tietze, C. & Dawson, D. A. (1973). Induced abortion: a factbook, *Reports on Population/Family Planning,* **14** (first edition), 1.
Tietze, C. & Murstein, M. C. (1975). Induced Abortion: 1975 factbook. *Reports on Population/Family Planning,* **14** (second edition), 1.
Moore-Čavar, E. C. (1974). *International Inventory of Information on Induced Abortion.* International Institute for the Study of Human Reproduction & Columbia University Press, New York.

1 Rongy, A. J. (1933). *Abortion: Legal and Illegal.* Vanguard Press, New York.

2 Lorimer, F. (1946). *The Population of the Soviet Union: History and Prospects.* League of Nations Publication, Geneva.

3 Gens, A. (1930). The demand for abortion in Soviet Russia. In *Sexual Reform Congress,* ed. N. Haire, p. 143. Kegan Paul, London.

4 Taussig, F. J. (1936). *Abortion, Spontaneous and Induced: Medical and Social Aspects.* Kimpton, London.

5 Muller-Dietz, H. (1964). Abortion in the Soviet Union and in the East European States. *Review of Soviet Medical Sciences,* **1**(2).

6 Herr, D. M. (1965). Abortion, contraception and population policy. *Soviet Studies,* **17**, 76.

7 Herr, D. M. (1968). The demographic transition in the Russian Empire and the Soviet Union. *Journal of Social History,* **1**, 193.

8 David, H. P. (1970). *Family Planning and Abortion in the Socialist Countries of Central and Eastern Europe.* Population Council, New York.

9 David, H. P. (1974). Abortion and family planning in the Soviet Union: public policies and private behaviour. *Journal of Biosocial Science,* **6**, 417.

10 Sadvokasova, Y. A. (1969). *Socio-Hygienic Aspects of Regulation of Family Size.* Meditsina, Moscow.

11 Berent, J. (1970). Causes of fertility decline in eastern Europe and the Soviet Union. *Population Studies, London,* **24**, 1 and 247.

12 Katkova, I. P. (1968). Some sociohygienic aspects of the childbearing functions among young women. Dissertation (in Russian). Quoted in David (1974); see note 9.

13 Sokolova, N. S. (1970). Statistical analysis of the outcome of pregnancies. *Zdravookhranenie Rossiiskoi Federatsii*, **14**, 38. Quoted by Steinhoff, P. G. (1972). Abortion data from the Soviet Union. *Abortion Research Notes*, Suppl. **1**(3).

14 Grods, L. (1971). Abortion in the Soviet Union. Quoted in David (1974); see note 9.

15 Muramatsu, M. (1971). Demographic aspects of abortion in Japan. In *Proceedings of the International Population Conference of the IUSSP*, vol. **2**, p. 1160. IUSSP, Liège.

16 Muramatsu, M. (1960). Effect of induced abortion on the reduction of births in Japan. *Milbank Memorial Fund Quarterly*, **38**, 153.

17 Ministry of Health and Welfare of Japan (n.d.). *Survey*.

18 Potts, M. (1967). Legal abortion in Eastern Europe. *Eugenics Review*, **59**, 232.

19 Tietze, C. (1967). Abortion in Europe. *American Journal of Public Health*, **57**, 1923.

20 Szabady, E. & Miltenyi, K. (1964). Problem of abortion in Hungary: demographic and health aspects. *Demografía*, **7**, 303.

21 Frejka, T. & Kaubek, J. (1968). Les avortemonts en la Tchécoslovaquie. *Population et Famille*, **1**, 1.

22 Mojić, A. (1969). Incidence of abortion and births in Yugoslavia in the last five years. *Ginekologiya i Obstetriciya*, **9**, 1.

23 Mehlan, K-H. & Falkenthal, S. (1965). Der legale Abort in der Deutschen Demokratischen Republik: Statistik der Jahre 1953–1962. *Deutsche Gesundheit*, **20**, 1163.

24 David, H. P. (1972). Personal communication.

25 Jureck (1966). *Demographie*, **1**. Quoted in Berent (1970); see note 11.

26 Hoffmeyer, H. & Norgaard, M. (1964). Investigations and calculations of incidence of illegal abortion since 1940. *Ugeskrift for Laeger*, **126**, 355.

27 Bruusgaard, C. (1961). Die Abortsituation in Norwegen. In *Internationale Abortsituation, Abortbekämpfung, Antikonzeption*, ed. K-H. Mahlan, Thieme, Stuttgart.

28 Ottensen-Jensen, O. (1971). Legal abortion in Sweden: thirty years' experience. *Journal of Biosocial Science*, **3**, 173.

29 Stamm, H. (1967). Statistische Underlagen zum Problem der Gerburtenkontrolle und der Familienplanung. *Ars Medici*, **11**, 748.

30 Stamm, H. (1971). Abortsituation in der Schweiz und Notwendigkeit sozialmedizinischer Massnahmen. *Geburtshilfe und Frauenheilkinde*, **3**, 241.

31 Diggory, P., Peel, J. & Potts, M. (1970). Preliminary assessment of the 1967 Abortion Act in practice. *Lancet*, **i**, 287.

32 Tyler, C. W., Bourne, J. P., Conger, S. B. & Kakn, J. B. (1972). Reporting and surveillance of legal abortions in the United States, 1970. In *Abortion Techniques and Services*, ed. S. Lewit, p. 192. Excerpta Medica, Amsterdam.

33 Weinstook, E., Tietze, C., Jaffe, F. S. & Dryfoos, J. G. (1975). Legal abortions in the United States since the 1973 Supreme Court decisions. *Family Planning Perspectives*, **7**, 23.

34 Institute of Medicine (1975). *Legalized Abortion and the Public Health.* National Academy of Sciences, Washington D.C.

35 Anonymous (1972). Family planning in the People's Republic of China. Report on the first official IPPF visit. *IPPF Medical Bulletin*, **6**(3), 1.

36 Chen, P. S. J. (1974). Singapore. In *Psychosocial Aspects of Abortion in Asia*, Proceedings of the Asian Regional Research Seminar on Psychosocial Aspects of Abortion, Kathmandu, Nepal, November 1974. Transnational Family Research Program, Washington D.C.

37 Lean, H. (1975). Personal communication.

38 Anonymous (1972). The care and treatment of therapeutic abortion patients in Canadian Hospitals January 1 – September 30, 1971. *Hospital Administration in Canada*, **14**, 25.

39 Cox, L. (1972). Personal communication.

40 Statistique de l'Association Tunisienne du Planning Familial (1971).

41 Marcoux, A. (1975). Tunisia. *Studies in Family Planning*, **6**, 307.

42 Bhatt, R. V. & Soni, J. M. (1974). Outpatient termination of pregnancy in India: scope and limitation. In *Transactions of Scientific papers by IFRP Contributors at the 17th All India Obstetrical and Gynaecological Congress*, ed. C. S. Dawn, p. 62. India Fertility Reseach Programme, Calcutta.

43 Seth, D. D., Maitra, S. K. & Sinha, B. N. (1973). *Abortion and Termination of Pregnancies in India.* Delhi Law House, Allahabad.

44 Cuban Ministry of Public Health (1974). *Obstetricia.* Havana. Quoted by Tietze, C. & Murstein, M. C. (1975). *Reports on Population/Family Planning*, **14**, (second edition), 1.

45 Hubinont, P., Brat, T., Polderman, J. & Ramdoyal, R. (1970). Abortion in Western Europe. In *Abortion in a Changing World*, ed. R. E. Hall, vol. **2**, p. 325. Columbia University Press, New York.

46 Desmeules, A. (1954). *L'avortment et le Contrôle des Naissances. Aspects Medico-socials et Legals.* Payot, Laussane.

47 Ajoon, G. (1973). Personal communication.

48 Bachi, R. & Matras, J. (1963). Contraception and induced abortion among Jewish maternity cases in Israel. *Milbank Memorial Fund Quarterly*, **41**, 207.

49 Bachi, R. (1970). Abortion in Israel. In *Abortion in a Changing World*, ed. R. E. Hall, vol. **1**, p. 274. Columbia University Press, New York.

50 Bickers, W. (1972). Serious complications of induced abortion in Lebanon. In *Induced Abortion: A Hazard to Public Health?*, ed. I. R. Nazer, p. 102, IPPF, Beirut.

51 Hathout, H. (1972). Looking at abortion material. In *Induced Abortion: A Hazard to Public Health?*, ed. I. R. Nazer, p. 216. IPPF. Beirut.

52 Tietze, C. (1970). United States: Therapeutic abortions, 1963–1968. *Studies in Family Planning*, no. **59**, 5.

53 Lewis-Faning, E. (1949). Family limitation and its influence on human fertility during the past fifty years. *Papers of the Royal Commission on Population*, vol. **1**. HMSO, London.

54 Elderton, E. M. (1914). *Report on the English Birthrate*. Part 1, *England, North of the Humber. Eugenics Laboratory Memoirs*, **19** and **20**.

55 British Medical Association (1936). Special Committee on Abortion. *British Medical Journal*, **1** (Supplement), 230.

56 Ministry of Health (1937). *Report on an Investigation into Maternal Mortality*. Ministry of Health, London.

57 Ministry of Health (1930). *Interim Report of Inter-Departmental Committee on Maternal Mortality and Morbidity*. Ministry of Health, London.

58 Glass, D. V. (1940). *Population Policies and Movements in Europe*. Clarendon Press, Oxford.

59 Parish, T. N. (1935). A thousand cases of abortion. *Journal of Obstetrics and Gynaecology of the British Empire*, **42**, 1107.

60 *Annual Report of the (London) Council* (1937), **3**(1), 18.

61 Pierce, T. V. (1930). 300 cases of abortion. *Journal of Obstetrics and Gynaecology of the British Empire*, **37**, 769.

62 Young, J. (1937). The part played by contraception and abortion. *Medical Press and Circular*, July, 72.

63 Cooke, R. G. (1938). An analysis of 350 cases of abortion. *British Medical Journal*, **1**, 1045.

64 Obeng, B. (1967). *500 Consecutive cases of abortion*. Ph.D. thesis, University of London.

65 *Irish Independent*, 16 February 1931.

66 Taussig, F. J. (1911). *The Prevention and Treatment of Abortion*. Mosby Co., St Louis.

67 Macomber, D. (1925). Etiology of abortion. *Boston Medical and Surgical Journal*, **193**, 116.

68 Kopp, M. E. (1934). *Birth Control in Practice*. McBridge, New York.

69 Stewart, R. E. (1935). Analysis of 1,772 abortions and miscarriages with a consideration of treatment and prevention. *American Journal of Obstetrics and Gynaecology*, **29**, 872.

70 Findley, P. (1922). Slaughter of the innocents. *American Journal of Obstetrics and Gynaecology*, **3**, 35.

71 Miller, W. M. (1934). Human abortion. *Human Biology*, **6**, 271.

72 Stix, R. K. (1935). Effectiveness of birth control. *Milbank Memorial Fund Quarterly*, **13**, 347.

73 Beebe, G. W. (1942). *Contraception and Fertility in the Southern Appalachians*. Williams & Wilkins, Baltimore.

74 Pearl, R. (1937). Fertility and contraception in New York and Chicago. *Journal of the American Medical Association*, **108**, 1385.

75 Pearl, R. (1939). *Natural History of Population*. Oxford University Press, London.

76 Gebhard, P. H., Pomeroy, W. B., Martin, C. E. & Christenson, C. V. (1959). *Pregnancy, Birth and Abortion*. Heinemann, London.

77 Abernathy, J. R., Greenberg, B. G. & Horvitz, D. G. (1970). Estimates of induced abortion in urban North Carolina. *Demography*, **7**, 19.

78 Tietze, C. (1949). Report on a series of abortions induced by physicians. *Human Biology*, **21**, 60.

79 Whittemore, K. R. (1970). The availability of nonhospital abortions. In *Abortion in a Changing World*, ed. R. E. Hall, vol. **1**, p. 212. Columbia University Press, New York.

80 Hall, R. E. (1971). Induced abortion in New York City. *American Journal of Obstetrics and Gynecology*, **110**, 601.

81 Tietze, C. (1954). Pregnancy wastage. In *Fetal, Infant and Childhood Mortality*, p. 12. United Nations, New York.

82 Peller, S. (1967). *Quantitative Research in Human Biology and Medicine*. Wright, Bristol.

83 Heiss, H. (1967). *Die Künstliche Schwangerschaftsunterbrechung und der kriminelle Abort*. Enke, Stuttgart.

84 Stamm, H. (1974). *Probleme des legalen Aborts in der Schweiz*. Verlag Ars Medici Ludin AG, Liestal.

85 Gardlund, T. (1934). Vissa uppgifter om preventivteknikens utbredning. *Betänkande i Sexualfrágan*, p. 325.

86 Sjövall, H. (1972). Abortion and contraception in Sweden 1870–1970. *Zeitschift für Rechtsmedizin*, **70**, 197.

87 Edin, K. A. (1934). *Undersukningau Abortforekomsten i Sverige under Senare AR*. Lund, Malmo.

88 Evang, G. (1936). *Mødrehygunenekontact i Oslo*. Quoted in Glass (1940); see note 58.

89 Kolstad, P. (1957). Therapeutic abortion: clinical study of 968 cases from a Norwegian hospital, 1940–53. *Acta Obstetricia et Gynaecologia Scandinavica*. **36**, Suppl. 6.

90 Berthélemy, H. (1917). *De la Répression de l'Avortement Criminel*. Paris.

91 Dourlen-Rollier, A. M. (1967). *L'Avortement en France*. Librairie Maloine, Paris.

92 Pressat, R. (1966). Sur le nombre des avortements en France. *Concours Medical*, **14**, 87.

93 Dalsace, J. & Dourlen-Rollier, A. M. (1970). *L'Avortement*. Casterman, Paris.

94 INED (1966). Report de l'Institute National d'Études Demographiques á Monsieur le Ministre des Affaires Sociales sur la regulation des naissances en France. *Population*, **21**, 645.

95 Cliquet, R. & Thiery, M. (ed.) (1972). *Abortus Provactus: Een Interdisciplinaire Studie met Betrekking tot Beleidsalternatieven in Belgie*. Der Nederlandsche Boekhandel, Antwerp.

96 Klein-Vercautere, E. (1961). Die Abortsituation in Belgien. In *Internationale Abortsituation, Abortbekämpfung, Anticonzeption*, ed. K-H. Mehlan, p. 23. Thieme, Stuttgart.

97 Doughe, G. (1971). Demografische aspecten van de abortuspraktijken. *Kultuurleven*, **38**, 27.

98 Cliquet, R. L. (1972). Knowledge, practice and effectiveness of contraception in Belgium. *Journal of Biosocial Science*, **4**, 41.

99 Treffers, P. E. (1967). Abortion in Amsterdam. *Population Studies, London*, **20**, 295.

100 Treffers, P. E. (1965). *Abortus Provocatus en Anticonceptie.* De Erven F. Bohn, Haarlem.

101 Muntendam, P. (1966). Socio-medical aspects of criminal abortion. *Nederlands Tijdschrift voor Geneeskunde*, **110**, 1337.

102 Van Emde Boas, C. (1967). Abortus provocatus. *Nederlands Tijdschrift voor Geneeskunde*, **4**, 169.

103 Borruso, V. (1967). *Practice of Abortion and Birth Control in Sicily.* Libri Siciliani, Palermo.

104 Potts, M. (1968). Abortion – Italian style. *Family Planning*, **17**, 12.

105 Quattrocchi, G. (1968). L'Aborto procurato. *Clinica Ostetrica e Ginecologica*, **70**, 163.

106 Figa-Talamanca, R. (1971). Social and psychological failures in the practice of induced abortion as a means of fertility control in an Italian population. *Genus*, **27**, 100.

107 Laufe, L. (1972). Personal communication.

108 Department of Demography, Australian National University, Canberra (1972). Australian Family Formation Project, Melbourne Survey. (Duplicated document.)

109 Claman, A. D., Wakeford, J. R., Turner, J. M. M. & Hayden, B. (1971). Impact on hospital practice of liberalizing abortions and female sterilization. *Canadian Medical Association Journal*, **105**, 35.

110 Facer, W. A. P., Simpson, D. W. & Murphy, B. D. (1973). Abortion in New Zealand. *Journal of Biosocial Science*, **5**, 151.

111 Werry, J. S., Pearson, A. S., Taylor, C. M. & Bonham, D. G. (1977). Extranuptial conception in New Zealand. In preparation.

112 Peled, T. (1974). Israel. In *Psychosocial Aspects of Abortion In Asia*, Proceedings of the Asian Regional Research Seminar in Psychosocial Aspects of Abortion, Katmandu, Nepal, November 1974, p. 53. Transnational Family Research Program. Washington D.C.

113 Bachi, R. & Matras, J. (1963). Contraception and induced abortion among Jewish maternity cases in Israel. *Milbank Memorial Fund Quarterly*, **40**, 207.

114 Halvei, H. S. & Brzesinski, A. (1958). Incidence of induced abortion among Jewish women in Israel. *American Journal of Public Health*, **48**, 102.

115 Valaoras, V. G. (1965). Control of family size in Greece – the results of a field survey. *Population Studies*, **18**, 265.

116 Valaoras, V. (1969). The epidemiology of abortion in Greece. In *Social Demography and Medical Responsibility in Family Planning.* IPPF, London.

117 Cominos, A. (1967). Criminal abortion and its complications. In *Preventive Medicine and Family Planning*, p. 112. IPPF, London.

118 Valaoras, V. G. (1970). Abortion in Greece. In *Abortion in a Changing World*, ed. R. E. Hall, vol. **1**, p. 284. Columbia University Press, New York.

119 Danezis, J. (1969). Induced abortion as an international and as a Greek problem. *Iatriki*, **15**, 195.

120 Armijo, R. & Monteal, T. (1965). The problem of induced abortion in Chile. *Milbank Memorial Fund Quarterly*, **43**, 265.

121 Stycos, J. M. (1968). *Human Fertility in Latin America*. Cornell University Press, Ithica, New York.

122 IPPF (1970). 'Induced Abortion in Latin America.' A preliminary study based on materials in the Library of the International Planned Parenthood Federation, Western Hemisphere Region, New York. (Duplicated document.)

123 Armijo, R. & Monreal, T. (1965). The problem of induced abortion in Chile. *Milbank Memorial Fund Quarterly*, **43**, 263.

124 Aldama, A. (1963). 'El aborto provocado problem de salud pública, Mexico, 1963.' Population Council, New York. (Duplicated document.)

125 Hall, M. F. (1965). Family planning in Lima, Peru. *Milbank Memorial Fund Quarterly*, **43**, 100.

126 Viel, B. (1969). 'Induced Abortion in Latin America.' WHO, Geneva. (Duplicated document.)

127 Hutchinson, B. (1964). Induced abortion in Brazilian married women. *America Latina*, **7**, 21.

128 Gall, N. (1972). Births, abortions and the progress of Chile. *American Universities Field Staff Reports*, no. **29**, vol. **2**, p. 1.

129 Tabah, C. (1963). A study of fertility in Santiago, Chile. *Marriage and Family Living*, **25**, 20.

130 Ferrarotti, N. G. & Varela, C. G. (1964). *Investigaciones Sobre Incidence del Aborto Criminal*. Quoted in Stycos (1968); see note 121.

131 Ferrarotti, N. G. & Varela, C. G. (1964). Encuesta Sobre et Aborto y sus Variables Incluyendo Métodos de Planificación de Familia. In *Revista de la Sociedad de Obstetricia y Ginecologia de Buenos Aires*, **611**.

132 Rosada, L. (1964). 'La Situación del aborto voluntario en el Uruguay, posibles soluciones.' IPPF, Western Hemisphere Conference. (Duplicated document.) Quoted in Stycos (1968); see note 121.

133 Stycos, J. M. (1971). *Ideology, Faith and Family Planning in Latin America*. McGraw-Hill, New York.

134 Hoyte, R. A. St Clair (1964). 'An analysis of abortion at the Central Hospital, Port of Spain.' Fourth Conference of the IPPF, Western Hemisphere Region, April 1964. (Duplicated document.)

135 Bhagwansingh, A. (1973). In *UJIN Conference, University of the West Indies, Jamaica Family Planning Association Limited, IPPF and National Family Planning Board*. Proceedings of a Conference, 15–16 December 1972, University of the West Indies. (Duplicated document.)

136 Williams, A. (1973). In *Ibid.* (Duplicated document.)

137 Arjoon, G. (1973). In *Ibid.* (Duplicated document.)

138 Awan, A. K. (1969). *Provoked Abortion amongst 1,447 Married Women*. Maternity and Child Health Association of Pakistan, Lahore.

139 Yaukey, D. (1961). *Fertility Differences in a Modernizing Country.* Princeton University Press, Princeton, N.J.

140 Bickers, W. (1962). Serious complications of induced abortion in Lebanon. In *Induced Abortion: A Hazard to Public Health?*, ed. I. R. Nazer, p. 102. IPPF, Beirut.

141 Özbay, F. & Shorter, F. C. (1970). Turkey: changes in birth control practices, 1963–68. *Studies in Family Planning*, no. **51**, 1.

142 Erenus, N. (1967). *Provoked Abortion.* Gürsoy, Ankara.

143 Fisek, N. H. (1972). Epidemiological study on abortion in Turkey. In *Induced Abortion: A Hazard to Public Health?*, ed. I. R. Nazer, p. 264. IPPF, Beirut.

144 Alavi-Naini, M. (1972). The incidence of induced and spontaneous abortion among high socio-economic classes in Iran. In *Induced Abortion: A Hazard to Public Health?*, ed. I. R. Nazer, p. 182. IPPF, Beirut.

145 Daneshbod, K., Borazjani, G. R., Sajadi, H. & Hamidzacheh, M. M. (1970). Survey of maternal deaths in South Iran, analysis of 96 autopsies. *Journal of Obstetrics and Gynaecology of the British Commonwealth*, **77**, 1103.

146 Larsen, T. B. (1972). Estimates of induced abortion in some Middle East countries. In *Induced Abortion: A Hazard to Public Health?*, ed. I. R. Nazer, p. 78. IPPF, Beirut.

147 Foda, M. S., Darwish, M. A., Shafeek, M. A. & Osman, E. (1972). Abortion in the UAR. In *Induced Abortion: A Hazard to Public Health?*, ed. I. R. Nazer, p. 122. IPPF, Beirut.

148 Kamal, I., Ghoneim, M. A., Talaat, M., Abdallah, M. & Eid, M. (1972). An attempt at estimating the magnitude and probable incidence of induced abortion in the UAR. In *Induced Abortion: A Hazard to Public Health?*, ed. I. R. Nazer, p. 106. IPPF, Beirut.

149 Toppozada, H. K. & Toppozada, M. K. (1972). Induced abortion: a comparison of its incidence and hazards with those of spontaneous abortion in private practice in Alexandria. In *Induced Abortion: A Hazard to Public Health?*, ed. I. R. Nazer, p. 168. IPPF, Beirut.

150 Thambu, J. A. M. & Marzuki, A. (1971). 'The problem of septic and criminal abortion?' IPPF, London. (Duplicated document.)

151 Puvan, I. S. (1974). Malaysia. In *Psychosocial Aspects of Abortion in Asia*, Proceedings of the Asian Regional Research Seminar on Psychosocial Aspects of Abortion, Katmandu, Nepal, p. 56. Transnational Family Research Program, Washington D.C.

152 Dabbas, H. (1972). Abortion in Jordon. In *Induced Abortion: A Hazard to Public Health?*, ed. I. R. Nazer, p. 201. IPPF, Beirut.

153 Bose, S. (1959). Abortion – a clinical review of 1,217 cases. *Journal of Obstetrics and Gynaecology of India*, **10**, 56.

154 Mukherjee, S. (1959). Abortion, A statistical survey. *Journal of Obstetrics and Gynaecology of India*, **10**, 77.

155 Anand, D. (1965). Clinico-epidemiological study of abortions. *Licentiate*, **15**, 208.

156 Rao, A. R., Belavalgidad, M. I. & Anand, D. (1968). A study on abortion. *Family Planning News, India*, **9**(12), 7.

157 Mohanty, S. S. P. (1968). Review of some selected studies on abortion in India. *Journal of Family Welfare*, **14**, 39.

158 Francis, O. (1969). Analysis of 1,150 cases of abortion from Government RSSM laying-in hospital, Madras. *Journal of Obstetrics and Gynaecology of India*, **10**, 62.

159 Sadashivaiah, K. & Rao, M. S. S. (1971). A study of the prevalence of foetal deaths. *Journal of the Christian Medical Association of India*, **46**, 164.

160 Srinivasan, K., Muthiah, A. & Krishnamoorthy, S. (1969). Analysis of the decline of fertility in Arthour Block. *Bulletin of the Institute of Rural Health and Family Planning Gandhigram*, **4**, 28.

161 Hong, S. B. (1966). *Induced Abortion in Seoul, Korea*. Dong-A Publishing Co., Seoul.

162 Hong, S. B. (1971). *Changing Patterns of Induced Abortion in Seoul, Korea*. Seoul.

163 Hong, S. B. & Koo, D. S. (1969). Studies in female deaths in the reproductive ages in Seoul. *Korean Journal of Obstetrics and Gynaecology*, **12**, 67.

164 Friedman, R., Jam, A. K. & Sun, T. H. (1970). Correlates of family limitation in Taiwan after IUD insertion. In *Taiwan Family Planning Reader*, ed. G. P. Cernada, p. 293. Chinese Center for International Training in Family Planning, Taichung.

165 Keeney, S. M., Cernada, G. P., Hsu, T. C., Sun, T. H., Hsu, S. C. & Chow, L. P. (1970). Population and program profile. In *Taiwan Family Planning Reader*, ed. G. P. Cernada, p. 3. Chinese Centre for International Training in Family Planning, Taichung.

166 Chow, L. P. & Liu, P. T. (1975). 'A new random response technique: multiple answer model.' (Unpublished.) Quoted in Tietze & Murstein (1975); see note 44.

167 Debhassom, A. (1973). Personal communication from survey available in Thai.

168 Rosenfield, A. G. & Somboosuk, A. (1971). 'An urban family planning centre.' IPPF, London. (Duplicated document.)

169 Ampofo, D. A. (1970). 330 cases of abortion treated at Korle Bu Hospital; the epidemiological and medical characteristics. *Ghana Medical Journal*, **9**, 156.

170 Larkeru, A. A. (1973). 'Abortion in Lagos – as seen at the Lagos Island Maternity Hospital, Nigeria.' Conference on Medical and Social Aspects of Abortion in Africa. IPPF, London. (Duplicated document.)

171 Pauls, F. (1973). Personal communication.

172 Ampofo, D. A. (1973). 'Epidemiology of abortion in selected African countries.' Conference on the Medical and Social Aspects of Abortion in Africa. IPPF, London. (Duplicated document.)

173 Moore-Čavar, E. C. (1974). *International Inventory of Information on Induced Abortion*. International Institute for the Study of Human Reproduction & Columbia University Press, New York.

174 David, H. P. (1974). Personal communication.
175 Fox, L. P. (1967). Abortion deaths in California. *American Journal of Obstetrics and Gynecology*, **98**, 645.
176 Laslett, P. & Oosterveen, K. (1973). Long term trends in bastardy in England: a study of the illegitimacy figures in the parish registers and in the reports of the Registrar General. *Population Studies, London*, **27**, 255.
177 Soonawalla, R. (1973). Personal communication.
178 David, H. P. (1974). India. In *Psychosocial Aspects of Abortion In Asia*. Proceedings of the Asian Regional Research Seminar on Psychosocial Aspects of Abortion, Katmandu, Nepal, p. 8. Transnational Family Research Program, Washington D.C.
179 Janmejai, K. (1963). Socio-economic aspects of abortion. *Family Planning News, India*, **4**(3), 55.
180 George, A. & Ramakumar, R. (1973). Reporting bias in pregnancy wastage. *Journal of Family Welfare*, **20**, 28.
181 United States Department of Economic and Social Affairs (1973). *The Determinants and Consequences of Population Trends*, vol. **1**, p. 133. United Nations, New York.
182 Langer, W. L. (1963). Europe's initial population explosion. *American Historical Review*, **69**, 1.
183 Suporn Koetsawang (n.d.). 'A study of patients with criminal abortion.' Family Planning Research Unit, Mahidol University, Bangkok. (Duplicated document.)
184 *Bulletin of the Hacettepe Institute of Population Studies* (n.d.). No. **15**.
185 Grujica Žarković (1976). The factors affecting the disposition of the natural population growth in SFR Yugoslavia. (In preparation.)
186 Potts, M. (1970). The White Plague: population control in Vojvodina. *World Medicine*, **6**(3), 31.
187 Simoneti, S. & Novak, F. (1972). 'Decline of birth rate and the influence of infant mortality. IPPF Western Hemisphere Region meeting, Ottawa. (Duplicated document.)
188 Beric, B. M. (1967). Quoted by Potts, M. (1967). Legal abortion in Eastern Europe. *Eugenics Review*, **59**, 232.
189 Weiner, J. (1973). Personal communication. See also Weiner, J. (1976). *Abortion: The Experience of a Freestanding Clinic in Melbourne*. Fertility Control Clinic, Melbourne. Victoria.
190 Weill-Halle, C. (1973). Personal communication.
191 Diamond, M., Steinhoff, P. G., Palmore, J. A. & Smith, R. G. (1973). Sexuality, birth control and abortion: a decision making sequence. *Journal of Biosocial Science*, **5**, 347.
192 Miro, C. & Rath, F. (1965). Preliminary findings of comparative fertility surveys in three Latin American cities. *Milbank Memorial Fund Quarterly*, **43**, 36.
193 Ingham, C. & Simms, M. (1972). Study of applicants for abortion at the Royal Northern Hospital, London. *Journal of Biosocial Science*, **4**, 351.
194 Soonawalla, R. (1973). Personal communication.

4
Demographic consequences of legal abortion

Analysis suggests that induced-abortion rate is correlated with urbanisation, socio-economic status, parity and marital status, but relatively independent of religion or cultural background. Evidence will be presented later (Chapter 13) to suggest that the probability of induced abortion and that of contraceptive practice are tightly linked, as two aspects of the single aim to control fertility.

Is the law a significant determinant of the total number of induced abortions in a country? Does a liberal law translate abortions from illegal to legal? Does a liberal law encourage pregnancies that might otherwise have gone to term to be terminated? Is a restrictive law a deterrent to induced abortion? Does awareness of a liberal abortion law undermine contraceptive practice? All these questions, and many others, are important and deserve answers.

The overall conclusion of this chapter is that the law does not appear to be a major determinant of the total number of induced abortions occurring in a community, although it may be a more important variable for some subgroups, such as the unmarried, than for others. There is considerable evidence that the major effect of a liberal abortion law is to transfer illegal operations to the legal sector, without any great alteration in the total rate.

Certainly, restrictive abortion laws are very rarely enforced. There are few 'crimes' where the prosecution rate is as low as in the case of illegal abortion, often less than one per 1000 illegal operations. In addition, those prosecuted may be acquitted, especially when trial is by a jury, or the police take bribes.

Consequences of liberal laws

Socialist countries

In Moscow the number of women reporting previous illegal abortions fell rapidly following the introduction of a liberal law in 1920[1] and the number of incomplete abortions admitted to hospital plateaued, suggesting that the switch from illegal to legal took perhaps five years (Fig. 11, p. 66). Roesle & Paevsky[2] estimated that the maternal mortality due to sepsis following childbirth and abortion in Leningrad was one-quarter that in Berlin (2.8 and 11 per 1000 deliveries and abortions, respectively). When Taussig[3] reviewed the Russian experience in 1936, he concluded there was 'evidence of a marked diminution in the number of secret abortions carried out by unscrupulous persons for money, under the worst possible conditions'.

No other eastern European country experimented with liberal abortion before World War II. Illegal abortion rates appear to have been high. In the 1930s Poland had a birth rate in the middle 20s per 1000 of the population. Statistics from the Charity and Hospital Commission of Warsaw showed a very high incidence of hospital admissions for abortion (Table 14). If the Latin American experience of one in three illegal abortions requiring hospital admission is taken as a yardstick, then the illegally induced abortion rate in Poland before World War II is comparable to the registered legal abortion rate today.

After World War II, the illegal abortion rate in eastern Europe rose further, as a result of the prevailing social disruption. The pressure to reform the law came in a significant part from a medical profession aware of the toll of ill-health created by a high illegal abortion rate. Before the law was changed in Czechoslovakia, a survey (1950–55) of women who had completed their families showed that one-quarter of all pregnancies ended in abortion. It was estimated that after the law was changed some 110000 to 140000 abortions would need to be performed annually (in fact the total reached 102600 in 1969). It is thought that the Czechoslovakian laws caused a 65–80 per cent reduction in the number of illegal abortions and, in the experience of doctors engaged in gynaecological practice, illegal abortions have become comparatively rare since the introduction of the new laws.[4]

Table 14. *Hospital admissions for abortion and delivery in Warsaw (1921–24)*

Year	Admissions for abortion (spontaneous and induced)	Hospital deliveries	Ratio
1921	1138	3403	1:3
1922	1100	5917	1:5.4
1923	1761	7108	1:4
1924	1843	7929	1:4.3

Major and minor changes in the law can be examined in relation to the number of legal abortions and births in Czechoslovakia (Fig. 13, p. 71). The law was altered to include social grounds in 1957. In 1960 a Government Decree (26 July) removed several hurdles to abortion, such as payment when the operation was performed on other than medical grounds. The number of legal abortions rose from 77000 in 1959 to 88000 in 1960 and 94000 in 1962. However, this increase in the abortion rate occurred at a time when the number of births was virtually unchanged (in fact births increased by 500 between 1959 and 1961). Therefore, the change in the number of registered abortions mainly seems to reflect transfers from illegal to legal. Under a Decree of 21 December 1962, payment under certain circumstances was reimposed and the Commissioners considering terminations were requested to apply stricter criteria. In 1963 the number of legal abortions fell to 70500, and the number of births increased from 217000 in 1962 to 235000 in 1963. What part of this rise was due to women carrying to term fetuses that might have been aborted and what part was an intrinsic rise in the birth rate is difficult to estimate. Certainly, by 1965 there had been a rise in the incidence of pelvic inflammation from illegal abortions and in the suicide rate among pregnant women, and the practice with regard to legal abortion was relaxed once again. This was followed by a rise in the number of legal abortions that by 1967 (96400) had surpassed the 1962 level. In 1969 the figures reached a new maximum of 102600, but some increase in the number of fertile women had taken place and the rate of 33.1 per 1000 women aged 15–69 and was no greater than that for 1959–61. The political upheavals of the late 1960s may account for some changes in abortion practice.

In Hungary there were no changes in legislation between 1956 and 1974 (Fig. 14, p. 72). The lowest birth rate in Hungarian history, and also for that date the lowest in European experience, occurred in 1962 (12.9 per 1000). Unlike those of most of the neighbouring countries, the Hungarian law then stated that termination must be granted 'if the applicant insists on the interruption of pregnancy after the commission has asked her to think it over'. The operation costs 300 forints ($12) when performed for social reasons although there remains a strong and binding tradition of giving the surgeon a present. An illegal operation by a physician costs approximately 1000 forints ($40), so that it is not surprising that some illegal operations persist for reasons of privacy. Hospital admissions for spontaneous and illegal abortions are registered and rose slightly from 34 300 to 43 100 in the five years before the law was liberalised, fell to 33 800 in 1960 and have remained within a thousand of that figure since then. It is impossible to estimate what would have happened to the illegal abortion rate, or the birth rate, if the law had not been altered, and the number of legal abortions registered each year gives no indication of how many babies might have been born if the law had been otherwise. In 1952 there were 185 000 live births and 1700 legal abortions; 12 years later, after the alteration of the abortion law, there were 184 400 legal abortions. However, the number of live births had not fallen correspondingly, but stood at 132 100. Contraceptive practice had improved (see Chapter 13). Some rise in conception rate as the result of a lowering of the age when sexual relations begin may also have occurred. Therefore, illegal abortion must have been common in 1952 and it is reasonable to surmise that a significant proportion of the legal abortions performed under the liberal legislation would have occurred as illegal abortions if the law had not been changed.[4]

Mehlan[5] has estimated that the combined total of legal spontaneous and criminal abortions taking place in East Germany declined from 150 000 in 1950 to 70 000–90 000 in 1962. The change was, however, unevenly distributed and in some groups (large urban communities, women under 21, and the unmarried) the rate rose despite the overall fall.

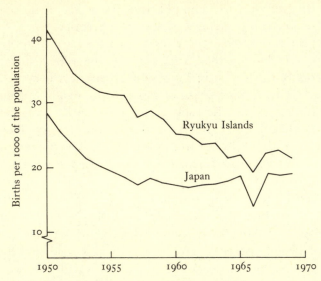

Fig. 28. Live birth rates per 1000 of the population in the
Ryukyu Islands and Japan (1950–69).

Japan

In Japan, as in parts of eastern Europe, it is possible to follow
changes in the legal abortion rate over extended intervals of time
and to demonstrate a fall in legal abortions with a concurrent
improvement in contraceptive practice (see Chapter 13).[6]
The vagaries of modern history have created a unique and informative control experiment for assessing the Japanese experience.
During the Pacific War, Okinawa and the other Ryukyu islands were
occupied by Allied forces shortly before the Japanese surrender and
the islands were requisitioned and administered separately until
their return to the Japanese in 1972. During this interval, the
abortion law followed the American pattern and the operation was
illegal except for strictly medical reasons. Culturally, Okinawa is
part of Japan, although Chinese influence is slightly greater and it
lags behind in income *per capita*. Nevertheless, the birth rate (Fig.
28) follows that of Japan accurately, including the same dip in 1966
– the year of the Fiery Horse – when it was said to be unlucky to
conceive a girl baby. A survey by the Okinawa Family Planning
Association found that, among 380 women using contraceptives, 61.6
per cent reported having illegal abortions. A parallel figure from

Japan is 65 per cent having legal abortions. The inference is that the liberal abortion law in Japan made evident a broad trend that would have occurred even if the law had never been liberalised.

It could be argued that the more rapid decline in the birth rate in Japan was the result of the 1949 Eugenics Protection Law but it is more likely that it was the result of economic factors (in 1971 the gross national product *per capita* of Japan was US $1190 and of the Ryukyu islands US $580).

Western Europe

Abortion is common: in eastern Europe and Japan, liberal laws, liberally interpreted, have led to abortion ratios of from 20 to over 100:100 live births. In Britain and Scandinavia the situation is different. The law and medical practice are not so liberal and ratios are nearer 10:100 live births. Contraceptive practice among married women is better than in eastern Europe, USSR or Japan, however, pregnancies to unmarried women make up half or more of the total terminated and in this group contraceptive practice is less effective. In addition, the abortion law in Britain was altered, and in Scandinavia practices became more liberal, at the very time that sexual practices among the young unmarried were changing, and this complicates the interpretation of the statistics. The British situation is further discussed in Chapter 8 (see also Table 15).

At the time when abortion reform first occurred in Denmark, Auken[7] conducted an investigation of abortion incidence among a sample of 315 women, collecting material over the years 1933–47. Half the reported pregnancies were unplanned, 9.5 per cent were said to have ended in spontaneous abortion, 1.4 per cent in legal operations and 2.6 per cent in self-induced abortion. An additional 11.5 per cent attempted to provoke an abortion but failed. Probably the survey underestimated the amount of illegal abortion. In Sweden, when the first abortion law was passed in 1938, there were thought to be 10000 to 20000 illegal abortions annually, that is 10 to 20 induced abortions per 100 deliveries. Thirty years after the law was first altered the legal abortion ratio reached 10:100 births and passed the 10000 mark annually. However, during this interval, contraceptive practices had improved (for example, up to 20 per cent of fertile women came to use oral contraceptives) so the total number of induced abortions might be expected to have declined. There have been some changes in population, but the main changes that have taken place are probably (1) a significant transfer from illegal to legal abortions, with (2) a possible decline in the total number (illegal and legal) of abortions among the married, and (3) an increase in the number of premarital pregnancies and a concomitant rise in the induced abortion rate among the young unmarried.[8]

In Sweden when most abortions were granted after application to a commission, those rejected could be followed up. Ottensen-Jensen[9] reviewed the literature for an aggregate of nearly 6000 women where applications were refused. The percentage who aborted spontaneously or illegally varied from 14 to 39. Presumably those accepted had what were considered stronger reasons for termination. Such reasoning presents indirect evidence that many of those who obtained legal abortions would have resorted to illegal ones.

United States

Rapid changes in law and practice which occurred in the USA, at a time of increasing economic stringency, combined with intense academic interest in the consequences of abortion, have created a uniquely informative situation, both with respect to the transfer of illegal abortions to legal practice and for the assessment of demographic effect.

The most complete analysis, by Tietze,[10] comes from New York City for the years 1970–72. It is a fortunate accident that the legal abortion figures were recorded for each 12 months from the implementation of the repeal situation in July 1970, so the 'abortion year' runs July–June. Birth statistics are available over the calendar year January–December. As most abortions occur in the first three months of pregnancy, the conceptions that gave rise to the 'abortion year' statistics also give rise to deliveries in the following calendar year. Records allow New York residents to be distinguished from out-of-state women.

Tietze calculated that, at the 1970 fertility rate and allowing for slight changes in population structure, 150700 deliveries would have taken place in 1971 to New York residents. In practice, there were 131900. The deficit of 18800 could have been because of the greater availability of abortion, or to an increased use of contraception (Fig. 29).

A total of 67400 legal abortions were registered in 1970–71. Before the law was repealed it is thought about 2000 legal abortions took place annually. It takes slightly more than one abortion to avert a

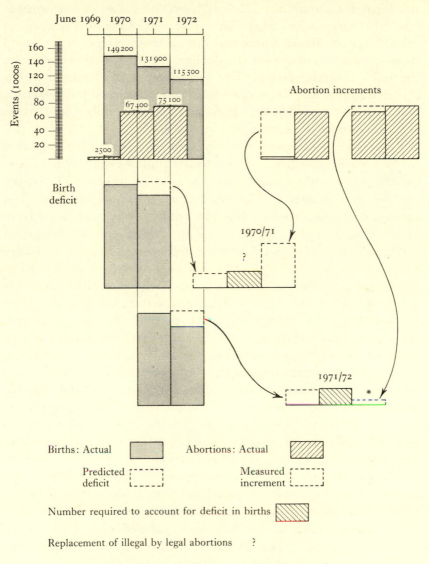

Fig. 29. Easily available legal abortion replaces previous illegal abortion and promotes effective contraceptive practice. Tietze's analysis of the New York City birth and abortion statistics (1970–72).

live birth in a community, such as New York, that has a reasonable level of contraceptive usage. Therefore, out of the total increase of 65 000 legal abortions, a maximum of 22 600 (or 35 per cent) would be sufficient to account for the decline in births, if abortions were the only changing factor. The remaining legal abortions either replaced previously illegal operations and/or represented a genuine climb in the conception rate because easier availability of abortion led to a decline in contraceptive practice.

Fortunately, a comparison of 1972 with 1971 allows the elimination of the second hypothesis. The estimated number of births in 1972 (at the 1971 fertility rate) would have been 134 500. The actual number of registered births was 116 400: a decline of 18 100. The number of legal abortions taking place only rose by 7000 (that is from 67 400 in 1970–71 to 75 100 in 1971–72). The maximum number of births this increment could have averted would be 6400. This leaves a deficit of 11 700 births which could only have been prevented or postponed by other changes in reproductive behaviour. There was a drop in the total number of marriages of 1000, but this would not account for more than a minority part of the births averted. Therefore, it seems reasonable to conclude that *there was a significant improvement in contraceptive practice* between the years 1971 and 1972. The only alternative hypothesis would be that the inhabitants of New York underwent a sudden change in patterns of sexual behaviour between 1971 and 1972. If contraceptive practice improved between 1971 and 1972 it seems unlikely that it had worsened between 1970 and 1971, so the second important finding of the Tietze analysis is that *the overwhelming majority of the legal abortions performed in New York replaced previously illegal operations.* An analysis of the figures for England and Wales, discussed in Chapter 9, reveals a similar situation (see Fig. 42, p. 319).

Looked at another way, nine-tenths of the effect of changing the New York abortion law appears to have been in transferring previously illegal abortions to the legal sector; one-tenth gave rise to direct demographic effect. Certainly, the law was repealed at a time of falling birth rates. In 1961 the nationwide birth rate in the USA was 23.4 per 1000, in 1970 it was 18.3. As always abortion played a major role in these changes *both* during the phase of restrictive legislation and after the reform and repeal laws were implemented. The exceptional liberality of the New York situation accelerated this trend by a modest degree. The pattern of birth rate change in New

Table 15. *Percentage change (annual average) in marital and illegitimate birth rates in the presence and absence of liberal abortion legislation*

USA	1965–1970[a]	1970–71
Legitimate births (women aged 15–44)		
All races		
Liberal states	−1.4	−7.8
Restrictive states	−1.4	−4.9
White women		
Liberal states	−1.0	−7.9
Restrictive states	−1.1	−4.9
Non-white		
Liberal states	−3.6	−7.1
Restrictive states	−3.3	−4.4
Illegitimate births (women aged 15–44)		
All races		
Liberal states	+2.9	−12.4
Restrictive states	+3.0	−1.9
White women		
Liberal states	+4.5	−16.9
Restrictive states	+4.4	−9.1
Non-white women		
Liberal states	+0.4	−8.6
Restrictive states	+1.0	+2.6
Illegitimate births (women aged 15–19)		
All races		
Liberal states	+5.7	−10.2
Restrictive states	+5.8	+0.3

UK	1967–69/70
Illegitimate births (women aged 15–44)	
Liberal areas[b]	−5.0
Restrictive areas	+2.4

[a] Until 1970, 15 US states had reformed laws. After 1970 five states practised abortion on request. The more socially advantaged began to cross state boundaries in large numbers.
[b] The British law was reformed in 1967. Some geographical areas adopted liberal policies, doing more than 6.00 legal abortions per 1000 women, while the most restrictive did less than 2.00.

York City and the USA is very similar, but New York has been in advance of the rest of the country since the repeal of the abortion laws.

As emphasised elsewhere, the behaviour of the young unmarried in relation to unwanted pregnancy is sufficiently different from that of married couples to warrant separate analysis – including speculation about possible demographic effects.

A higher proportion of premarital conceptions end in induced abortion, but the exact level is subject to various sociological pressures. In California the availability of legal abortion began by replacing previously illegal abortions,[11] but it is thought that from 1972 it began to have a demonstrable effect on the birth rate. However, the effect fell unevenly on marital pregnancies (which fell by 10.3 per cent in 1971 and 10.1 per cent in 1972) and illegitimate pregnancies (which fell by 16.3 per cent in 1971, but only by 2.7 per cent in 1972). In other words, some women appear to have chosen to continue an illegitimate pregnancy. Both marital and non-marital fertility rates are higher among black than among white women in California but the gap between the two has narrowed (general fertility rates per 1000 women aged 15–44: 1966, white 85, black 107; 1972, white 67, black 78) and the black rates overall and for each parity follow the white trends.

In the USA as a whole, three-quarters of all births to women in the 15–19 age group are conceived premaritally. Analysis of birth rates per 1000 women for the years 1965–71, when legal abortion was unequally available in different states (see Chapter 10), shows that the states with liberal laws and practices were subject to a slightly more rapid decline in fertility, especially among the unmarried, than states then retaining restrictive legislation (Table 15).[12]

Deaths due to abortion

In industrialised nations with a fairly reliable death certification, the number of deaths registered as due to illegal abortion is a possible indicator of the transfer of abortions from illegal to legal services, although there are obvious pitfalls in handling the data (p. 24).

After the change of law in Poland (1956), the number of deaths thought to be due to illegal abortion dropped from 79 in 1956 to 26 in 1959. (The number of prosecutions for illegal operations fell in parallel.) In Western societies, change in abortion legislation came when maternal mortalities were already low. The effect in Britain is discussed in Chapter 9 and that for the USA as a whole is illustrated on p. 349 (Fig. 44).

In California, the numbers of hospital terminations rose logarithmically in the late 1960s, while septic-abortion admissions and maternal deaths due to abortion (1967, 8 per 100000 live births; 1968, 5 per 100000; 1969, 3 per 100000) fell. Analysis of the effects of liberal abortion attitudes on illegal abortion rates is always open to criticism, but the Californian evidence is valuable because it includes data from different geographical regions within the state. In the San Francisco Bay area many legal abortions were performed and abortion-related maternal deaths decreased more rapidly than in Los Angeles, where fewer hospital abortions were operating at this time.[13,14]

In New York City the maternal mortality rate (including deaths from legal and illegal abortion) fell from 5.2 per 100000 in 1970 to 2.3 in 1971. Admissions for incomplete abortions in two large municipal hospitals fell by 48 per cent, comparing the records for 1 July–31 December, 1970. In Maryland, for the first time in history, there was only one abortion death in 1970. One illegal abortionist approached the President of Planned Parenthood/World Population and asked what he should do now he was unemployed.

In Romania, during the years of liberal abortion, deaths attributed to all types of abortion were registered at a rate of well under 100 a year. After the imposition of a restrictive law in 1966 they rose to 170 for the calendar year 1967 and to 364 by 1972 (Fig. 30).

The restriction of previously liberal laws

Another way to gain insight into the relationship between illegal and legal abortion is to follow events after liberal laws are made restrictive, as happened in Russia in the 1930s, in Bulgaria and Romania in the 1960s, and is currently happening in Hungary.

The Russian experience can only be followed in broad outline.[15-17] The birth rate rose from 32.6 per 1000 in 1936 (the last year of liberal legislation) to 37.7 in 1937. The effect was greatest in the cities where abortion had been most used. The absolute number of births in Moscow rose from 35107 in 1936 to 68279 one year later (82 per cent increase) and in Leningrad from 63129 to 79261 (82 per cent). The change in abortion practice coincided with the rise of Stalin, his political purges and the aftermath of collectivi-

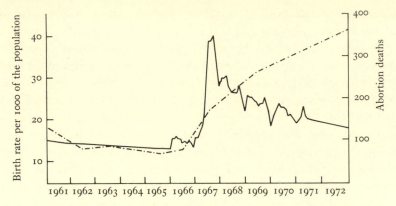

Fig. 30. Romanian birth rate per 1000 of the population (—)
and deaths attributed to abortion (–·–) (1961–72). (Note that
the birth rate is plotted monthly for the years 1966–71.)

sation, all of which probably added to the decline of the birth rate.
The birth rate subsequently fell rapidly back to the level before the
change and by 1940, on the eve of the giant social dislocations of
World War II, it was 31.2 per 1000. There is anecdotal evidence,
which it seems reasonable to accept at its face value, that illegal
abortion rates rose, and one Leningrad gynaecologist claimed 70
per cent of his beds were filled with the complications of illegal
abortion during the period of restriction.

In November 1955, shortly after the end of the Stalinist era, all
legal restriction on abortion was removed for a second time (p. 388).

The Bulgarian experience was little more than a legal sideshow.
In December 1968 the Central Committee of the Communist Party
restricted the then existing abortion-on-request situation to 'facilitate better conditions for population growth in Bulgaria'. The
changes were mild, still allowing easy abortion for any woman over
45, or with three or more children, in fact they seem mainly to have
been aimed at the childless couple. The restriction was not followed
consistently. And in April 1973 the instructions were changed to
permit elective abortion to any woman with two children and to those
under 18 years of age. In practice, the legal abortion rate rose
steadily during this period from 11.8 per 1000 of the population in
1967 to 15.4 in 1971.

Romania introduced liberal abortion legislation in September 1957
and reversed it on 1 October 1966.[18-20] During these nine years, a
very liberal policy of abortion on request was followed and high

numbers of operations performed.[21] In the mid 1960s women seeking abortions in Bucharest had an average of 3.9 prior operations. In 1965 induced abortions in the whole of Romania exceeded 1 100 000:[22,23] in 1967, after the law was restricted, 52 000 were performed (a 20-fold fall).

The Romanian changes were much more fundamental than the Bulgarian. With little contraception, heavy pressure for small families and an uncertain tradition of *coitus interruptus*, Romania used abortion as the predominant method of fertility regulation. Even so, some contraception must have been practised because, if abortion had been the *sole* method of fertility regulation, the calculated rate for 1966, in order to have achieved the observed birth rate of 14.3, would have had to have been 72–108 per 1000 of the population, instead of the 59 per 1000 observed. The Romanian net reproductive rate was down to 0.91 by the mid 1960s.[19]

The 1966 law limited abortion to women over 45, those with four or more children, cases of rape, where there was risk of congenital defect and for serious medical grounds. The adjustment was from freely available abortion to something like the Scandinavian legislation of the early 1960s. (Interestingly, the total number of terminations under the revised law runs at half the English number for a nation a quarter the size.)

Additional strong pro-natalist policies accompanied the change in the abortion law. Men and women without children, whether married or not, over the age of 26 were taxed, while couples with three or more children had their taxes cut by 30 per cent. Divorce legislation was tightened. Contraceptive sale and import were regulated. But the imposition of anti-contraceptive legislation has been irregular. Condoms are still available. Pills and intrauterine devices are not allowed officially, although their sale is not prohibited and informal enquiries in Bucharest suggest that physicians give off-duty consultations on family planning and pass over Pills and devices imported from neighbouring socialist countries.

The October 1966 legislation produced the single most dramatic change ever recorded in human birth rates. Between December 1966 and September 1967 the birth rate more than tripled (12.8–39.9 per 1000). However, within a year the birth rate had fallen to under 30 and in two years to near 20. Illegal abortion services opened up. The revised law was more liberally interpreted in relation to legal abortion, in particular the mental health indications are probably being widened as the continuing need for abortion becomes more apparent and evidence for a climbing illegal abortion rate accumulates.

David summarised the Romanian experience with two statements: 'A review of Romanian health trends and statistics suggests that the long standing preference for a small family was not seriously affected by the shifting legislation . . . Romanian experience suggests that well established behavioral patterns of fertility control are resistant to significantly prolonged changes by government edict alone.'[24]

By 1972–73 admissions for incomplete abortion to hospital in Bucharest were running at about one-third of the total number of legal abortions previously performed. (Of course, most of the admissions resulted from illegal abortion and required inpatient care, while the legal operations had been done as outpatient operations.) Formidable changes in the structure of the Romanian population have occurred with bewildering consequences for education and subsequent employment of the offspring produced in the bulge years.

Analysis of the birth changes following the law show that women over 25 having second to fifth children contributed most to the bulge.[19]

In Russia in the 1930s and in Romania in the 1960s the demographic effect of restricting liberal legislation was more marked than in the case of switching from restrictive to liberal legislation. The two situations are not simply sociological mirror images of one another. The restriction of previous laws involves some novel additional elements. Under a liberal law, the number of hospital terminations takes several years to build up; when a liberal law is reversed, the cessation of hospital operations can be instantaneous. Likewise, although the criminal abortionists' work will be slowly curtailed, as women learn to take advantage of a liberal law, the illegal network, with its web of subtle relations between clients, takes some years to form.

Summary

All known societies use a mixture of contraception and abortion to control their fertility.[25] The factors that influence the relationship between these two variables and their possible separate and combined impact on the birth rate have been discussed in Chapter 1. Further consideration of the relationship between induced abortion and contraception is given in Chapter 13. The quantitative evidence set out in the previous chapter and the qualitative data presented in the next chapter lead to the conclusion that the relative roles of contraception and induced abortion vary between different countries and in the same country at different times, but that both are essential components of fertility regulation.

It is well known that contraceptive practice by an individual couple improves with the duration of use; it is also apparent that, at the community level in Western developed countries, contraceptives are more readily available and being more widely used in the last third of the twentieth century than they were previously. The witness of history is that abortion was very common in the late nineteenth century and early twentieth century in Europe and North America.

The simplest hypothesis to construct is that (1), when the demographic transition begins, induced abortion plays a relatively more important role in fertility control than it does later; and (2), with the passage of time, contraceptive practices improve and the resort to abortion is reduced, although never eliminated.

The available evidence goes a long way to confirm this hypothesis. Abortion was common in nineteenth-century Britain (and several other European countries) as the demographic transition began and contemporary commentators reflected upon an apparent increase in frequency. The more quantitative data available for the twentieth century show a continuation of this trend. Unfortunately, all data on illegal abortion are based on local, non-random samples but the evidence from most observers is consistent, and some additional checks are available. It is an often overlooked fact that during the Depression the birth rate in many Western countries was as low, or lower, than it was in the 1960s. Yet contraceptives are more effective and more widely used than a generation ago. For example, in Britain by 1970 over one million women, or one-seventh of all fertile women, were using oral contraceptives. There had been some decline in the age of marriage since the inter-war period and possibly an increase in the prevalence of premarital sexual relationships, but these changes were unlikely to have boosted the conception rate to such an extent as to absorb all the effects of the undoubted improvements in contraceptive practice that had taken place.

Summarising the evidence from several sources it is possible to map out a crucial, but changing, role for induced abortion in the pattern of fertility control in the Western world over the past century or more. However, no single item of available evidence is sufficient by itself to establish a watertight case. Evidence from other areas of the world would be useful and, conversely, the pattern that is apparent in the western European data may assist the interpretation of changes taking place elsewhere.

Within any given society, the remarkable consistency in socio-economic correlates among women resorting to abortion in all continents, and the equally striking *lack* of correlation with religio-cultural background, reinforces the supposition that it is reasonable to attempt to fit the experience of induced abortion in most, or all, countries into a common pattern.

In this chapter the effect of liberal legislation in eastern Europe and Japan has been considered. Legal abortion appears to have largely replaced the previously illegal practice of induced abortion in these countries. (The same inference may apply to Russia, but paucity of published statistical data, together with the poverty of contraceptive practice, makes caution even more necessary than usual.) It is true that Japan and eastern Europe, during the period that legal abortions have been freely available, have undergone a more rapid demographic transition than occurred in western Europe. But there are sufficient socio-economic pressures to account for the speed of change.

Liberal abortion laws seem to have given little more than a modest acceleration to inevitable changes. What the liberalisation of abortion legislation has done is to highlight the part played by induced abortion in the regulation of fertility. In other words, a procedure that has been recognised and registered by the hundred thousand, and even by the million, in the hospitals and nursing homes of Hungary or Japan took place at a similar rate in the back streets and on the kitchen tables of Britain and the USA during the comparable phase of their demographic transition.

A community appears to wish to control its fertility most powerfully, and resorts to abortion with the greatest readiness, when it perceives a decline in living standards, as did the British middle classes after 1860. When it undergoes a real decline, as in Japan and continental Europe in the later war and immediately post-war years, the pressure to control fertility is very strong indeed. It seems that in Japan a liberal law was introduced both at an earlier stage in the demographic transition than in Britain and at a time of unusually powerful social pressures directed towards the control of fertility.

Japan and certain countries in eastern Europe also exemplify the beginning of the second stage of the demographic transition, when contraceptive practice begins to gain on the resort to abortion. A falling abortion rate with increasing usage of contraceptives, and a falling or constant birth rate probably occurred earlier in western Europe and the USA – at least among married women – before, during and shortly after World War II. While western Europe and North America have moved fairly far into the situation where contraception is replacing abortion, the magnitude of the need for induced abortion in contemporary North America is vividly illustrated by the New York experience.

Most developing countries are at an earlier phase in the evolution of abortion practices. The rising use of contraceptives, *combined* with a climbing use of abortion now found in certain developing countries such as Korea, may well have taken place in Europe and America in the late nineteenth and early twentieth century. Statistics on hospital admission for abortion, and data based on the histories of women seeking family planning advice, are strikingly similar for Europe in the first half of the twentieth century and contemporary developing countries.

It seems that the two populations are undergoing a similar travail, the one later than the other, but with many of the characteristics in common – including the fact that many of the abortions are being carried out illegally. However, it seems possible that the recognition of the problem and the initiative to tackle it may be more rapid in the countries of Third World (see Chapter 12) than they were in the developed world.

A case has been made in the present chapter for believing that the law is a relatively unimportant variable determining the total number of abortions occurring in a country. The irresistible tides of history, of economic development and of social change set the level of desired family size and of abortion, which is an intrinsic part of fertility regulation. The law is not a major determinant of the total number of embryos being destroyed, although it is often the key to safe, cheap and dignified care for women.

Tietze,[26] commenting on the effect of abortion legislation in

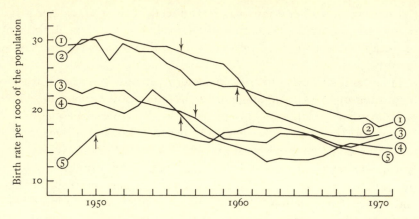

Fig. 31. Birth rates per 1000 of the population for selected
eastern European nations (1948–72). Note that the birth rate
began to fall prior to the liberalisation of the abortion laws
(arrows), which occurred at different times during the post-war
trend towards lower fertility. 1, Poland; 2, Yugoslavia; 3,
Czechoslovakia; 4, Hungary; 5, German Democratic Republic.

Europe, wrote: 'The difference in natality between the two groups
[*eastern and western Europe*] of countries have been sufficiently
striking...to justify the conclusion, without more vigorous analysis, that the legislation of abortion has had a depressant effect on
the birth rate in most countries concerned.' This is a statement to
which few will take exception.[27] However, it is important to note
that it cannot necessarily be read the other way, to imply that if the
abortion laws had *not* been changed the birth rates in eastern and
western Europe would have remained similar. Eastern Europe has
been subject to some emotional and economic restraints on fertility
not found in the West. Limited housing and female employment
(the number economically active in Hungary increased by a third
between 1960 and 1968) are correlates of low fertility that are particularly marked in eastern Europe.

Even if the abortion laws had not been liberalised in eastern
Europe before they were in western Europe, eastern European births
would probably have been lower, and the role of induced abortion
– whether legal or illegal – even more marked (Fig. 31).

To appreciate the weight of social forces over-riding the fragile
barriers of law and overt medical practice is not to deny that liberal
abortion policies do not have some effect on achieved fertility. Van

der Tak concludes her review of legal abortion and demographic change as follows:

> The most dramatic recorded decline in fertility over relatively short time periods appear to have generally occurred where elective abortion has been introduced to a population already strongly motivated to control family size and practising only traditional or no contraception at the time of legalistion: eastern Europe, the USSR, Japan, and, according to some reports, the People's Republic of China, where free abortion and contraception were introduced and made available simultaneously.[28]

Population changes, like a battleship at speed, have great inertia and some trimming of the course set in one generation will be important in determining where the next generation finds itself. Kapotsy[29] has looked at the long-term consequences of the population changes that have taken place in Hungary since reform of the abortion law. In 1958 the United Nations estimated the 1970 population of Hungary at 11.1 million. The actual population reached 10.35 million and the 1958 over-estimate was probably partly the result of failure to allow for the effect of the liberalisation of abortion a year previously. Population projections from 1965 to 1990 suggest an upper limit of 13.4 per cent growth over these years and a lower limit of 1.5 per cent total increase in Hungarian population over the 25 years. In Czechoslovakia, where abortion practice has been somewhat more restrictive, the estimates of population growth 1965–90 are 3.5 to 16.1 per cent.

At a global level, current rates of population growth pose threatening problems for the generations that will follow – perhaps even problems that may be insoluble in any civilised way (Table 48). Any contribution which changed attitudes to induced abortion may make in steering the *Dreadnought* of human population on to a safer course will be much appreciated by future generations.

If we look to the past, it is clear that relatively low birth rates and falling family size have been essential ingredients of the socio-economic advances that have occurred between the reigns of Victoria and Elizabeth II, or the presidencies of Lincoln and Carter. The illegal abortionist has played a much abused, but essential, role in providing a framework in which these changes might occur. In Europe and North America the medical profession has stumbled on to the stage late, pushed on by the legal prompter and still largely uncertain of its lines.

References

Many of the arguments set out in this chapter are reviewed by van der Tak in a book published as part of work of the International Reference Center for Abortion Research.

van der Tak, J. (1974). *Abortion, Fertility, and Changing Legislation: An International Review.* Lexington Books, Lexington, Mass.

1 Gens, A. (1930). The demand for abortion in Soviet Russia. In *Sexual Reform Congress*, ed. N. Haire, p. 143. Kegan Paul, London.

2 Roesle & Paevsky, quoted by Gens (1930); see note 1.

3 Taussig, F. J. (1936). *Abortion, Spontaneous and Induced. Medical and Social Aspects.* Kimpton, London.

4 Potts, M. (1967). Legal abortion in Eastern Europe. *Eugenics Review*, **59**, 232.

5 Mehlan, K-H. (1966). Combating illegal abortion in the socialist countries of Europe. *World Medical Journal*, **13**, 84.

6 Muramatsu, M. (1971). Demographic aspects of abortion in Japan. In *Proceedings of the International Population Conference of the IUSSP*, vol. **2**, p. 1160. IUSSP, Liège.

7 Auken, K. (1953). *Undersøgelser over unge kvinders sexuelle adfaerd.* Rosenkilde & Bagger, Copenhagen.

8 Sjövall, H. (1972). Abortion and contraception in Sweden 1870–1970. *Zeitschrift für Rechtsmedizin* **70**, 197.

9 Ottensen-Jensen, O. (1971). Legal abortion in Sweden: thirty years' experience. *Journal of Biosocial Science*, **3**, 173.

10 Tietze, C. (1973). Two years experience with a liberal abortion law: its impact on fertility trends in New York City. *Family Planning Perspectives*, **5**, 36.

11 Jackson, E. W. (1971). California's abortion legislation and its demographic effects. In *California's Twenty Million: Research Contributions to Population Policy*, ed. K. Davis & F. G. Styles. University of California, Berkeley.

12 Sklar, J. & Berkov, B. (1974). Teenage family formation in postwar America. *Family Planning Perspectives*, **6**, 80.

13 Stewart, G. K. & Goldstein, P. J. (1971). Therapeutic abortion in California. *American Journal of Obstetrics and Gynecology*, **37**, 510.

14 Seward, P. N., Ballard, C. A. & Ulene, A. L. (1973). The effect of legal abortion on the rate of septic abortion in a large county hospital. *American Journal of Obstetrics and Gynecology*, **115**, 335.

15 Heer, D. M. (1968). The demographic transition in the Russian Empire and Soviet Union. *Journal of Social History*, **1**, 193.

16 Mace, D. & Mace, V. (1963). *The Soviet Family.* Hutchinson, London.

17 David, H. P. (1974). Abortion and family planning in the Soviet Union: public policies and private behaviour. *Journal of Biosocial Science*, **6**, 417.

18 Teitelbaum, M. S. (1972). Fertility effects of the abolition of legal abortion in Romania. *Population Studies, London,* **26**, 405.
19 Teitelbaum, M. S. (1974). The de-legalization of abortion in Romania. *Family Planning,* **23**, 38.
20 Wright, N. H. (1975). Restricting legal abortion: some maternal and child health effects in Romania. *American Journal of Obstetrics and Gynecology,* **121**, 246.
21 Anonymous (1971). *Revista de Statistica,* **12**, 57.
22 David, H. P. & Wright, N. H. (1972). Abortion legislation: the Romanian experience. *Studies in Family Planning,* **2**, 205.
23 Romanian Communist Party Central Committee. Analiza starii de senatate a popolatiei si masurile privind prefectionarea organizani retelei sanitare se imbunatatirea asistentei medicale in Republic Socialista Romania. *Scinteia,* 27 Oct. 1968.
24 David, H. P. (1972). 'Psycho-social research in fertility regulating behavior.' Paper prepared for presentation at the Center for Population Studies, Harvard University, Cambridge, Mass.
25 Potts, D. M. (1970). Postconceptive control of fertility. *International Journal of Gynaecology and Obstetrics,* **8**, 957.
26 Tietze, C. (1964). The demographic significance of legal abortion in Eastern Europe. *Demography,* **1**, 119.
27 Brackett, W. (1971). Demographic consequences of abortion. In *Abortion Obtained and Denied: Research Approaches,* ed. S. H. Newman, M. B. Beck & S. Lewit, p. 97. Population Council, New York.
28 van der Tak, J. (1974). *Abortion, Fertility, and Changing Legislation: An International Review.* Lexington Books, Lexington, Mass.
29 Kapotsy, B. (1971). *The Demographic Effects of Legal Abortion in Hungary.* Contribution to the Second European Population Conference, Strasbourg. IPPF, London.

5
Abortion in the nineteenth century

Induced abortion is recorded in all societies with written histories,[1] just as it is known in nearly all contemporary primitive societies.[2] For example, in 1590, a vicar was accused before an ecclesiastical court in Chester, England, of 'committeeinge adulterye with dyvers and sundrie women. He is also an instructor of yoong folkes how to comyt the syn of adultrie or fornication and not to beget or bring forth children'.[3] However, the resort to abortion was probably insufficient and the evidence is too fragmentary to assemble any useful historical picture of the situation prior to the nineteenth century. Then the scene changes for a number of reasons. As industrialisation and urbanisation gathered pace so the real battle to control human fertility began. There is the witness of literature, of the lay press and of medical observation to fill in some details, even though large gaps remain. As the tide of illegal abortion first spread through society, public comment was muted and medical interest minimal – except to condemn in near-joking terms of unrealism. Yet the references to induced abortion in industrialised nations in the nineteenth and early twentieth centuries establish its presence beyond doubt. The scale of activity is more difficult to judge, but even about this occasional insights exist.

Infanticide, as an alternative to abortion in the eighteenth and nineteenth centuries, is discussed in Chapter 13. The role of the present-day illegal abortionist, which frequently mirrors that of his historical antecedents, is reviewed in Chapter 7.

Therapeutic abortion

Certain elements of the history of technical developments and of legal and political attitudes are discussed in Chapters 6 and 8.

Abortion for strictly therapeutic reasons was accepted by early nineteenth-century obstetricians. In an era when Caesarean sections were performed without anaesthesia, when cutting the symphysis pubis to break open the pelvic ring was a treatment for obstructed labour and when fetal destruction was relatively common, the need for induced abortion was appreciated. For example, in 1849 Oldham described a case of induced abortion in a woman of 34 with a past history of recto-vaginal fistula.[4]

The *Theory and Practice of Obstetrics* by Gazeux & Tarnier was first published in Paris in 1840 and translated and issued in many editions in Britain and North America.[5] The authors claim that induced abortion for cases of pelvic deformity was approved by William Hunter (1768) in Britain, and by Fodéré (1813), Mare (1821) and Velpeau (1829) in France. They write:

> Too many imposing authorities have pronounced in favour of
> producing abortion to make it necessary for us to stop in order
> to discuss the moral, religious and medico-legal questions
> which this operation has raised. Like premature delivery, it is
> now received as an obstetrical operation, and it only remains
> for us to determine indications, and the most expeditious and
> least dangerous means of accomplishing the object.

In addition to a degree of pelvic contraction which would manifestly make delivery impossible, Gazeux & Tarnier allowed the possibility of first-trimester abortion for inoperable pelvic tumours, a past history of life-threatening haemorrhage at delivery, and 'obstinate vomiting which threatens a speedy termination of life'. However, they only had personal experience of three cases and make the point, 'it is no longer sufficient that the mother's life is *probably* compromised, it should be almost certain that death is imminent'.

Medical attitudes towards all matters relating to human reproduction evolved with painful slowness and were rapidly left behind in terms of social needs and clinical opportunities. Sixty years after Gazeux & Tarnier, Edgar's *The Practice of Obstetrics* was a popular British text.[6] Although contraception had been a social talking point since the Bradlaugh–Besant trial in 1878, and was by 1900 a demonstrable factor in a declining birth rate, Edgar would only allow it on the grounds of danger to the mother's life or for eugenic reasons. Outside these reasons 'the prevention of impregnation is justly regarded as a violation of the moral law, an injury to the State, and to a certain extent a detriment to the health of the participants [and] a violation of the criminal code'. The doctor 'must insist that conception shall not occur. Much further than this he can hardly go.' Except for restricting intercourse to the last part of the cycle, Edgar goes on to condemn all forms of contraception. In a textbook of over 1000 pages, three lines are devoted to criminal abortion. By contrast there are 29 figures of perforated and unperforated hymens, a long section on rape and a recurrent interest in corsets. One can only conclude that medical teaching related to human reproduction involved a desire to escape from reality, bordering on perversion. And Edgar is not alone: Kelly's two-volume treatise on gynaecology relegates the treatment of incomplete abortion to one page, adding that the operator should never use his finger nails 'to scrape tissue off the uterine walls, as such a practice would often introduce sepsis'.[7]

The nineteenth-century technology for bringing-on delayed periods is reviewed in Chapter 7.

Illegal abortion

At first glance, it would appear that in the nineteenth century there were neither the means, the wish nor the need to resort to illegal abortion on a large scale. But buried, like fragments of an almost totally destroyed building in an archaeological site, are the outlines of a problem which was to become increasingly important as the century proceeded.

For some, especially among the unmarried, the pressures not to bear a child were stronger than today, and many women may have perceived that the future for their children was bleak indeed. William Acton, who wrote the first objective account of prostitution in Britain in 1857, commented:

> It is grievous that children should be born dependent for
> support on the caprice or good feelings of the father...the
> offspring of unlawful love is to the mother, instead of a source
> of joy and an object of loving care, an intolerable burden and
> cause of shame. Her natural desire is to hide her reproach from

the world, and to rid herself of the burden; hence the
concealment of birth, baby farming and infanticide. The
procuring of abortion might perhaps be added to the list, but
need not be considered, as it is likely to be practised most by a
class far removed from the very poor; it is also a crime
recognised as such by the law and by the law adequately dealt
with.[8]

The lesser role which Acton ascribes to illegal abortion may be partly
true, although it was to alter as the century advanced – and for many
groups other than prostitutes. Perhaps, also, abortion was difficult
to describe because there was not the intellectual machinery to deal
with it. As noted elsewhere (p. 281) the 1861 Abortion Act in Britain
despite its rigorous prohibitions against abortion, was not the result
of passionately debated, strongly felt emotions within the country,
but of seemingly uninvolved parliamentary draftsmanship. As late
as 1931, when Mr Justice McCardie first raised the issue of abortion
law reform (p. 286) the *Weekend Review* commented,

> Like euthanasia, abortion is a subject which is only just
> beginning to be mentionable. Evolution was at the same stage
> in England two generations back, and still is in Tennessee. It
> took most of the nineteenth century to win recognition for
> biology in the fields of philosophy and religion: it may take
> much of the twentieth to win it a place in politics and
> business.[9]

Quantitative evidence

In the year 1845–46, Whitehead[10] questioned 2000 women
attending the Manchester Lying-In Hospital on several aspects of
their reproductive life involving a past history of abortion. He
provides a uniquely objective and detailed account of several aspects
of reproduction which many commentators over the next 100 years
were to prove much less able to handle. Whitehead recorded a wider
range of data than usual. The average age of the menarche proved
to be 15.5 years and of the 'final menstrual crisis' (or menopause)
47.5 years. He defined actual fertile life as from 21.5 to 41.5 years
of age and concluded that a woman might have 12 pregnancies in
that interval, including abortions and 'false conceptions' (pseudo-
cyesis). The women reporting abortions (Table 16) had a higher
average age and considerably higher parity than those not reporting
abortions. Whitehead, with unusual thoroughness for the mid-
nineteenth century, broke down the original 2000 cases into 10 groups

Table 16. *Abortion admissions at the Manchester Lying-in Hospital* (*1845–46*)

	Number of women	Average age	Number of preg-nancies	Average number pregnancies/abortions
Total	2000	30.00	8681	4.34
Women not reporting abortions	1253	28.62	3900	3.11
Women reporting one or more abortions	747	32.88	4775	6.39
Total number of abortions reported			1222	1.64

of 200 consecutive admissions and re-analysed age and parity. The result showed no obvious trend over time, or unexpected discontinuities. The age–parity profile could reflect some induced abortions among women attempting to control fertility after numerous pregnancies, but it is not totally incompatible with the pattern to be expected from spontaneous abortion. The nature of the sample, based on case histories at a lying-in hospital, would have excluded any young unmarried women having provoked abortions.

Whitehead made a direct effort to determine etiology in two ways. He interviewed the whole sample (Table 16), and also one subsample in particular detail. 'In interrogating poor, uneducated women, respecting their personal history' commented the author, 'great caution must necessarily be exercised to avoid being led into error'. Today, we have the additional problem of interpreting the validity of the original nineteenth-century diagnoses. Induced abortion *per se* is not a recorded diagnosis. Accidental causes are frequent, yet, as Whitehead notes, are likely to be under-reported as they are 'seldom brought to the notice of the medical man'. In a subsample, 44 cases of 378 were assigned to accidental cases and 275 to 'diseases of the lower part of the uterus'. This latter cause and 'inward weakness' (Table 17) referred to what Whitehead described as 'vaginal discharges vulgarly denominated the "whites"'. This diagnosis is probably much more closely linked to the fact that Whitehead happened to be about the first British gynaecologist to

Table 17. *Reported etiology of 1222 cases of abortion at the Manchester Lying-in Hospital (1845–46)*

Cause given	Number
'Inward weakness', impaired state of general health and acute disease	911
Accidents, mental perturbations, etc.	222
No assignable cause	90

Table 18. *Duration of gestation at time of termination at the Manchester Lying-in Hospital (1845–46)*

Months	Number of women
2	35
3	275
4	147
5	30
6	32
7	55
8	28

use a vaginal speculum than to any pathology relating to the aetiology of abortion, spontaneous or induced.

More revealing is the fact that only half the terminations occurred in the first trimester (Table 18). If most of the abortions were spontaneous then there is a deficit of early cases. This could be because some women failed to report some of the induced abortions they had had early in pregnancy. Individual accounts of abortion at this time often describe rather late procedures, as the technology for mechanically inducing premature labour in the first 12 weeks of gestation was rather more advanced than that for emptying the uterus. Certainly in the 1860s, Greaves, addressing the Manchester Statistical Society, used Whitehead's figures as evidence of a high incidence of induced abortion. His approach was more moral than epidemiological,

I have known a married woman, a highly educated, and in other points of view most estimable person, when warned of the risk of miscarriage from the course of life she was pursuing, to make light of the danger and express her hope that such a result might follow. Every practitioner of obstetric medicine must have met with similar instances, and will be prepared to believe that there is some foundation for the stories, floating in society, of married ladies whenever they find themselves pregnant habitually beginning to take exercise, on foot or on horseback, to an extent unusual at other times, and thus making themselves abort. The enormous frequency of abortions (amounting, according to one high authority (Dr Whitehead) to one miscarriage in seven conceptions, and to another (Dr Granville) to one in three), cannot be explained by purely natural causes. It makes one almost tremble to contemplate the mischief which such laxity of principle, on the part of those who ought to be the leaders of society, must produce upon their inferiors and dependants, and especially in the class of female domestic servants.[11]

Greaves' use of Whitehead's study may be little more than a person with a strong impression that there were a lot of induced abortions looking for figures to quote, but the Manchester Statistical Society was one that responded to the public health problems of this large, rapidly growing industrial city and perhaps the use of Whitehead's statistics was at least partially justified. In the 1840s, Manchester was to England what Chicago was to America in the 1890s. On historical grounds it is one of the places where the induced abortion rate might be expected to rise first. The city fascinated writers like Disraeli, Engels, Mrs Gaskell, Dickens and the travel commentator Alexis de Tocqueville because of its industrial and social change and tension. *The Report on the Sanitary Conditions of Labouring Population of Great Britain* (1842) quoted the average age at death for tradesmen in Manchester as 20 and of labourers and their families as 17. The corresponding figures for Rutland were 41 and 38. 'There is no town in the world where the distance between the rich and poor is so great or the barrier between them so difficult to be crossed', wrote a clerical commentator in 1839.[12]

Industrial Europe probably behaved in a moderately homogeneous way with regard to the sociology of fertility control in the nineteenth century, as it does in the twentieth. Fifteen years after Whitehead found a ratio of one abortion to seven births, Hegar in Germany estimated one abortion to eight or ten term-deliveries.[13]

The birth rate in Britain began to decline in the 1870s, following the already noted Bradlaugh–Besant trial. Charles Bradlaugh and Annie Besant had intervened in the case of a Bristol bookseller who had been found guilty, under the Obscene Publications Act, of publishing C. K. Knowlton's remarkable book *The Fruits of Philosophy*. The attention that the trial attracted made the early nineteenth-century American doctor's book famous throughout Britain and within three months 125000 copies were sold. However, while the public learnt of the possibilities of contraception they also discovered in their private lives about the defects of the available methods – *coitus interruptus*, douching, spermicides, and the use of what were then poor-quality sheaths. One would expect the induced abortion rate to rise at this time and late nineteenth-century writers did indeed have an impression that this was taking place.

The situation was summed up by Rentoul in 1889:

> everyone must notice that, although the number of marriages is on the increase, the number of births to each couple is decreasing, and also that no satisfactory explanation is forthcoming. Instead of the number of cases of abortion undergoing a diminution an enormous increase is taking place and this is all the more strange since our knowledge of maternal, paternal and foetal causes of abortion being investigated is steadily growing large. It is not too much to suppose that for every arrest for this crime at least one thousand cases escape public notice.[14]

France appears to have undergone a similar evolution. As early as 1868 Professor Tardieu[15] claimed that abortion in France had grown 'into a veritable industry' and by the end of the century several writers commented upon the explosive rise in hospital admissions for abortion. In 1905 Dóleris reported: 'Seven years since, at the Boucicaut Hospital, the proportion of abortions to deliveries was 7.7; it is now 17.7. The progression is met with at Tenon, Beaujon, Lariboisière, and above all at the Hospital Saint-Antoine, where the proportion has grown from 6.66 to 18.49.' Some doctors complained that they could no longer accommodate expectant mothers because of the abortion load.

The trend set in the late nineteenth century seems to have continued into the first quarter of the twentieth. Rongy[16] quotes German figures on this subject, but without references and they may be no more than intelligent guesses. More meaningful records come from a limited number of hospitals (Table 4, p. 84). When

considering hospital admission it is important to remember that
only a minority of criminal abortion cases are ill enough to warrant
hospital treatment and that women suffering from the consequences
of illegal abortion have always been unpopular hospital admissions
because of the risk of sepsis and the appreciation that abortion was
a criminal act.

In summary, the least that can be said about nineteenth-century
numerical estimates of induced abortion is that they prove that the
problem existed on a measurable scale, the most that it was a major
social problem. If a trend is to be discovered, it is that induced
abortion became more common as the century drew to its close.

Qualitative evidence

'A shudder and a loathing came over us,' reads the *British
Medical Journal* in 1868, 'when we looked back on the matter-of-fact
details in our late numbers on baby-farming and its allied trades'.
During the year the *Journal* had run a series of editorials built on
information gained by replying to advertisements for ladies who
were 'temporarily indisposed' (Advertisements which one abortionist noted, disgruntledly, were refused by *The Times* and
Express).[17] Visits were made to a number of establishments that took
women in for delivery and arranged for the 'adoption' of the child.
It is implied that the writer posed as a worried husband or friend.
Over half the advertisements answered also offered abortions and
the articles were headlined 'Baby-farming and Baby Murder'.

All the elements of illegal abortion services, as observable in
contemporary developing countries or witnessed in developed
countries without law reform, were already fully established – high
prices, frequent physician involvement, fee splitting, a high degree
of freedom from prosecution, advertisement by innuendo, use of
medical methods before surgical, self-imposed time limits when it
becomes 'too dangerous', and even the earthy realism of some of
the operators. Snippets of conversation were reported verbatim from
one woman aged 55–60 who claimed to have been in the business
27 years (that is back to the early days of Victoria's reign) and she
said she had clients who 'came back six or seven times'; 'I'm a
jokelar [*jocular*] person, I am; and I says funny things and cheers
'em up. She needn't mind and mustn't fret, and I'll see her all right.
I'm the old original, I am, and have had hundreds.' Not all the
women were as relaxed. One house of baby-farming was run by a

mother of 12 children who was pregnant yet again. She did 'not hold with bringing on abortion', although she had 'applications every day'. She appears to have approached her job in a particularly pedantic way throughout and helped women who were to 'adopt' babies to have mock confinements bringing bottles of bullock's blood from the slaughterhouse, sometimes even obtaining a placenta, and encouraging the women to make 'as much mess' as they liked.

The *British Medical Journal* writer comments repeatedly on the 'neat' appearance and 'respectability' of the houses where abortions and deliveries were performed. Even the frequent presence of a pianoforte in the parlour is noted, although the writer adds, 'There are uglier instruments in the cupboard.' The nature of the investigation, a follow-up of newspaper advertisements, meant that it was mainly middle- and upper-class services that were visited. Indeed, the *Journal* says that it did not attempt to penetrate the poorer establishments, although it implied that they existed. Consequently the prices quoted were all high and ranged from £10 to 50 guineas ($20–$101) or more, for delivery and farming out the baby. One woman, who claimed to have been in the business for 12 years, 'without mishap', offered that if the 'lady [was] not far gone, the affair could be managed for a much larger sum than charged for confinement only'. She claimed women often stayed for 10 days, but the *Journal* writer observed that 'it was not uncommon for a lady to be taken to the house of this person in her carriage, the doctor to be fetched, and after a short interval the same lady to be *carried* to her carriage'.

A sample pamphlet put out by an illegal abortionist was printed in the *Journal*:

> Mr —— Consulting Accoucheur No. ——
> *after many years devoted to the practice of*
> *midwifery in its most intricate forms, is*
> *enabled to afford immediate relief in all cases*
> *of female irregularity however difficult.*
> *Early applications preferred. Twenty per cent*
> *allowed for recommendations.*

Such a circular would be immediately understood in contemporary Manila, or Bogota. Then (as now) the indignation which social élites adopt concerning illegal abortion seems to be inversely proportional to their desire to stop it. The 1868 articles in the *British Medical Journal* aroused comment in parliament, but everyone from the

Home Secretary and *British Medical Association* downwards piously claimed it was someone else's responsibility to prosecute. When the *Journal* experimented with a sham baby-farming advertisement itself, it had 353 replies in one week. Another illustration of the underground demand for fertility regulation came later in the century from the trial of two brothers called Chrimes, who were convicted and sentenced in 1898. Their trial gives a vivid indication of the extent of the problem of illegal abortion at that time. The brothers had tried to blackmail their former clients and in a period of three or four days, which appeared to be representative of their practice, £800 ($1600) changed hands. The prosecution claimed 12000 women had applied to them for abortifacients.[18]

Even the fee of £10 ($20) quoted on some occasions must have been beyond the reach of most of the population. The year of the passage of the Offences Against the Person Act also saw the publication of Isabella Beeton's famous *Book of Household Management*.[19] This jumbo-compendium is usually recommended for its ambitious recipes but it also happens to provide a vivid insight into mid-Victorian social history. A family with an income of £1000 a year is recommended to have a cook, upper housemaid, nursemaid, under housemaid and man servant. For a lower middle-class family with an annual income of £100–£200 ($200–$400) a maid-of-all-work (£9–£14 ($18–$28) per annum) and 'a girl occasionally' were reckoned to be sufficient. Beeton describes the maid-of-all-work as 'perhaps the only one of her class deserving commiseration . . . subject to rougher treatment than either the house or kitchen maid, especially in her early career, she starts in life, probably a girl of thirteen, with some small tradesman's wife as her mistress, just a step above her in the social scale'. Perhaps the maid-of-all-work and her sisters were too busy to conceive a pregnancy – wanted or unwanted – but in 1850 there were over 900000 women in domestic service in Britain and their morals seem to have been a source of concern to many, including Dr Greaves, quoted above. Cheaper abortions were available and law court reports of criminal cases quote midwives charging £3–£4 ($6–$8)[20, 21] (a quarter to one-third of a maid's annual disposable income). Cheaper still, although still representing perhaps a fortnight's wages, was recourse to abortifacients (see also p. 256). A criminal case of 1867 quoted 7s 6d (75 cents) for the purchase of savin.[22] Margaret Powell,[23] who worked as a parlourmaid in a London home in the 1920s, tells of a fellow maid who became pregnant and describes a scene which was probably common throughout at least the second part of the nineteenth century, although it went unrecorded at that time: 'She bought bottles of pennyroyal pills which were supposed to be very good at getting rid of it, Beecham's pills and quinine. But all they did for Agnes was to make her spend half the day in the lavatory.' A further misfortune befell another one of her colleagues during World War II, although the outcome was probably less representative. 'Grandad...lit a couple of fireworks – jumping jacks, they were – and slung them under the [lavatory] door...two penny fireworks were cheaper than a £1.50 abortion!'[24]

Queen Victoria's reign saw a rapid evolution in the definition of medical tasks. The General Medical Council was constituted in 1858, but unregistered practitioners continued to work in a number of ways. Pharmacists, herbalists and shopkeepers shared in medical care by providing medicines, advice and surgical goods, and many entered into the illegal abortion system. In 1889 Rentoul accused physicians, midwives and 'monthly nurses' of performing many illegal abortions.[12] The drafting of the 1902 Midwives Act suggests a similar problem existed in Britain.

Experience in the USA duplicates that in Victorian Britain and what little comment there was was often shared on both sides of the Atlantic. The moral stance was the same and a US judge of the 1870s verbally counterpoised the 'unblushing effrontery, unchastity, and utter heartlessness' of a woman who sought abortion against the 'delicacy, refinement, and chastity of American maidens' who carried their children to term.[25]

As in Europe, American writers comment upon the frequency of abortion. Reese,[26] writing in the second half of the nineteenth century, recounts how 'The ghastly crime of abortion has become a murderous trade in many of our large cities, tolerated, connived at and even protected by corrupt civil authorities.' In the 1860s it was said that abortionists were engaged in a 'large and lucrative business' and were 'never in want of engagements'.[27] One cache of abortion instruments included spoons 'bent in different directions to suit the operator', 'several penholders with wire attached' and 'one hair curling tongs, altered to resemble a placenta-forceps'.[28] And medical writers agreed, 'Every physician must have been approached by persons of upright motives with solicitations to prescribe remedies or employ means which would terminate an early pregnancy.'[29]

Unfortunately physicians did not always show the greatest sagacity in relation to human sexuality. In 1872 the Gynecological Society of Boston, Massachusetts, not only solemnly discussed whether the use of a sewing machine could effect menstruation, but a Dr Perry reported that he 'had known of two or three cases of severe uterine disease, in one of which death occurred, that were due to the use of a sewing machine'. Despite this there is an unusual ring of truth in the most direct observations concerning abortion, some of them betraying attitudes still extant. In 1861, Dr Toner from Philadelphia was approached by a merchant's wife seeking an illegal abortion, shortly after he had attended a near fatal illness in another woman who had succeeded in obtaining a termination.

'I wish to speak with you professionally, and to know if I can rely upon you keeping the matter of the consultation sacredly secret?'

'Certainly, madam, in everything that is proper in the profession or personal to yourself.'

'Well, I can trust you, I suppose, and it is this. I am about three months gone in pregnancy, and I have made up my mind that I will not slave myself to death with another child.'

As she spoke her eyes flashed and her voice and manner evinced her positive determination to do as she said. Looking her steadily in the face, I said 'Madam, are you aware that wilfully to cause an abortion is a criminal offence – murder to all intents and purposes?'

'Nonsense, doctor, there is no life yet, and a great many persons do so and think it not harm, nor do I; you need not be afraid. Do you see this arm?'

'Yes, certainly.'

'Well, rather than speak one word that would get you into trouble, I would cut it off at the shoulder.'

'You mistake your man,' I replied; 'I have not the slightest intention to put myself in any danger of the kind, as I firmly believe it to be murder, whether you destroy life at the age of one day or fifty years.'

'Doctor, I do not believe it is a crime, for God cannot wish to afflict us with the suffering and denials that it compels a woman of my age and tastes and position to undergo. But, crime or no crime, I am fixed in my resolution not to have another child; so you may as well make a good fee, and be henceforth our family physician.'

I answered very positively that no consideration would

induce me to become a party to her criminal designs, and I
moreover assured her that I would closely watch her course,
and, if need be, appear as a witness against her if she persisted
in her scheme of folly and crime. She left my office without
evincing the slightest change in her wicked determination.
What has been the result I cannot say, but I fear the worst. I
can recall ten similar applications within the last three years,
about one-half of them being made by married women, and
some of them by husbands on behalf of their wives; and I have
no doubt but that this will accord with the experience of other
physicians in practice.

All large cities have dens of wickedness and crime, where
premature labour with its concomitant evils is frequently
produced. In fact, it has become a regularly established, money
making trade – carried on by both sexes.[30]

Toner could not buttress his granite opposition to abortion with
embryological descriptions, because observations on early human
development were non-existent at this time. Instead he adopted
philosophical supports: 'Morally considered, it is of no importance
whether the murderous hand is raised to destroy the seed of man
in its incipient germination, or in its etherial or more refined
existence, or when it is physically mature.' Like some twentieth-
century commentators, Toner was particularly offended by trivial
events reported as reasons for abortion: 'Married women who wish
to travel, or enjoy the freedom of society, either with or without
the consent of their husbands, determine on abortion'.

In 1871 Ely van de Warkle addressed the Boston Obstetrical
Society on the 'Detection of criminal abortions'.[31] Like Toner he
adopts a pious attitude: 'The married woman who gives to society
the womanhood she ought to give to humanity seeks the abortionist
and by the outlay of a few dollars shirks the high destiny of a mother.'
Unlike Toner he does not threaten to enforce the law. He describes
the case of a physician's wife who sought an abortion. She had had
one previous termination without her husband's knowledge and,
although he had been a surgeon in the American Civil War, he did
not notice or wish to notice his wife's menstrual irregularity. Van
de Warkle rejected the woman's petition: 'I watched her from the
window of my office and saw her enter the den of a notorious
abortionist, nearly opposite, I have no doubts of her success in again
deceiving her husband.' Van de Warkle tried to obtain a general
overview of abortion practices in Syracuse, his hometown: 'Having

taken considerable trouble to ascertain the most common method, I believe injection of water into the cavity of the womb is the means generally relied on by the abortionist.' He described 'women who have achieved the difficult feat of auto-catheterism of the uterus cavity'. The American practice, then as now, appeared to encourage early abortion and he comments upon women who sought abortion 'at the expiration of the first month, if the menses are tardy in their return'. Van de Warkle comments on costs: 'The luxury of an abortion is now within the reach of the serving girl. An old man in the city performs this service for $10 and takes his pay in *instalments*'. [Original italics.] His interest in the subject led him to attempt some complicated estimates of certain aspects of illegal abortion. He collected 21 newspaper reports of death due to abortion and noted 10 due to abortifacient drugs; 5 'implicated medical men' but in the remaining cases it was not possible to categorise the means that had been used.

The stubborn persistence of abortion in the face of noisy minority condemnation or aloofness still comes across in nineteenth-century writing. The Boston Obstetrical Society in the 1870s frequently returned to the problem, calling upon the evidently more pragmatic brethren to cease, 'their notorious harborage of the habitual abortionist' and to 'take immediate and decided action'. The bulk of the medical and lay community appears to have been a little difficult to rouse and the zealots were warned not to 'stir a dunghill'. Clearly, passions over abortion ran high in Massachusetts a hundred years ago as well as today. When one doctor was expelled from the Gynecological Society, its journal editor gleefully commented, 'A ball has been set in motion which should not cease rolling, a movement has been inaugurated which should not be arrested until it has overthrown the grim Moloch to whom our children are being sacrificed yearly in numbers that would seem incredible to one not familiar with the statistics of the horrible rite'.

But the Molochs of illegal abortion were found in all western nations throughout the second half of the nineteenth century and undoubtedly played a major role in the demographic transition which has been a necessary prelude to modern civilised living.

Outside the developed world there are no qualitative accounts of abortion, although nineteenth-century colonial expansion was bringing increasing numbers of Western physicians into contact with other cultures. In the British *Obstetrical Transactions*, which was published for over half a century, there was only one entry referring to illegal abortion and that dealt with India: 'The natives fully understand the enormity of the crime, and its punishment when detected; but their moral views on such subjects are so distorted that they prefer having recourse to criminal abortion, at risk to their lives, to facing the disgrace of expulsion from the caste.'[32]

Briefly, the qualitative evidence in the nineteenth century confirms a well-established illegal abortion service with a variety of components. Verisimilitude is given to the picture by the continued existence of similar services into contemporary societies (see Chapter 7). The American records, in particular, suggest that physicians were becoming more and more involved as the century wore on. Certainly, the evidence that does exist confirms the commonsense assumption that the market was partially segmented by income and that midwives (probably using mechanical techniques) and herbalists (purveying do-it-yourself medicines) were the groups to which the poorer, most numerous, part of the population would first turn.

Emmenogogues and abortifacients

While the formal literature on induced abortion is sometimes scanty, the folk literature is voluminous. The vacuum of political debate and the deficiencies of the medical literature are made good by the inside-page advertisements in the lay press, the entries in the books of herbal remedies and volumes on home medicine.

A great many products were marketed as emmenogogues – products to bring on delayed menstruation. Sometimes they appeared as 'correctives', or were described as relieving 'obstructions'; sometimes they were explicitly labelled, and on other occasions their purpose was so well known that no explanation was needed. Many emmenogogues were also abortifacients – that is they were claimed to abort an established pregnancy.

Some remedies were probably useless. The careful Whitehead[10] commented 'Although...what are commonly denominated emmenogogue medicines may sometimes be followed by abortion. I believe need to be a very unusual occurrence.' The appearance of beetroot, raspberries and potassium permanganate in emmenogogues may be for no better reason than that they are red. Records of solutions of gunpowder being drunk[33] show that ideas of sympathetic magic were not uncommon in this field. But ergot, for example, has demonstrable effects and remains an important drug in gynaecology. Whatever the pharmocology of the situation, sociologically the description and the trade in emmenogogues was, and still is in many developing countries (see p. 259), the smoke above the fire of induced abortion. Deaths from ergot, lead and other poisons recur in nineteenth-century medical journals.[34] One case in 1864 excited an editorial in the *British Medical Journal* and the prescriber confessed that 'he was in the habit of largely dispensing the medicine ergot... [and] was fully aware of its effects. He has known it to be given for three weeks.'[35]

Savin

A recurrent theme in nineteenth-century herbal remedies is the use of savin-oil of juniper. Davis[36] has unravelled much of this tortuous story using a range of source material.

Juniper is a plant native to the Mediterranean, well known to the Greeks and Romans for its pharmacological properties and deliberately introduced into transalpine Europe. Nicolas Culpeper (1616–1656) in his great work *The Complete Herbal*[37] says 'To describe a plant so well known is needless, it being in almost every garden.' Of its properties Culpeper comments 'but inwardly it cannot be taken without manifest danger, particularly to pregnant women and to those subject to flooding'. John Dryden (1631–1700) mentions savin (savix) and is unequivocal about its use:

> Help her make manslaughter let her bleed
> And never want for savix for her need.[38]

Even earlier Spenser wrote in *The Faerie Queene*:[39]

> 'But th'aged Neurse... had gathered Rew and Savine.'

Savin (or sabin) oil was a component of innumerable 'female remedies' and, of course, an additive to gin. In 1891 Taylor, in England, described how to identify the tips of the pine needles in the stomachs of women who die as the 'indirect result of its use as a popular means of procuring abortion'. In New York in 1869, Ellington[40] discussed illegal abortion induced by savin and another common abortifacient, pennyroyal.

Potter and Clarke Limited (English drug merchants established in 1812) sold fresh savin at 28s ($2.80) a hundredweight and dried at 9d (7 cents) a pound in their 1872 wholesale catalogue. (Slippery elm (p. 262) incidentally, sold at 100s ($10) a hundredweight or 10d (8 cents) a pound.) In 1898 they were selling 'Wind and Water Pills' with juniper oil, and the catalogue, under 'unofficial pills' offered twelve 'corrective' preparations including S1 Corrective (wholesale 5s 9d (57 cents) a gross) which contained both ergot and savin ('only supplied to registered chemists, or with signed order form from doctor or hospital').[41]

Perhaps the most renowned domestic preparation of this type is Beecham's Pills. Some contemporary (1974) varieties of Beecham's Pills still contain 0.7 mg *oleum juniperi*. An advertisement of 1897 in the Queen Victoria Diamond Jubilee Number of the *Christian Herald* is typical

> '*Worth a guinea a box.*'
> *Beecham's Pills for all bilious and nervous*
> *disorders such as Sick Headache, Constipation,*
> *Weak Stomach, Impaired Digestion, Disordered*
> *Liver and Female Ailments. The sale is now*
> *6 million boxes per annum*

Florence[42] writing in 1930 about the first five years' experience at the pioneer family planning Cambridge Women's Welfare Clinic, describes one patient thus: 'She often took gin and Beecham's Pills to bring about a miscarriage and thinks some of her children were born frail and weakly for this reason.' She had 12 pregnancies and two abortions. The descriptions by Margaret Powell have already been noted (p. 164).

Van de Warkle tested his collection of nineteenth-century emmenogogues on himself – and on his dog. His description of savin is particularly vivid: 'A violent pain in the abdomen, vomiting and powerful cathartic action, with tenesmus, strangury, heat and burning in the stomach, bowels, rectum and anal region; intoxication, flushed face, severe headache...salivation is often present. Its odour is clearly evident in the urine, which is increased in quantity and passed more frequently... distressing hiccup is very generally present.'[31]

One of the constituents of savin is podophyllin, which is toxic to the cell nucleus. It is used locally on warts – just as it was recommended by Culpeper 'to clean out filthy ulcers and fistulae' – and has been studied as an ovicidal and abortifacient agent in animals.

In rats, given as a pure preparation at 5 mg/kg body weight (one-third of the lethal dose for the adult) it causes 90 per cent fetal death at 11–12 days of pregnancy and in lower doses correspondingly low abortion rates, with stunting, but no obvious malformations, in fetuses that survive.[43,44]

The effect of savin in humans, particularly within a few days of the missed period (which appears to have been the common time for administration) has never been scientifically evaluated. Perhaps all that can be said of it is that no other therapeutic agent has been so widely used, for so specific a therapeutic purpose and yet so little studied in animals and never once scientifically investigated in man – or woman.

Instruction and sale

The widely read nineteenth- and twentieth-century do-it-yourself home manuals of medicine were nearly always helpful and explicit about delayed menses – or 'stoppages', as they were often classified. From T. J. Graham's *Modern Domestic Medicine: The Whole Intended as a Comprehensive Medical Guide for Use of Clergymen, Heads of families and Invalids* (4th edition, 1829) to W. Fox's *The Working Man's Model Family Botanic Guide or Everyman his own Doctor* (22nd edition, 1920), there are instructions about the treatment of 'suppression of the menses'. Fox's work has a non-conformist coyness mixed with a north-country directness: 'emmenagogues or forcing medicine must not be given', it counsels under 'delayed periods', but adds in the next sentence 'but the treatment recommended for painful menstruation will be found to have the desired effect'. Among the remedies producing the 'desired effect' was ground pine or savin oil. A comparable American work, the Vitalogy Association of Chicago's *Vitalogy an Encyclopaedia of Health and Home* (1930), has a predictable passage on delayed and suppressed menses.

The information, which was on many people's bookshelves (a book of home remedies being the next acquisition after the Bible for many families), was backed up by advertisements that arrived on millions of breakfast tables with the local and national press. As with the manuals, the message was a constant one for well over a century. For example, a typical early nineteenth-century advertisement in *John Bull*, mixed in among the remedies to cure toothache, reads:

> *Dr Fothergill's Female pills – These pills have*
> *been in Public estimation for a very considerable*
> *time, and are found particularly serviceable in*
> *removing Obstructions and other Diseases, to which*
> *Females more especially the younger part are liable...*
> *Sold in boxes at 1s 1½d and 2s 9d by Butler*
> *Chemist Cheapside*[45]

Early twentieth-century advertising copy still contained the same elements and even the same prices. An example from the *Hull News* in 1903 read:

> *For more than twenty years*
> *Thousands of ladies have derived*
>   *great benefit from*
> *Dr Davis's Famous Female Pills*
>   *They are the best-known remedy for*
>   *Anaemia, giddiness,*
>   *Loss of appetite, palpitation of*
>   *the heart,*
> *fullness and swelling after meals,*
>   *hysteria, debility,*
> *irregularities, depression, etc.*
> *Boxes 9½d, 1s, 1s½d, 2s9d, and 4s9d at all Chemists,*
> *or direct from the Proprietor, 309 Portobello Road,*
> *Notting Hill, London.*
> *Dr Davis's little book for married people (most*
> *invaluable) sent free on receipt of a stamped*
> *addressed envelope.*[46]

At the turn of the century, Potter and Clarke (*vide supra*) issued their own trade newspaper, *Potter's Bulletin*. It is obvious that the sort of preparations they sold, and in particular their herbalist outlets, were under pressure, not on moral grounds but as part of the war between the registered medical practitioner and the unregistered 'botanic' doctor. They reported herbal doctors diagnosing diphtheria, fighting prosecutions by the Medical Defence Union and the Pharmaceutical Society and aggressively using the title *doctor*. The Medical Acts Commission on the 1858 Medical Act considered it 'undesirable to attempt to prevent unregistered persons from practising'. It is an issue that remains real in contemporary developing countries. From the point of view of the sociology of abortion, it seems that the professional group which is closest to the consumer is the most important provider of service, and abortion too easily becomes tangled up with restrictive practice and disputes between professional groups.

Folk remedies and self-medication are most important when society is least affluent. The trade in 'female correctives' continues in all countries, but most especially in the poorer countries of the world (see also p. 259). The *Jamu* remedies of Indonesia are the counterpart of Beecham's Pills and Potter and Clarke's preparations. They meet a large, persistent market. Sometimes they have an underground, illicit aura, innuendo replaces direct advertisement, the packaging may be deliberately old-fashioned, the great majority of outlets are *outside* the medical profession and the profession is often quick to condemn, but slow to study, the biological properties – and more important the sociological significance – of this type of product.

The trade in emmenogogues and abortifacients continued in full flood until the 1967 Abortion Act in Britain (see also p. 258) and even today women ask pharmacists for remedies for late periods. The confidence of salesmen of emmenogogues testifies to the desperation of the purchaser more than to the certainty of the outcome. A typical advertisement appeared in the *Hull Times* in 1914:

> *TO LADIES*
>
> *You want a guaranteed remedy. You want something infinitely superior to Steel and Pennyroyal, Bittle Apple, and all English Preparations. Then send for Nurse Grey's Renowned American Compound Tablets. Never fail to give relief, frequently in a few hours. A lady writes: "Your remedy is absolutely reliable." Prices, 1/3 and 2/9 (treble quantity), or a stamped addressed envelope for sample. – Nurse Grey, The American Drug Stores, 90 Hazelbourne Road, London S.W.*[47]

The final picture

Some attempt to understand induced abortion in the nineteenth century is essential to any overall perspective of the role of abortion in the demographic transistion and assists in (and is itself assisted by) an understanding of abortion in the contemporary Third World.

Among women marrying in Britain in 1860, a quarter were to bear eight or more surviving children. Among their great-grandchildren marrying in 1925, over two-thirds were to have two, one or no children.[48,49] This represented a change of profound social, economic and political significance. It was achieved by the use of *coitus interruptus*, seedy corner-shop contraceptives and by the illegal abortionist. He or she was classified as a criminal, but without their help history would have taken a different course.

References

1 Himes, N. (1936). *Medical History of Contraception*. Reprinted 1963. Gamut Press, New York.

2 Deveraux, G. (1960). *A study of Abortion in Primitive Societies*. Thomas Yoseloff, London.

3 Wrigley, A. (1969). *Population and History*. Weidenfeld & Nicolson, London.

4 Oldham, H. (1849). Criminal lecture on the induction of abortion in a case of contracted vagina from cicatrisation. *London Medical Gazette*, **44**, 45.

5 Gazeux, P. & Tarnier, S. (1885). *Theory and Practice of Obstetrics*. Blakiston, Philadelphia.

6 Edgar, J. C. (1911). *The Practice of Obstetrics*. Robman, London.

7 Kelly, J. (1898). *Operative Gynaecology*. Kimpton, London.

8 Acton, W. (1857). *Prostitution Considered in its Moral, Social and Sanitary Aspects in London and other Large Cities*. Churchill, London.

9 *Week-end Review*, 21 October 1931.

10 Whitehead, J. (1847). *On the Causes and Treatment of Abortion and Sterility, the Result of an Inquiry into the Physiological and Morbid Conditions of the Utertus with Reference to Leucorrheal Affliction and the Diseases of Menstruation*. Churchill, London.

11 Greaves, G. (1862). Observations on some causes of infanticide. *Transactions of the Manchester Statistical Society*, 1862–3.

12 Parkinson, R. (1839). Quoted by Briggs, A. (1963), *Victorian Cities*. Oldham Press, London.

13 Hegar, A. (1863). *Beiträge zur Pathologie des Eies und zeim Abort*. Enke, Stuttgart.

14 Rentoul, R. R. (1889). *The Causes and Treatment of Abortion*. Pentland, Edinburgh & London.

15 Tardieu, P. (1868). Quoted by Scharlieb, M. (1925). *Towards Moral Bankruptcy*. Constable, London.

16 Rongy, A. J. (1933). *Abortion: Legal and Illegal*. Vanguard Press, New York.
17 *British Medical Journal* (1868), **1**, 127, 175, 197.
18 *British Medical Journal* (1899), **1**, 14 January. Quoted by Banks, J. A. (1954). *Prosperity and Parenthood*. Routledge & Kegan Paul, London.
19 Beeton, I. (1861). *Book of Household Management*. S. O. Beeton, London.
20 *British Medical Journal* (1866), **2**, 668.
21 *British Medical Journal* (1863), **2**, 629.
22 *British Medical Journal* (1867), **2**, 432.
23 Powell, M. (1968). *Below Stairs*. Peter Davis, London.
24 Powell, M. (1970). *The Treasure Upstairs*. Peter Davis, London.
25 *British Medical Journal* (1870), **1**, 189.
26 Reese, D. (1910). *Report on Infant Mortality in Large Cities*. Quoted in Sanger, W. W. (1913). *History of Prostitution*. Medical Publishing Co., New York.
27 *British Medical Journal* (1863), **1**, 17.
28 *British Medical Journal* (1863), **1**, 197.
29 *British Medical Journal* (1863), **2**, 460.
30 *Journal of the Boston Obstetrical Society* (1861), p. 1037. See also Toner, J. H. (1861). *Criminal Abortion in the United States*. Philadelphia Medical & Surgical Press, Philadelphia.
31 van de Warkle, E. (1870). The detection of criminal abortion, *Journal of the Boston Obstetrical Society*, **4**, 292; **5**, 229; **5**, 350.
32 Shortt, J. (1868). On criminal abortion. *Obstetrical Transactions*, **9**, 6.
33 Parry, L. A. (1932). *Criminal Abortion*. John Bale, Sons & Daniellson, London.
34 *British Medical Journal* (1866), **1**, 346.
35 *British Medical Journal* (1864), **2**, 446.
36 Davis, G. (1974). Interception of pregnancy – a new dimension in world fertility control. World Population Society First Annual Conference: A Global Dialog of Disciplines of Population, Washington D.C. See also Davis, G. (1974). *Interception of Pregnancy*. Angus & Robertson, Sydney.
37 Culpepper, N. (1923). *Culpeper's Complete Herbal*, 15th edn, London.
38 Dryden, J. (1693). *Juvenal*, **vi**, 775.
39 Spenser, E. (1590), *The Faerie Queene*, III (ii), 49.
40 Ellington, G. (1869). *Women of New York*. New York Book Company, New York.
41 Wills, D. (1974). Personal communication.
42 Florence, L. S. (1930). *Birth Control on Trial*. Allen & Unwin, London.
43 Thiersch, J. E. (1963). Effect of podophyllin (P) and podophyllotoxine (PT) on the rat litter *in utero*. *Proceedings of the Society for Experimental Biology and Medicine*, **113**, 124.
44 Kelly, M. G. & Hartnell, J. L. (1954). The biological effects and the

chemical composition of podophyllin: a review. *Journal of the National Cancer Institute*, **14**, 967.
45 *John Bull*, 31 October 1824.
46 *Hull News*, 16 May 1903.
47 *Hull Times*, 27 June 1914.
48 Potts, M. (1972). Models for progress: United Kingdom (1919–1939) and China People's Republic (1957–1971). In *New Concepts in Contraception*, ed. M. Potts & C. Wood, p. 213. Medical & Technical Publishing Co., Oxford & Lancaster.
49 Peel, J. & Potts, M. (1969). Demographic aspects of abortion in Britain. *International Population Conference* of the IUSSP, p. 1174. IUSSP, London.

echniques of therapeutic abortion

Doctors have always been conservative but surgeons and gynae-cologists seem to have been particularly slow to accept new devel-opments and techniques. For example Paracelsus noted the anaesthetic properties of ether more than 300 years before Morton first used it in Boston in 1846. Even in the mid-nineteenth century, the eminent American obstetrician Meigs refused to use anaesthesia in labour on the grounds that the pain of childbirth was 'a desirable, salutary and conservative manifestation of the life-force'. The tragic history of Semmelweis' unsuccessful attempt to use statistics to overcome the impressions of his colleagues concerning the cause and treatment of child-bed fever is well known. The celebrated British gynaecologist Lawson Tait refused to recognise the need for aseptic operative techniques until well into the 1870s and continued to operate in a frock coat (with the cuffs rolled up) in a room with an open fire and with the woman tied to the operating table.[1]

The combination of medicine with anything concerning sex appears to have a particularly paralytic effect upon human resourcefulness. This has been especially true in the field of abortion where the interaction of a hostile sociological milieu halted all progress for a century. The relaxation of attitudes, which has taken place within the last decade, has released and brought to the surface several important surgical advances which are only now becoming accepted, just at the very time when they may well be overtaken by the development of effective drugs that could possibly make surgery redundant for the termination of pregnancy.

The evolution of surgical techniques

Performing an abortion is a relatively simple task; it is necessary to gain entrance to the uterus and then to totally remove the products of conception. Performed with moderate skill, and with appreciation of all the problems involved, the procedure can have a very high degree of safety. However, the pregnant uterus is particularly intolerant of bad technique. It is vascular and can bleed severely; the venous sinuses in the placental bed are particularly susceptible to the creation of emboli; the raw areas of the endometrium, and especially any placental debris inadvertently left behind, form an ideal site for infection, to which they are, anatomically, peculiarly exposed. Finally, the relatively inaccessible position of the uterus and the extremely soft wall of the pregnant organ make perforation a distinct possibility, unless particular care is taken.

The cervical canal is a narrow passage with thick muscular and fibrous walls. It permits sperm to pass upwards into the uterus and it dilates to allow the passage of the baby at the time of delivery, or of the fetus at the time of spontaneous abortion. When closed, and in a healthy state, it is the guardian of the upper reproductive female tract against the spread of bacterial infection. The vagina and the cervix are constantly subject to bacterial invasion, but the remarkable mucous plug, or operculum, which fills the cervical canal, is resistant to the passage of infecting organisms, and the upper cervical canal, uterus and tubes are normally bacteriologically sterile.

The techniques of dilating the cervix in order to pass instruments into the uterus have remained unchanged for two and a half millennial.[2] Hippocrates (*c.* 460–370 B.C.) has long been regarded as an anti-abortionist, from the oath associated with his name. In fact it is uncertain how much of this oath can accurately be ascribed to the physician and how much is subsequent embroidery on the mantle of his fame. Edelstein sees the oath as an expression of conflict between the absolutes of the Pythagorean school of philosophers and the general liberality of the rest of the Greek world.[3] Moreover, in a work ascribed to Hippocrates there is a description of a graduated set of dilators essentially similar in shape to those devised by Hegar in Germany only a hundred years ago and still widely used. The dilators described by Hippocrates were made of tin, lead or pine. The metal ones could be slipped on and off a common handle –

a device reinvented by Lawson Tait and others in the nineteenth century. In classical times, once entry had been gained to the uterus, it seems to have been emptied by using the probes and instruments borrowed from other surgical procedures. As with the criminal abortionist of today, advantage was taken of the fact that, once instruments had been passed through the cervix and the membranes surrounding the embryo or fetus had been ruptured, natural expulsion of the products of the conception almost invariably occurs.

Archaeological excavation has confirmed textual evidence that the ancient Greek and Roman world knew how to terminate pregnancy and was well equipped to do so. In a collection of surgical instruments from Herculaneum and Pompeii, there are several types of vaginal speculae (whose use must have made it relatively easy for Roman doctors to visualise and manipulate the cervix), together with apparatus designed to irrigate the intrauterine cavity with fluids. Interestingly, in the light of modern techniques, a syringe that could have been used for suction was recovered. A uterine sound, for probing the cavity, which would not be out of place in a modern operating theatre has been unearthed from an archaeological site in England. A poem attributed to Ovid (43 B.C.–A.D. 18) provides the poetic counterpart to the archaeological evidence:

> Now she that wishes to seem beautiful harms her womb
> And rare in these days is the one who would be a parent.[4]

The immediate ancestor to the uterine sound used today is to be found in late eighteenth-century France and this instrument was described before the Academy of Medicine in Paris by Samuel Lair in 1828.[5]

The curette – a spoon-shaped instrument originally devised to enable the surgeon to scrape a wound clean – was also a French invention and the name is derived from the French verb *curer*, viz. to cleanse.[6] It was invented in 1723 by Réné-Jacques Croissant Jarengeot. Curettage of the uterus is said to have been introduced in 1842 by another Frenchman, J. C. A. Recamier, who also reintroduced the vaginal speculum into gynaecological practice. Simpson in Britain and Marion Simms in the USA adopted it and elaborated their own modifications. In 1874, Alfred Hegar brought it to the attention of German gynaecologists and the operation of 'dilatation and curettage' gained worldwide acceptance.[7] Often the curette was used to treat uterine pathology but its use in inducing abortion, or in treating incomplete abortions, was obvious, and in 1887 a New York gynaecologist stressed the value of curettage to 'clean the post-abortal uterus of its retained products of conception'.

From time immemorial, dilatation of the cervix has been achieved by inserting into it various substances, such as asparagus steeped in alcohol or more recently dried compressed seaweed (the basis of the modern laminaria tents), that absorb moisture from the cervical glands and swell, thereby slowly and evenly dilating the cervix over a period of up to 24 hours.[8] Until recently it was difficult to sterilise materials of plant origin and in any case the introduction of a foreign body into the cervical canal dislodges the operculum and leaves an open route for infection to spread upwards from the vagina into the cavity of the uterus. For this reason, the technique was associated with infection and fell into disrepute. The use of dried compressed seaweed as a means of inducing premature labour was first described by Simpson in England in the latter half of the nineteenth century. Guerney's *The Application of the Principles and Practice of Homeopathy to Obstetrics*, published in 1881, introduced the techniques to American readers. Laminaria tents can now be effectively sterilised by irradiation and are currently widely used in Japan and Korea for the induction of abortion; they are also used by some gynaecologists in England and Europe, but are less well known in the USA.

The disadvantages of procuring an abortion merely by passing instruments or foreign bodies along the cervical canal are that infection may occur before subsequent reactive abortion is complete, and serious haemorrhage may accompany the expulsion of products of conception. For these reasons, in the eighteenth and early nineteenth centuries, abortions were often treated either by irrigating the intrauterine cavity with various caustic liquids or by packing it with sticks of silver nitrate. Subsequently, it was realised that the risks of bleeding and of infection could be more effectively reduced if care were taken to ensure that the products of conception were completely removed by curettage at the time of operation.

In 1863 in a series of *Clinical Lectures on Diseases of Women*, the Edinburgh surgeon, Sir James Young Simpson described a number of techniques 'for the restoration of catamenial [*menstrual*] function'.[9] He was responsible for introducing chloroform to surgery in Europe and gave it to Queen Victoria during childbirth. He wrote:

> Direct Stimulants applied to the Uterus or Uterine Cavity itself are undoubtedly the most certain means at our command for recalling its suspended function. The irritant may be nitrate of silver, or cantharides, or iodine. They may be applied to the lining membrane of the uterine cavity by means of such an instrument as that I now show you. This is simply a Lallemand's portecaustique of sufficient length to pass readily into the interior of the uterus – curved so as to adapt it to the uterine inclination – and furnished with a knob, like that of a uterine sound...charged with some powdered nitrate of silver...it is introduced, about the period when a menstrual discharge is expected, into the interior of the uterus, and the stylet being then pushed forward and subsequently rotated twice or thrice, the irritant is thus sprinkled over the mucous membrane, or dissolved out so as to come in contact with it. I have often known this form of irritant application to produce menstruation in a few hours.[9]

History of vacuum aspiration

Simpson also described a process of 'dry-cupping the interior of the uterus'. Dry-cupping was a procedure in which alcohol was burnt in a vessel placed against the skin thus raising a bleb as a vacuum developed. The method was quoted as 'bringing on menstruation during early intervals of amenorrhoea'. Later Simpson changed the vacuum source:

> I have made frequent use of a tube resembling in length and size a male catheter, with a large number of thickly set small orifices stretching along for about two inches from its extremity, and having an exhausting syringe adapted to its outer lower extremity, by which air could be withdrawn after it had been introduced into the cavity of the uterus. The use of this instrument is in some cases attended with striking results.

Barnes referred to the dry-cupping method 'without approval' in 1873.[10]

Simpson's technique was rediscovered by the Russian Bykov in 1927.[11] He was also familiar with the injection of intrauterine irritants: 'Whereas we know that intrauterine injections of iodine, as a contraceptive, are widely used by the population and particularly by accoucheurs. The demand for this method is extraordinarily great and great is the supply' and also went on to experiment with glass and metal syringes of 100 to 200 ml. He also used a water jet pump. The operation took 3 to 10 minutes. He used the syringe to evacuate the uteri of 25 women over a number of months, '5–7 days before menstruation'. Subsequently, the technique seems to have been lost once again in the swing against liberal abortion which took place in the USSR in the 1930s (p. 379).

Historical 'ifs' can be dangerous, but it does seem reasonable to point out that the rational possibility of vacuum aspiration must have been apparent to many people. It was probably reluctance to devote thought to the problem of abortion, rather than anything intrinsically complex in the idea, that impeded progress. While it might be frivolous to suggest that vacuum aspiration could have been invented at any moment since the famous experiment of Von Guericke with the hollow metal hemispheres and the teams of horses, it is not unreasonable to emphasise the simplicity of the method. It is not a technically demanding process, and one surgeon acting extra-legally is known to have terminated pregnancy by simple oral suction, using a collecting bottle between the cervix and his mouth.

The most recent rediscovery of vacuum aspiration was by Wu & Wu in China in 1958.[12,13] Many Japanese doctors had worked in China during World War II and seem to have known the method – in fact it may even have been re-invented by the Japanese rather than the Chinese. Certainly by the late 1950s and early 1960s it had spread to Japan, to Russia and to eastern Europe, although it did so only slowly. Czechoslovakian doctors found that the skilled glass workers of Bohemia could make excellent suction curettes. Enthusiastic reports were published in eastern Europe but progress stopped, partly because travel between eastern and western Europe at that time was less common than, say, across the Atlantic, but also because many Western observers were suspicious and distrustful of evidence which came from the other side of the Iron Curtain.

In 1967 Kerslake began to use suction termination in Britain and together with Casey she published a survey of vacuum aspiration which introduced the method to much of the English-speaking world.[14] By 1969 one-third of all terminations in England and Wales were performed by vacuum aspiration or 44.9 per cent of all those of less than 12 weeks of gestational age. A similar evolution occurred in Scandinavia and North America.[15] In the USA, for the period mid-1970 to mid-1972, of 402000 abortions, 321500 were at 12 weeks of gestational age or less and, of these, 81 per cent were performed by vacuum aspiration.

However, probably the most significant development related to vacuum aspiration was the ability it bestowed on the operator to perform safe, simple, outpatient termination of early pregnancy.

Daycare abortion

In 1937 M. B. Beric (Yugoslavia) published the first paper on outpatient termination of pregnancy using local anaesthesia to block pain caused by cervical dilation.[16] This paper was presented in Yugoslavia at a National Congress on the health and treatment of village women. In 1966 his son, B. M. Beric, combined his father's paracervical block technique and vacuum aspiration.[17] He soon established the advantages of the method, from the point of view of safety, simplicity, ease of operation and ability to be used in a health service giving total care to the community.

In 1961 Harvey Karman, a Californian lay psychologist, who was appalled by the misery he found amongst girls unwillingly pregnant, began to abort them extra-legally. Not being conditioned by a formal medical training he approached the problems of abortion with an open mind, and, lacking the facilities and training to give general or even local anaesthetics, he sought to apply the principle of vacuum aspiration using only a very small-bore tube so that he did not dilate the cervix. Having ready access to plastic technology, he deliberately chose a soft and pliable tubing. The suction curettes, used by Kerslake and others, all incorporated a single opening and it was found that, when they were made from small-bore tubing, invariably they became blocked. Consequently it became accepted that suction curettage was impracticable using a diameter of tubing small enough to avoid the need for cervical dilation. But Karman made two openings (Fig. 32) in his curette. The fortuitous advantage of this choice became apparent later when it was found that such small, pliable tubes tend to be deflected and to curl up inside the uterine cavity rather than to perforate the wall of the uterus, as a rigid instrument may do. Therefore Karman was able to overcome at a stroke the triple problems of curettage without blockage, dilatation and anaesthesia.

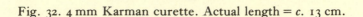

Fig. 32. 4 mm Karman curette. Actual length = *c.* 13 cm.

This simple, small-bore, flexible abortion catheter, allowing very early abortion to be performed with only local cervical anaesthesia (or even without any anaesthesia at all)[18] has spread to many countries and its simplicity and safety has become accepted. It has reduced the cost of early abortions, thus allowing the poorer members of the community ready access to abortion, which previously was open only to the more affluent.

Second-trimester abortions

Techniques for terminating pregnancies of more than 12 weeks' duration are quite different from those applicable to earlier abortions. Most of them evolved in the late nineteenth or early twentieth centuries, but the most basic method, the passage of a foreign body through the cervix and between the membranes that surround the fetus and the wall of the uterus itself, may be assumed to have a much longer history. The introduction of a length of rubber (a bougie), or a rubber tube (sometimes a male urinary catheter), is described in nineteenth-century obstetric textbooks both in Europe and America. It was used in the induction of premature labour and its application before the fetus was viable must have been obvious. In the years 1945–65 one London gynaecologist carried out several hundred late abortions by introducing, with aseptic precautions, one or two firm male catheters, always curetting the uterus after the reactive abortion had occurred. In the latter years he changed from rubber catheters to plastic ones, having become convinced that they carried a lower incidence of infection. More recently Harvey Karman produced the *Supercoil* a much larger edition of a plastic intrauterine contraceptive coil that he used for the induction of abortion in much the same way.[19]

The injection of fluids between the uterine wall and the fetal membranes also dates back to the nineteenth century. Its invention at that time was ascribed to Professor Lazarewitch, who used it for the induction of labour. Special medicated soaps were invented as abortifacients in Germany during the 1920s. They still sell in large quantities with unchanged formula, particularly in the Far East. In the late 1940s and 50s one London teaching hospital used to prepare

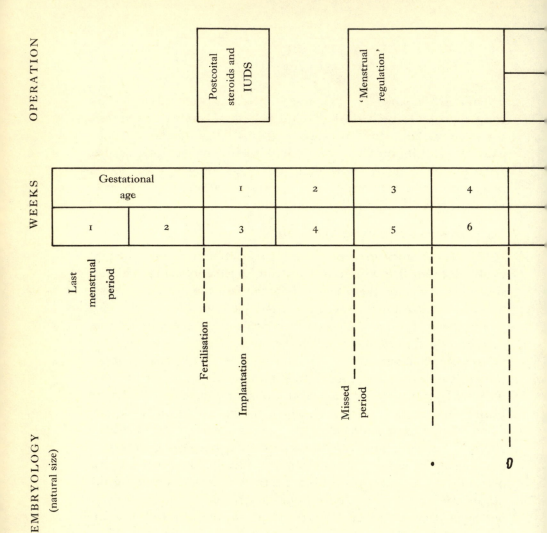

Fig. 33. Growth of the human embryo (natural size) with appropriate abortion techniques. Early growth is extremely rapid, but mainly concerned with the placenta (not shown).

Vacuum aspiration

Dilation and curettage

6	7	8	9	10	11	12
8	9	10	11	12	13	14

such abortifacient pastes to its own formula in large quantities.[20] Today, the use of pastes as abortifacients has been largely abandoned in Britain, because of associated infection.[21] Characteristically, little scientific attention has been given to the design and improvement of pastes.

It was observed in the 1930s that the injection of X-ray-opaque liquids into the amniotic cavity for diagnostic purposes sometimes induced premature labour. Such an injection is *inside* the fetal membranes and thus unlike the technique previously described. Aburel in Italy in 1934 exploited this accidental discovery and used it to induce abortion. In 1935 Buero published and described a variation of the technique using 40 per cent formaldehyde,[22] but there the matter rested until the 1950s when there was a resurgence of interest,[23] largely stimulated by the liberalisation of abortion laws in Scandinavia and Japan. Brosset, in 1958,[24] described the injection of 50 per cent glucose, and Bengtsson & Stormby the use of hypertonic (20 per cent) saline solution.[25] In 1971 Greenhalf & Diggory improved the safety of this technique by using intra-amniotic urea instead of hypertonic saline.[26]

Hysterotomy, i.e. the operation in which the uterus is opened and the fetus and placenta removed, developed out of experience with Caesarean operations carried out at term. The vaginal approach was known in the nineteenth century, and the famous British gynaecologist Victor Bonney described the modern abdominal operation in 1918.[27]

Contemporary techniques

Abortion techniques are sharply divided. Operations performed after the twelfth week of menstrual age require a much higher level of surgical skill and more sophisticated facilities than first-trimester operations. They present profoundly different physical and emotional risks to the woman. It is misleading that the two different categories are both known by the same name 'abortion'. The early procedure is safer than normal childbirth and the latter more dangerous than a forceps delivery.

In the descriptions which follow we have tried to present the technique according to the sequence of events usually facing a woman seeking abortion. We have therefore started by discussing the examination, choice of type of anaesthesia and methods of dilating the cervix, before describing techniques for emptying the uterus according to the duration of pregnancy. Next, the effect of menstrual extraction and of current developments in possible medical methods on those who provide abortion services, and on those who use them, are considered. Finally, the short- and long-term effects of abortion are reviewed.

The preliminary examination

As with any other operative procedure, careful preliminary examination is essential. A general examination should be sufficiently thorough to exclude any significant medical disease not disclosed by the medical history. With one or two fingers of the operator's prime hand in the woman's vagina and the other hand firmly on her abdomen, it is possible to assess the pelvic organs with reasonable accuracy, even without an anaesthetic. The first need is to confirm that a pregnancy exists and to estimate its duration for comparison with the woman's menstrual dates; a discrepancy may suggest multiple pregnancy, molar pregnancy (a disease of placental tissue) or uterine fibroids, in which case the uterus is likely to be irregular in outline. The operator also needs to consider the possibility of ectopic pregnancy (pregnancy within one of the fallopian tubes) and to exclude it as well as pelvic tumours, such as ovarian cysts. The version (forward or backward tilt) of the uterus must also be established.

In the first 12 weeks of pregnancy, careful bimanual assessment, as described above, is by far the most reliable guide to the duration of the pregnancy. The skill and experience of the doctor who carries out this assessment are crucial. Relatively junior and inexperienced personnel can be trained to perform vaginal abortions safely in early pregnancy. Indeed, in some parts of the world auxiliaries perform these minor operations, but the preliminary clinical assessment with reliable exclusion of advanced pregnancies is critically important. Wherever possible, the person who first examines and assesses the woman seeking abortion should also perform the operation. It has been found that, in units where the first examination and acceptance for abortion are separated from the procedure, even experienced gynaecologists are surprisingly overoptimistic in accepting that the pregnancy is suitable for the procedure proposed. On the contrary, a skilled doctor, first in contact with the woman, is best placed to decide whether or not she is early enough for vaginal termination and, if so, whether she is suitable for local anaesthesia and whether best aborted as an outpatient or inpatient.

Anaesthesia

The most important categorisation of vaginal techniques of abortion depends upon the type of anaesthesia selected rather than on the surgical technique. It is stretching of the cervix that gives rise to pain in abortion. The nerves supplying the cervix pass along the broad ligament which runs from the side of the pelvis. They enter the cervix just above the vault of the vagina, and local anaesthetics, such as 6–10 ml of two per cent lignocaine, if injected through the vault of the vagina at two or three sites around the cervix, can effectively block such pain impulses.[28-31] The choice between general and local anaesthesia is partly determined by the availability of skilled anaesthetists. In many developing countries the operating surgeon is responsible for his own anaesthetics and in such situations a local anaesthetic must be used. Thus, by the time the American abortion laws were liberalised there was already a mass of evidence showing that local anaesthesia was not only acceptable, but probably safer than general anaesthesia. For this reason local anaesthetics have been much more widely used in the USA than in Britain. However, with modern techniques of general anaesthesia, involving pre-medication followed by intravenous tranquillisers and analgesics in conjunction with a low dose of general anaesthetic, these procedures can also be quick, safe and suitable for daycare use. The use of deep anaesthesia, particularly with inhalation anaesthetics such as Halothane, can result in loss of uterine tone and of the reflex contractility which normally occurs when the conceptus has been wholly or partially removed and heavy bleeding may result.

Abortion up to about 8–10 weeks can be performed without any anaesthesia, if a small (4–6 mm) Karman curette is used and cervical dilatation avoided. For such procedures it is essential that the woman fully understands what is being done. She therefore needs careful pre-abortion counselling.

Most gynaecologists are used to performing dilatation of the cervix and curettage of the uterus under general anaesthesia. Indeed, examination of the pelvic organs under anaesthesia is essential where pelvic abnormalities have to be excluded. Because they are familiar with general anaesthesia, they tend to be reluctant to perform abortions under local anaesthesia even though they will agree that coincidental gynaecological abnormality is highly unlikely. Many experienced surgeons will claim that the use of general anaesthetics permits abortion to be performed safely by the vaginal route at a later stage than is possible with local anaesthetics. General anaesthesia is also appropriate when sterilisation, by use of the laparoscope, small abdominal incision or by posterior colpotomy (incision in the vault of the vagina) is to be performed at the same time as abortion.

Dilatation of the cervix

Dilatation of the cervix is a prerequisite of the conventional *D & C* abortion and is necessary for all vacuum aspiration operations requiring the use of a cannula of more than 4–6 mm external diameter.

In pregnancy the cervix is peculiarly soft and tears easily so it is essential that the Volsellum, or other forceps that need to be applied to hold the cervix, has an adequate bite. In passing rigid dilators the danger of accidental perforation exists. The safeguard against such an accident is constant manual uterine palpation. The operator's abdominal hand should always be in close contact with the uterine fundus. In this way, not only will perforation be avoided but the exact position of the intrauterine instrument is easily felt and the thickness and tone of the uterine wall appreciated.

It is the internal cervical os which is the crucial source of resistance to dilatation and it is a tear at this point that may be followed by subsequent cervical incompetence, with recurrent miscarriages or premature delivery in the future. Hulka has measured the force required to dilate the cervix.[32] Dilatation should always be slow and gradual and the cervix should never be dilated beyond 14 mm in diameter in a multiparous woman, nor beyond 12 mm in a nulliparous girl. Experiments with vibrating dilatation systems have not been successful.[33] The possibility of using prostaglandins to assist cervical dilatation is being explored.[34]

Dilatation beyond 14 mm, permitting vaginal termination, is acceptable when concurrent sterilisation by laparoscopy or culpotomy is to be performed. There is a group of British surgeons who will use vaginal termination for a pregnancy of up to 20 weeks, even when reproductive function is to be preserved. They first gently dilate the cervix to 12–14 mm diameter (anticipating cervical tearing and stopping before it occurs), passing the dilators only just through the internal cervical os so as to preserve the membranes. The dilated cervix is then packed with three to five laminaria tents, which are left *in situ* for a minimum of 12 hours. During this time the tents absorb moisture and their expansion induces gradual further dilatation of the cervix. When they are removed the internal diameter of the cervix will be about 18 mm and, by careful intrauterine crushing (a task requiring expert skills), advanced pregnancies can be successfully removed. So far, the technique has not been shown to be associated with cervical incompetence.

Early abortion

The vaginal approach is almost always used. The only exceptions being where there is gross uterine pathology or occasionally when sterilisation is simultaneously carried out. The surgeon may then chose hysterotomy, although this is not nowadays considered as safe as vaginal termination and concurrent laparoscopic sterilisation if the facilities exist.

DILATATION AND CURETTAGE

Dilatation and curettage was the established way of treating incomplete abortions and of performing first-trimester therapeutic abortions for many years.[35–37] It can be carried out under local anaesthesia, but the operator has to learn a somewhat more gentle technique. It is now largely being replaced by vacuum aspiration, which is much more effective in completely emptying the uterine cavity.

Operators differ in whether they prefer to introduce a curette or a pair of gripping forceps into the uterus first, once dilatation of the cervix is complete. In either case, the aim is to reduce the volume of the uterine contents and induce a contraction of the muscular wall. The stroking action of the curette is, itself, a stimulus to such a contraction. Before the tenth week, forceps may fail to dislodge the placenta and preliminary curettage is preferable. The detached placental tissue is then removed with forceps.

It used to be taught that a blunt curette should be used exclusively within the pregnant uterus for fear of perforating its soft wall. In practice, uterine perforation almost invariably occurs as the instrument, be it sound, dilator, forceps or curette (Table 19), is being

Table 19. *Perforation of uterus according to type of instrument and method used*

Instrument	Total perforations	Currettage (14261 cases)	Vacuum aspiration with para-cervical block (22909 cases)
Cervical dilator	11	4	7
Curette	8	6	2
Uterine sound	7	4	3
Ovum forceps	6	6	0
Suction cannula	1	—	1
Total	33	20	13

introduced. Perforation almost never occurs during the return or truly 'curetting' action. Therefore, the sharp curette, which is lighter, more sensitive and more efficient, is actually safer for these very reasons.

A completely emptied uterus normally has good tone and the blood vessels that used to supply the placenta will be constricted and closed by the strongly contracted uterine wall. Once fully emptied the uterus should not bleed. A well-contracted state can easily be confirmed by bimanual examination, and if there is any doubt the cavity must again be explored thoroughly.

VACUUM ASPIRATION

Apart from the thin, pliable Karman curette, other vacuum aspiration cannulae are made of metal or hard plastic, and have a variety of end-openings. For other than the Karman curette it is usually recommended that the cannula selected should have a diameter in millimetres equal to the duration of the pregnancy in weeks. When the cannula has been fully introduced into the uterus, suction is switched on. At first the cannula moves freely, but, as the negative pressure rises, the operator can feel tissue being pulled into the opening and resistance to movement occurs. The cannula is constantly moved in and out and simultaneously rotated about its own axis.

The signs of completed evacuation are, first, the appearance and amount of the evacuated products, secondly the presence of a slight froth in the aspiration bottle, and, most significant of all, a feeling that the aspiration curette is being gripped by the walls of the uterus so that, on moving it in and out, a slightly gritty sensation is appreciated by the operator.

The greater the vacuum the quicker and more successful the operation. Custom-made electric suction pumps are available and are convenient. Various forms of cannula and receptacles have been devised to be used with other sources of negative pressure. Very simple pumps, including a bicycle pump with reversed valve, can be used and such devices are becoming increasingly important as legal abortion becomes more widely practised in developing countries.[38-46] The Chinese have experimented with a fire-bottle in which the oxygen is burnt and the resultant partial vacuum used for uterine aspiration.[42] A steam-filled bottle that is cooled to create a partial vacuum has been described in the USA.[43] Karman curettes can be cut from off-the-shelf plastic tubing using a simple practical 'cottage industry' machine devised by Clifford.

Vacuum aspiration is a more rapid procedure than D & C and causes less blood loss, as well as being associated with fewer perforations.[44-49] It is aesthetically more acceptable to the professional personnel involved. It is particularly useful in the abortion of pregnancies of less than 10 weeks' menstrual age. Conversely, D & C has the advantage of being feasible in selected mid-trimester abortions.

Many gynaecologists already familiar with D & C find it difficult to adapt their operative technique so as to obtain comparable sensitivity using the vacuum curette. Clearly the advantages of the vacuum technique, while real, are not overwhelming. It is interesting to note that the D & C remains the commonest procedure in most of eastern Europe and in Japan. As with most procedures involving manual dexterity, the experience and commitment of the operator can over-ride differences in technology.

DAYCARE ABORTION

As reported elsewhere (p. 353) a large experience of daycare (ambulatory outpatient) abortion has now been built up in the USA and the technique is being used increasingly in Europe (especially Holland and France), Australia, India, Singapore and elsewhere.[17,50-58] In Britain the regulations imposed by the Department of Health and Social Security slowed its adoption and indeed totally prohibited it except within the National Health Service (NHS) until 1976. This is regrettable because daycare abortion is quick, cheap and has proved remarkably safe. It enables a woman to return home usually within three or four hours of the operation and, because only such a short stay is required, the organisation can be extremely flexible and utilise nurses and operators working part-time sessions. When inpatient procedures are used there is inevitably a delay between the decision to operate and finding the bed for the termination. This delay increases the risk of the operation.

The performance of outpatient abortion under local anaesthesia calls for some specialised training and for constant awareness of the associated risks and pitfalls, but it does not require the skill of a fully trained gynaecologist. Even non-medically qualified personnel have been trained to do outpatient abortions and the preliminary results suggest that a very satisfactory standard can be reached. The concentration of a repetitive procedure in the hands of a limited number of well-practised operators further reduces the hazard facing the patient. Senior gynaecologists who perform relatively few abortions may prove a good deal less skilled at this operation, and have a much higher morbidity and complication rate than more junior colleagues who are in constant practice (Table 20).

Outpatient abortion, particularly in conjunction with abortion counselling, has completely changed the image of the procedure in lay eyes. From experience so far in the USA and Holland, it would seem that outpatient abortion is an acceptable procedure preferred by the majority of women to hospital admission. But it is not possible to argue this case conclusively from the American and Dutch experience, since financial factors may play an important part. It will be interesting to see the acceptability of outpatient abortion under the NHS in Britain, when hospital admissions and daycare operations are freely and widely available. Probably the most important single improvement that the widespread usage of outpatient abortion has promoted is that terminations are being done at ever earlier stages. Eastern Europe and America are now catching up with Japan (Fig. 21, p. 107) in this respect although Britain and the rest of western Europe still have some way to go. In a series of over 13000 outpatient abortions performed in association with

Table 20. *Comparison between high and low volume abortion facilities*

	Outpatient facilities: high volume, specialist unit (USA 1970–72)		Inpatient facilities: low volume, mixed specialist gynaecology unit (UK 1968–70)	
Total legal abortions	26 000		1 182	
Percentage performed at less than 12 weeks	100		78	
Complications	Number	Rate per 1000	Number	Rate per 1000
Trauma				
Perforations only (no *sequelae*)	36	1.4	14	12.0
Laparotomy necessary	13	0.5	6	5.0
Hysterectomy necessary	1	0.03	2	1.6
Infection				
Pyrexia (38 °C or more for 24 hours)	391	15	321	270

American hospitals, only 100 (0.8 per cent) required hospital admission and only 50 needed to stay more than 24 hours. Even when matched for duration of gestation, this series of outpatient abortions was associated with a lower complication rate than inpatient operations.[48]

Abortion counselling has been a specifically American contribution to the development of modern abortion techniques. If a comprehensive and intelligible explanation of exactly what will happen to the woman during the process of abortion under local anaesthesia is given, and if the counsellor takes adequate time, answers all questions and remains with the woman (perhaps literally holding her hand during the procedure), then sophisticated and Westernised women are able to accept early termination of pregnancy with no anaesthesia, or with only a cervical block. Women used to lower standards of anaesthesia and analgesia for medical procedures tolerate the procedure readily and probably with less counselling.

However, the rapport established between the counsellor and the woman is also of value because it can allow discussion of sexual problems and future contraception, making the abortive procedure an educative process.

Outpatient abortions are only responsible if they are limited to the first 12 weeks of pregnancy and if women with complicating gynaecological or medical conditions are rigorously excluded. The performance of abortions within a specialised clinic with few facilities requires well thought-out back-up facilities in a fully equipped gynaecological department, preferably in the same hospital or very near by. Concentration of the facilities within one unit also ensures that all the members of the team are sympathetic to abortion and experienced in the handling of any women at risk for emotional trauma. Provision of abortion counselling and of future contraception help is normally accepted as a routine part of the work of such a clinic.[59]

Daycare units remove abortion from the wards, where it may cause some emotional distress to young trainee nurses and where the woman may otherwise lie next to someone who has just lost a much-wanted pregnancy, or is in hospital for the investigation of infertility. Clinically, day units have no real disadvantages. Experience shows that the complications of abortion occur either during the operation itself, or are those of secondary haemorrhage or infection, which manifest themselves some days later. Amongst 16000 consecutive cases operated upon as inpatients by the Pregnancy Advisory Service, London, only one suffered a moderately severe complication occurring during the overnight stay after the day of operation. It was considered that even she could well have been treated at home by an emergency medical service, such as is normally available. In Vojvodina, Yugoslavia, by the 1970s tens of thousands of consecutive cases had been treated as outpatients without a single death. The Centre for Reproductive and Sexual Health in New York began work on 1 July 1970 and 13 months later 26000 abortions had been performed as outpatient procedures, without a known death.[55] The total procedure usually took less than 15 minutes and the average blood loss was 35 ml. The woman paid $150 and approximately one in four had this amount further reduced. Thirty-six (0.14 per cent of total) definite perforations occurred and 13 of these required laparotomy. In 90 cases (0.35 per cent) repeat curettage was necessary. A total of 391 patients developed a temperature of 38 °C or over on two successive days or more. In 49 of these (0.19 per cent), the infection was serious enough to warrant hospital admission. One hysterectomy is known to have occurred in the series: 46 women were admitted to a nearby hospital from the outpatient clinic and 136 are known to have been admitted elsewhere within a few days of the procedure. This would represent a total hospital admission rate of 0.7 per cent but follow-up could not be perfect and additional unrecorded admissions probably took place. Nevertheless, the record of this centre, doing up to 100 outpatient abortions per day, is impressive (Fig. 20, p. 197).

Late abortion

Late abortion can be dangerous and is always disagreeable. The surgical risks rise steeply after 12 to 13 weeks,[58] the emotional cost to the woman becomes higher and many people feel that the operation is ethically more challenging. Late abortions carry a high political as well as surgical complication rate.

It is a recurrent theme of this book that early abortion is in every way preferable to late. Those who write laws, set standards of medical practice and create services must do all in their power to ensure that most operations are performed early: women will come early given the ready availability of a realistic service (Fig. 21, p. 101). However, even with good, well-publicised facilities, there will always be some women who present late. These include the very young, who have concealed their pregnancy from parents or guardians, and women with menstrual irregularities at or around the time of the menopause, some of whom may have been falsely reassured that they were panicking unnecessarily. There will also be unfortunate women for whom the diagnosis of a fetal abnormality is only established late in pregnancy.

Late terminations can be divided into two groups. Those which can be completed in one step and those which require two stages: an initial induction of abortion and its subsequent completion (spontaneous or as a separate surgical procedure) 24 to 48 hours later.

ONE-STEP PROCEDURES
Vaginal dilatation and curettage

Vaginal termination is technically feasible up to about the twentieth week of pregnancy, but requires such a degree of dilatation of the cervix that the internal sphincter, or os, is liable to be torn and rendered incompetent so that in future pregnancies a relatively late spontaneous abortion may occur. If the woman, or her husband, is accepting sterilisation at the time of the abortion then deliberate overstretching of the cervix is acceptable and vaginal termination, though requiring a high degree of skill, is preferable since it will require only a very short stay in hospital with quick full recovery. As described earlier, the use of laminaria tents permits cervical dilatation with a much reduced risk of damage.[60, 61] In women who have already borne children, such techniques allow intrauterine crushing of the fetus and curettage up to about the sixteenth week of pregnancy, even when further childbearing is contemplated. The technique is suitable only for experienced surgeons. The risks include partial separation of the placenta with resultant haemorrhage, which can be brought under control only when the placenta has been completely separated, and possible damage to the cervix by sharp parts of the fetal skeleton as it is extracted.

Even when late dilatation and curettage with fetal crushing is undertaken, many surgeons employ vacuum curettage at the end of the procedure to ensure that no small pieces of placental tissue have been left *in utero*.

Hysterotomy

Hysterotomy is the surgical opening and emptying of the uterus. It is normally performed through an abdominal incision as a miniature Caesarean section, but it can be done through the vagina by deliberately cutting (and later resuturing) the cervix. Vaginal hysterotomy is equivalent to a late vaginal abortion and has no advantages because once the cervix has been cut, resuturing rarely restores functional competence. Neither can vaginal hysterotomy be easily combined with sterilisation. Therefore it has little formal place among abortion techniques.

Until the development of the modern two-stage techniques for late abortion, hysterotomy was the only way such procedures could be performed. When reproductive function has to be preserved, a special technique of incising the uterus transversely in its lower segment (the part of the uterus, immediately above the cervix, that passively relaxes and stretches to allow the baby to pass into the vagina under the powerful contractions of the rest of the uterus in labour) is used. This technique requires far higher technical expertise than merely opening the upper part of the uterus – a procedure still used when concurrent sterilisation is performed. Nowadays, hysterotomy is rarely performed unless sterilisation is to be done at the same time.

Hysterectomy

When a termination is performed in the presence of known uterine disease, particularly if this was causing symptoms before the woman became pregnant, the total removal of the uterus and pregnancy can be performed.[62] In early pregnancy the procedure is feasible, but there is an increase in vascularity and careful haemostatis is essential. Abdominal hysterectomy is indicated in the presence of fibroids and vaginal hysterectomy in the presence of prolapse. Statistical evidence is needed to determine if it is safer to perform termination first and hysterectomy some weeks later, or to combine the procedures.

TWO-STEP PROCEDURES
Davis method

Davis has used a method that appears to have been invented by illegal abortionists in Australia and that is simple and straightforward. Under sterile conditions, the cervix is dilated to approximately 10 mm in diameter and the umbilical cord is pulled down (a vacuum curette will suck out a length of cord before any other product of conception). The cord is cut, but nothing else is done. The aim, as with other two-stage methods, is to destroy the placental function because, when it ceases to act, abortion will follow spontaneously. Unlike some other second-trimester abortion procedures, the method does not leave the physician or nursing staff with the possibility of having to deal with a living fetus and it deserves wider trial. The potential dangers of infection have apparently not so far been of significance, but where possible most operators would combine the technique with an intravenous Syntocinon drip, or with prostaglandins, to accelerate the abortion process. As with all the two-stage procedures the resultant abortion may be incomplete and many surgeons routinely perform curettage to ensure that the uterus is finally empty. The method is perhaps potentially most useful for developing countries.

Injection techniques

Intra-amniotic. A needle is passed through the abdominal wall (after local anaesthesia) and into the amniotic cavity. A portion of the amniotic fluid surrounding the fetus is removed and replaced by a chemical that will kill the placenta and therefore induce an abortion. Several substances have been used, but most present certain hazards: formalin[22] is absorbed from the amniotic cavity and has toxic effects; glucose[24] has been associated with intrauterine infections and hypertonic saline[25,63,64] has been responsible for maternal death, both from changes in salt concentration in the blood and cerebral haemorrhage in the base of the brain.[65,66] More recently, urea has been introduced, which is at least as effective and has no dangers if it accidentally enters the maternal blood stream or peritoneal cavity.[26]

With all intra-amniotic injection techniques, there is a delay between injection and the onset of abortion and the abortion itself may be incomplete, especially prior to the eighteenth week. A dead placenta retained in the uterus for many hours can cause fibrin (which normally circulates in the blood as one of the important factors in blood clotting) to become exhausted, probably because of clot formation in the placental sinusoids, leaving the blood stream deficient and the woman in danger of having severe haemorrhage. The more advanced the pregnancy the more likely is this complication, but fortunately it is rare.

There is considerable discomfort to the patient, not at the time of amniocentesis but later when uterine contractions begin and she experiences all the pain and discomfort of mid-trimester abortion, comparable to that of full-term labour. Pain can be relieved by the use of an epidural anaesthetic or a liberal use of opiates and tranquillisers. These can be used in much larger doses than during childbirth, since there is no concern for the survival of the fetus.

In the case of saline induction, fetal death (which can be monitored by following the fetal heartbeat) usually takes place within three hours. Death or damage to the placenta is more difficult to detect but is associated with a fall in the level of the hormone progesterone in the blood.[67-69] This fall invariably precedes a rise in the pressure within the uterus that heralds the abortion process. With urea, fetal death takes longer than with hypertonic saline.

Intra-amniotic injections of prostaglandins have proved effective in late abortion.[70, 71] Used alone, the injection may have to be repeated, but one of the most effective techniques in current use is to combine prostaglandins with urea. Unfortunately the more the process of uterine emptying is accelerated, the greater the risk of incomplete evacuation and the higher the probability of a need for surgical evacuation.[72]

EXTRA-OVULAR INJECTION

Instead of passing a needle directly into the fetal sac or amniotic cavity, effective irritants can be introduced through the cervix into the extra-ovular space (the space between the uterine wall and the fetal membranes).[20, 72–77] The use of pastes and medicated soaps to induce abortion in this way was first evolved in Germany and Denmark between the world wars. *Utus paste*, the patent of which was taken by Britain from Germany at the end of World War II, is still manufactured and sells in developing countries. Between 10 and 40 ml of the paste are injected, according to the duration of pregnancy. The tube of paste is screwed into a 3 mm diameter metal applicator, which is passed through the cervix, and the paste spreads round the fetal sac within the uterine wall. Abortion normally takes place within 48 hours. The physiological processes may be similar to those following intra-amniotic injections, but no scientific studies have been carried out. *Utus paste* fell into disfavour in Britain after several cases of intrauterine infection were reported. Rivanol (ethacriedine lactate) has been used as an alternative in Russia, Japan and Israel.[78–80] This compound is itself an antiseptic and if current trials are satisfactory it may gain wider use. use.

Nowadays prostaglandins (*vide infra*) introduced into the extra-ovular space are used for the induction of labour or for abortion. Self-retaining bladder catheters are designed with a small-bore tube running through the central lumen of the main catheter and ending in a balloon. Once introduced, the balloon is inflated with sterile water, thus holding the catheter in place. The use of such a device allows dilute solutions of prostaglandins to be dripped continuously or injected repeatedly into the extra-ovular space. The technique is free from the dangers of introducing toxic irritants, which could be absorbed through the placental vessels into the maternal blood stream. The rate of injection can be varied in individual cases according to the progress of the abortion or delivery.

Neither urea nor prostaglandins have found much favour in America, where the induction of late abortion by hypertonic saline is still preferred, despite the greater dangers. The reason is probably that the less toxic alternatives are more likely to produce an abortion where the fetus may still show some signs of life. One is then dealing with late abortions that are not only aesthetically offensive, but also raise the ethical problem as to whether or not resuscitative measures should be attempted, even though the possibility of survival is remote (see also p. 207).

MECHANICAL IRRITANTS

Reference has already been made (p. 185) to the use of pliable, plastic urinary catheters introduced via the cervix to induce late abortion by mechanical irritation. Modifications of the technique, using such household substitutes as lengths of draught-excluding rubber strips, have been used by illegal abortionists for a very long time. Mechanical techniques can be effective, but they carry an appreciable risk of introducing infection and they are less certain than injection methods.[81] It seems unlikely that they have a place any longer, except possibly in remote situations in developing countries where there are no facilities for producing hypertonic saline or urea solutions in sterile form.

MEDICAL AND HORMONAL TECHNIQUES
Quinine hydrochloride

In high dosage this drug was frequently effective if, until abortion was established, use was continued in the highest dose the woman could tolerate. About 300 mg were taken one- to two-hourly until toxic manifestations of severe dizziness and tinnitus (ringing in the ears) occurred. Until recent years it was used therapeutically, in less drastic dosage, for the induction of labour when the fetus had died. Cases have occurred where, after taking the quinine, the woman had permanently impaired hearing or damaged the fetus, and the method has no place in responsible services.

Ergometrine

Ergometrine produces severe contractions of the uterus at term, but it is ineffective in producing abortion in early pregnancy.

Pituitary extract and synthetic analogues

Pituitary extract is more effective in inducing uterine contractions in early pregnancy than ergometrine. The synthetic analogue *Syntocinon*, given intravenously using a mechanical pump, which allows a variable and controlled rate of administration, has proved very effective in accelerating the effects of intra-amniotic injections. Oxytocic drugs have proved effective in inducing second-trimester but not first-trimester abortions.

Irradiation

Between the world wars it was demonstrated that X-ray irradiation of the pelvis could result in abortion.[82, 83] Women with access to X-ray therapy machines have used the technique extra-legally: one 19-year-old student achieved her abortion by using such an overdose that she damaged her ovaries and became menopausal at the same time. The teratological effects should abortion fail, and the long-term dangers of genetic mutation in the ovaries, render the method unacceptable today.

Chemotherapeutic (anti-cancer) drugs

There is a range of drugs that will destroy the embryo in experimental mammals.[84–89] Certain drugs used in the treatment of cancer will cause abortion. Nearly 200 case histories of pregnant women being treated with anti-mitotics have been collected from the world literature.[90] Among 127 who received drugs in the first trimester, 54 aborted. Six abnormal babies were delivered. The women concerned were mainly cases of leukaemia and it is a serious reproach to the medical profession that they had neither received adequate contraceptive advice nor were offered routine abortion. In 1952 Thiersch conducted a clinical trial of the anti-metabolic aminopterin, a folic acid antagonist, as an abortifacient.[91] In his series, and in subsequent illicit usage of the drug, serious congenital abnormalities occurred in cases where abortion failed (see also p. 260).[92–94]

Hormones given at the time of a late period

Tablets containing oestrogen/progesterone mixtures (sometimes simply one or other alone) are widely used as pregnancy diagnostic agents, shortly after the first missed menstrual period. In many cases both the consumer and provider hope, or expect, an abortifacient effect. The first study of the efficiency of these hormones as abortifacients has been completed.[95] In a series of women seeking uterine evacuation within 14 days of the first missed period, Vengadasalam and his co-workers in Singapore randomly assigned women to a treatment group (receiving a proprietary 'hormonal pregnancy test' (intramuscular 50 mg progesterone and 3 mg oestrogen) and an untreated control group. All women were offered a menstrual regulation at the end of seven days if bleeding had not occurred and the contents of the uterus were examined histologically for evidence of pregnancy. Hormone treatment was ineffective in diagnosing pregnancy and when uterine bleeding did occur it began later in the untreated group. In view of the failure to demonstrate a useful effect and the undesirability of exposing the embryo to exogenous hormones, the use of 'hormonal pregnancy' tests cannot be recommended.

Prostaglandins

This family of long-chain fatty acids were, as the name suggests, first identified by von Euler in 1935[96] in extracts of the prostate gland. They are, in fact, found widely throughout the body and in significant amounts in the female and male reproductive tracts. Their function in the male remains mysterious, but in the female naturally occurring prostaglandins play an important part in menstruation, spontaneous abortion and in the process of labour. Their physiological functions and their potential role in fertility control are subjects of intense scientific interest[97,98] and, currently, probably an average of two scientific papers on prostaglandins are published every day.

In 1957 Bergström and associates at the Karolinska Institute first isolated pure crystalline extracts, and by 1962 the stereochemistry had been determined; in 1968 true synthesis of certain prostaglandins had been achieved, and effective analogues are now appearing and undergoing biological and clinical trials.

Prostaglandins have been used since the early 1960s to empty the uterus.[99–101] Karim showed in 1971 that they can be administered by the vaginal route, but their side effects include contraction of gut as well as uterus, and troublesome vomiting and diarrhoea. Contraction of the bronchioles can give rise to an asthma-like attack. The earlier they are used in pregnancy the higher the dose required and the worse the side effects. Early abortion can be procured by intravenous infusion of prostaglandin $F_{2\alpha}$ or E_2. The procedure is unpleasant but Karim & Filshie[100] have shown that there are no adverse effects upon blood-clotting mechanisms, renal function or a number of other parameters. Placental function appears to remain normal until shortly before abortion and almost certainly until uterine contractions have sheared the placenta from the uterine wall. The main drawback to the use of prostaglandins in early abortion is that the abortion is often incomplete, requiring surgical evacuation, and tends to be delayed, subjecting the woman to pain and worry and consuming expensive hospital space and services. At present the drugs have little to offer in comparison with the very excellent results that can be obtained surgically in first-trimester abortions (see also p. 191). (They may have a role in reducing cervical resistance to dilatation.)[34]

In late abortion, extra-ovular prostaglandins, or a combination of prostaglandins and urea, injected into the amniotic sac are now standard techniques widely used and far less dangerous than conventional surgical techniques. Prostaglandins are also much used in the labour wards for induction at, or near, term.

Abortion and sterilisation

Techniques of female sterilsation have advanced markedly in the last decade. It has become possible to offer to a woman undergoing abortion sterilisation with minimal extra time in hospital, or even with discharge home the day after the operation, as is normal practice in Britain for abortion cases. Initially, in British experience of abortion, hysterotomy was widely used when sterilisation was proposed, even in early pregnancy. Nowadays vaginal termination, even up to quite late stages, is preferred and hysterotomy is only used by surgeons with little experience and expertise in abortion. Laparoscopic sterilisation is readily combined with either one- or two-stage vaginal abortions. The technique is the same as for the non-pregnant woman. It is normally performed under general, but is possible under local, anaesthesia. A small incision is made within the confines of the umbilicus and a special needle with a spring-loaded device (which, freed from resistance, protects the sharp point from damaging the bowels) is introduced into the peritoneal cavity. Either carbon dioxide or nitrous oxide gas is introduced to expand the cavity and form a large space above the bowels and under the abdominal wall. A trocar and cannula is now pushed through the umbilical incision into the gas space and the trocar removed. This leaves the hollow metal tube, or cannula, leading from the exterior into the peritoneal cavity. A tightly fitting, lighted telescope or laparoscope is introduced through this cannula and the abdominal contents viewed. A fine-bore instrument is used either to coagulate and destroy, or to put occlusive rings or clips onto, the fallopian tubes. When the tubes are coagulated by electro-diathermy (effectively a technique of destruction by local heating) there is always a slight risk of injury to adjacent bowel and also the amount of other tissue damage is difficult to control, a factor that, recent work suggests, may cause subsequent menstrual problems if the damage is too great.

Instead of using laparoscopy, early vaginal abortions can be combined with vaginal sterilisation by entering the peritoneal cavity through the posterior vaginal fornix and seeking each tube in turn, ligating and partially excising it. The technique demands considerable skill, but causes minimal trauma and can be performed without special instruments. It is much practised in Bombay and all patients are allowed home in 24 hours. English experience confirms the value of the technique, but there may be cases where it is technically difficult and the alternative of mini-laparotomy needs to be kept in mind.

The term 'mini-laparotomy' has been coined for the use of a very small abdominal incision used, combined with manipulation of the uterus using special instruments, so as to bring each fallopian tube in turn under the incision, whereby the surgeon is able to seize the tube and perform sterilisation with minimal disturbance to the abdominal contents. In order to use very small incisions, expertise, training and practice are necessary, but it is possible for a woman to be discharged the same day as the operation, merely returning for removal of skin sutures. Statistical comparisons are needed, but the mini-laparotomy technique would seem to be marginally safer than laparoscopy.

The ambivalent and restrictive regulations made by the British Department of Health and Social Security, insisting upon the provision of resuscitative equipment on hand whenever late abortion is attempted, in case the fetus shows signs of life, are causing some British surgeons to revert to hysterotomy despite the known additional hazards. Local factors, such as the willingness of the nursing staff to supervise and support women undergoing late two-stage vaginal abortion may also be important. Major pelvic surgery in pregnancy, be it Caesarean section at term or hysterotomy or hysterectomy for abortion, always carries a higher than average risk of thrombo-embolism.

Abortion counselling

The special place of the counsellor in daycare abortion has been discussed above. Abortion is a situation that manifestly calls for sympathetic and supportive attitudes from all the professional staff with whom the couple come into contact. There are cultural differences between America and Britain with regard to the acceptance of formalised counselling by women and to its provision by the medical and allied professions. This partly reflects the different legal situations in the two countries. In America, abortion is a legal operation like any other. In Britain, two doctors must consider the specific grounds for abortion and formally certify that these grounds justify the operation; inevitably these doctors are involved in a counselling situation with the woman or couple and good ethical standards compel British doctors and nurses to accept this role. The majority of British women who are legally aborted are referred to the doctor who finally performs the abortion by their own family doctor, who remains in clost contact with them. In America the woman often has a more transitory relationship with the medical profession.

Madeleine Simms has pointed out that, whatever the detailed differences, the aims of abortion counselling are the same on both sides of the Atlantic and wherever abortion is freely available.[102] They are to provide psychological support during a crisis situation, to ensure that all the options open to the woman and her consort are fully understood and that they have mutually and/or separately considered any alternatives. Thence it is to extend sympathetic support throughout the abortion procedure, subsequently aiming to help the woman (or the couple, as the case may be) to plan for a more satisfactory contraceptive life in the future. Finally, it is to help those involved to accept the abortion, without guilt and remorse, as a rational decision. In Britain the woman's family doctor is ideally placed to fulfill all these functions – if he is temperamentally able to do so.

There are many unwanted pregnancies where the need for abortion counselling is minimal. For example, the older woman, whose family is complete, and where the pregnancy arises from a failure of reasonable contraception. Even in such a case, however, there is the need to point out that neither partner will be entirely happy to return to the contraceptive technique which has let them down. Sterilisation of one or the other may be the solution they will select and the counsellor's task is to ensure that the question is discussed between all interested parties and that the solution is freely chosen.

Conversely there are many situations where the need for close and sustained counselling is likely: pregnancy in young girls; women who have already had a previous unwanted pregnancy, whatever its outcome; women who show obvious signs of severe stress: women with a history of psychiatric breakdown; women who may not have had an overt breakdown but who have always failed to stay long in any job and whose personal relationships appear to have been transitory; women who have been sexually assaulted; women who have recently been bereaved by death or desertion; and women with insecure marriages, particularly if they are personally ambivalent about abortion.

Once abortion has been performed the counsellor, medical or lay, aims to help the woman to avoid finding herself once more unwantedly pregnant. The abortion experience is usually followed by improved contraceptive usage but it is impossible to assess to what extent, if any, formalised abortion counselling is responsible for this. Clearly the counsellor in the 'free standing' abortion clinic in America has a greater responsibility in this respect than any member of the team in Britain, because in the British NHS around 90 per cent of women are seen again, either at the gynaecological clinic or by their own general practitioner. In America a smaller proportion attend for formal medical check-up. The great differences in the frequency with which sterilisation is performed at the same time as abortion in Britain, as compared with the USA, reflects two factors. First, when sterilisation and abortion are performed under the NHS there is no cost to the woman, while in America the cost of the abortion is necessarily greatly increased by accepting sterilisation at the same time. Secondly, the British doctors, who have certified the need for this abortion may feel considerable responsibility to do all in their power to prevent a recurrence. In extreme cases gynaecologists, themselves emotionally disturbed by the abortion situation, have refused abortion unless the woman consents to sterilisation at the same time. Their attitudes contain a punitive element. Fortunately such situations were always rare and are further decreasing as the medical profession educates itself to deal more logically and effectively with the problems of the unwanted pregnancy.

Both in Britain and America the need for counselling in its widest sense, as an integral part of good abortion services, was rapidly accepted when liberal conditions had been established. In Britain the responsibility has remained primarily with the medical and nursing professions, together with social workers in hospitals and the community at large. In America there has been a tendency for a new profession of 'abortion counsellors' to develop. In both countries the needs and scope of counselling have changed and continue to change. Initially, women seeking abortion approached the situation, culturally imbued with the image of abortion as a secret and sordid act, and looked upon the doctors who provided abortion as separate from, and at odds with, their other medical colleagues. At this time the main need was to relieve anxiety about the dangers of life and health that seemed to threaten, and to establish the professional competence and ethical probity of those whose services were needed. Nowadays, few women fear the physical dangers of abortion but they still need information and support. The counsellor's role is rapidly changing to an educative one, constantly attempting to ensure that the woman who has had an abortion will for the future be able to cope with her sexual and emotional problems and will be less likely to find herself unwillingly pregnant again.

Adverse side effects

Mortality

According to British figures, therapeutic abortion is the third most commonly performed surgical operation, surpassed only by tonsillectomy and diagnostic D & C, and well ahead of appendectomy in frequency. Abortion is compulsorily notifiable and mortality is known accurately, whereas the total incidence of comparative surgical procedures is obtained only by estimate (Table 21).

The latest available figures for England and Wales are for 1968–73 and the mortality rate for abortions without sterilisation performed

Table 21. *Risk of death for selected operations*

Operation	Mortality rate (no. of deaths per 100000 operations)
Legal abortion	
First trimester	1.7
Second trimester	12.2
Tonsillectomy without adenoidectomy	3.0
Tonsillectomy with adenoidectomy	5.0
Ligation and division of fallopian tubes	5.0
Partial mastectomy (simple mastectomy)	74.0
Lower section Caesarean section	111.0
Abdominal hysterectomy	204.0
Appendectomy	352.0

in the first eight weeks of pregnancy was 1.7, for 9–12 weeks 3.8, and for second-trimester abortion 24 per 100000 operations.[103]

When comparing statistics from different countries some caution is necessary. In a number of countries where abortion has been liberalised in recent years, notification procedures have been instituted that require reporting of all deaths associated with abortion, including deaths which really resulted from the pre-existing disease for which the abortion was performed. Although no nationwide reporting system exists in America, data have been available since 1972 from the Center for Disease Control (US Department of Health Education and Welfare).[104] Many countries report deaths directly attributable to abortion, excluding, thereby, deaths due to concurrent disease.

The most important factor in abortion mortality is the duration of the pregnancy at the time of abortion. The earlier the abortion is done the safer it is (Table 22).

Both from the point of view of the individual operator and at a national level, there is an element of learned improvement as more abortions are performed. The individual learns to improve his technique and dexterity. Nationally, it comes to be realised by the medical profession and by the public that *early* abortion is safest, and facilities are developed to encourage the woman to present

Table 22. *Death rate for legal abortions in the USA, by week of gestation* (1972–74)

Menstrual age	Deaths	Cases[a]	Number per 100 000 operations	Relative risk[b]
≤ 8	3	747 550	0.4	1.0
9–10	13	581 002	2.2	5.5
11–12	12	330 537	3.6	9.0
13–15	12	129 536	9.3	23.3
16–20	27	147 160	18.3	45.8
≥ 21	6	30 282	19.8	49.5
Total	73	1 966 067	3.7	—

[a] Based on distribution of 1 459 495 abortions (74.2 per cent of total) in which gestational age was known.
[b] Relative risk based on index rate for ≤ 8 menstrual weeks' gestation of 0.4 per 100 000 abortions.

herself and for the abortion to be done as early as possible. This improvement of statistics with experience is readily demonstrated by comparing mortality from abortion in a few selected countries after reform of their abortion laws (Table 23).

These figures are for deaths following abortion at all stages. The high mortality shown in the Swedish and Danish figures resulted from the legal delays and consequent late abortion in those countries. The low mortality rate of the eastern European countries reflects the fact that the great bulk of all abortions are performed in the first trimester. The rapid improvement in mortality rates in America and in Britain does not imply solely improved surgical skill, but rather that women in a liberal atmosphere present early: the legal differences between the two countries are reflected in the extremely rapid adjustment to early abortion in America.

Only in Britain have we seen the widespread use of sterilisation procedures combined with abortion. The early experience has given irrefutable evidence of the dangers of indiscriminately combining the two operations. In 1969 no fewer than 20.3 per cent of all British women aborted were sterilised at the same time. The mortality of these combined procedures was 107.9 per 100 000 operations whereas

Table 23. *Abortion deaths for selected countries*

Country	Legal abortions	Deaths	Mortality rate (deaths per 100 000 legal abortions)
Denmark			
1956–60	19 900	18	90.5
1961–65	21 800	9	41.3
1966–70	34 700	2	5.8
Sweden			
1949–53	28 000	27	96.4
1954–63	35 200	21	59.7
1964–71	87 900	7	8.0
Czechoslovakia			
1957–61	330 400	19	5.8
1962–66	400 900	9	2.2
1967–70	398 600	9	2.3
Hungary			
1957–69	421 400	23	5.5
1960–63	669 700	21	3.1
1964–67	739 000	9	1.2
1968–70	787 600	8	1.0
USA			
1963–68	9 700[a]	7	72.2
1972	586 800	20	3.4
1973	615 803	22	3.6
1974	745 400	24	3.2
England and Wales (including foreign visitors)			
1969	54 819	17 (12)[b]	31.0
1970	86 565	14 (8)	16.2
1971	126 777	14 (6)	11.0
1972	167 884	6 (7)	9.4
1973	167 149	6 (2)	3.6

[a] Hospitals participating in the Professional Activity Survey.
[b] Figures in parentheses represent abortions where sterilisation was performed at the same time.

during the same year when abortion alone was performed the mortality rate was only 11.4. By 1973 only 7.1 per cent of British abortions were combined with sterilisation, the mortality rate for the combined procedure was 16.8 per 100 000 whereas abortion alone carried a mortality rate of only 2.6 per 100 000 abortions. We lack reliable data on the dangers of the various techniques of sterilisation, but the majority of British gynaecologists have been convinced that it is, in general, safer to perform abortion alone and carry out the sterilisation later where it is desired.

Morbidity

Much that is written about the consequences of induced abortion is more an affirmation of belief than an objective evaluation of reliable data. Unfortunately it has to be admitted that reliable data even today are not as readily available as they should be. Collection of such data is fraught with pitfalls.

Some forms of morbidity are sufficiently common for an individual practitioner or team to study their frequency, but there are special problems. Immediate complications such as perforation of the uterus may not be detected at operation, indeed many perforations may go undiagnosed, bleeding or infection may occur only after an interval of some days and be treated by another doctor, and because of the aura of secrecy which still tends to surround abortion, the patient may refuse permission for the operating surgeon to be informed. Long-term complications, such as infertility, are least likely of all to be reported back to the surgeon. When presenting elsewhere with complications, patients may deliberately conceal the fact that they had had an abortion.

Retrospective studies of presumed long-term complications are exceedingly difficult to evaluate because an element of case selection is inevitable, even in case-control studies. Nevertheless such studies are important until prospective trials are published. Studies on the randomised use of two similar technical procedures – such as the use or non-use of oxytocic drugs – could be important and ethically acceptable.

The psychological consequences of induced abortion are the most difficult of all to assess. This is both because of interaction between the observer and the woman observed and because the basic philosophy of the observer must inevitably colour his methodology and therefore his results: like the electron, the exact simultaneous position and velocity of which can never be measured by the physicist, so the true emotional consequences of abortion for an individual woman can never be known to her physician. Comparison by series of different observers inevitably means comparing the unlike and no large-scale results are available, so we cannot emulate physicists and use statistical techniques.

Individual experience can be shown to be very important. Buckle *et al.* in England recorded two uterine perforations in 409 consecutive suction abortions and both these cases occurred early in the series.[105] Diggory had three definite, and one further possible, perforations in his first 1000 consecutive recorded cases but only one further perforation in the next 800 cases.[21] In a co-operative study[49] between the National Institutes of Health, Washington, and the University Teaching Hospital, Ljubljana, Yugoslavia, it was found that operators performing less than 100 abortions in a 24-month interval inflicted more injuries (0.92 per cent) than those doing 200–300 operations (0.41 per cent). However, for those doing *more* than 300 abortions the injury rate rose (0.71 per cent). The complication rate was also higher for pooled observations on operations performed eighth or later in an operating list. As in most human affairs, familiarity improves performance until it begins to breed contempt.

The most important study of abortion complications was sponsored by the Population Council, under the direction of Tietze, and co-ordinated the findings of 66 institutions (60 teaching hospitals and 6 abortion clinics) from 1 July 1970 to 30 June 1971.[48] Almost 73 000 abortions were surveyed, which represented about one-seventh of all legal abortions carried out in America during the 12 month period. This Joint Project for the Study of Abortion (JPSA) computed complication rates for *total patients* and also separately for *local patients with follow-up*. The complication rate for total patients is a minimum estimate of complications because follow-up was not achieved for all patients. There are good reasons for assuming that the complication rate found for local residents who attended for follow-up represents a reasonable estimate of the maximum complication rate. This is because patients will include a much higher proportion of non-private patients and these can be shown to have a higher complication rate than private patients. Also it seems likely that, for those living locally, patients with complications are more likely than those free of all complaints to attend for follow-up care. Fig. 34 summarises the JPSA findings. The slight rise in

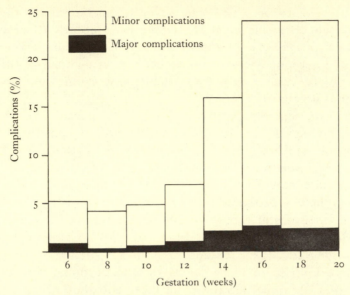

Fig. 34. Range of total and major (e.g. blood transfusion, 3 days of fever) complications per 100 operations by duration of gestation. (Women undergoing concurrent sterilisation omitted). Based on 67697 cases in the JPSA survey.

complications below eight weeks is probably partly the result of incomplete evacuation of the uteri. With newer techniques and more experience this problem appears to be becoming less frequent.

When complication rates found in the JPSA study are analysed by the place in which the abortion was performed, it is found that fewer complications occurred in clinic patients than in either out-patients or inpatients in hospitals. To some extent this difference, which is mimicked when comparing the private sector against the NHS in Britain, may be explained by the fact that more patients with pre-existing complications are handled by hospitals. Also clinic doctors tend to perform larger numbers of abortions and therefore possibly have more experience and skill than their hospital colleagues.

IMMEDIATE MORBIDITY

Tietze has drawn attention to the need to separate the medical complications of abortion into early (within 30 days) and late. The early complications can also be usefully considered as immediate complications occurring (though not necessarily discovered) during the operation or within a few hours, and delayed complications within the 30 days.

Uterine perforation

The incidence of this complication has already been discussed (Table 19). It should be remembered, however, that the JPSA study took place early in the evolution of American practice and with increasing experience individual operators unquestionably encounter this complication less frequently. The seriousness of the complication depends upon the likelihood of the instrument, which has passed into the peritoneal cavity, damaging the bowels, or the blood vessels supplying the bowels. In this respect, perforation of the uterine wall by suction curette, whilst aspirating, is more dangerous than a simple scraping curette. However, most studies have suggested that perforation is rare with a suction curette and very rare with the soft plastic Karman curette.

Haemorrhage

Inexperienced surgeons tend to fear haemorrhage, but in practice it is a rare complication.[17] In his first 1000 consecutive cases, Diggory gave six blood transfusions, five in cases of hysterotomy and one to a very anaemic girl who was transfused pre-operatively.[21] In his next 800 cases he required blood only once – in the case of an elderly and anaemic woman. Very few British NHS hospitals cross-match blood for first-trimester abortion procedures; nor is it necessary to do so any more than in dentistry, given the low rate of complications.

Haemorrhage may occur either at the time of operation, or within the next few weeks. In the latter case it is usually the result of retained tissue, normally placental tissue, within the uterus. In other words the uterus was incompletely emptied at operation. This latter complication is less frequently encountered after suction than conventional curettage. Very occasionally, prolonged uterine bleeding follows abortion, and subsequent menstrual periods are exceptionally heavy for several months. Again this is usually because of incomplete emptying of the uterus and may occur as secondary anaemia detected as a late complication of the operation.

Infection

Pyrexia and infection are generally said to have occurred if, on two successive occasions, a woman has a temperature of over 37.8 °C. High vaginal swabs and specimens of mid-stream urine are usually taken in an attempt to identify the infecting organism. But administration of antibiotics is often started without awaiting the results, since an intrauterine infection may spread rapidly to the fallopian tubes and could result in their permanent blockage. Diggory found 30 cases of pyrexia in his first 1000 cases and, in 17 of these, no pathogenic organism was isolated. In only one case was intrauterine infection established and this was severe staphylococcal infection. Since the original publication appeared the woman has reported the birth of a daughter. On the whole, genital tract infection is less of a problem than might be expected.

Infections can be reduced by the prophylactic use of antibiotics. When women attending Preterm Inc. in Washington were randomly allotted either to no treatment or to a four-day course of tetracyclines beginning immediately before the operation, the treated group had only two-thirds of the complications and one-quarter of the hospital admissions.[106] While the prophylactic use of antiobiotics is rightly questioned in many cases, the size of the differential in this trial suggests that their use may have a real place in abortion care.

Embolism

Venous thrombosis (clotting of blood within a vein) is usually associated with trauma, infection and venous stasis. Pulmonary embolism occurs when a detached blood clot passes through the venous system to the right side of the heart and round to the lungs, where the clot is finally arrested by the smaller blood vessels. Such an embolus may be fatal, since the oxygenation of the blood is obstructed. Embolism may follow any surgical procedure, particularly if complicated by infection. Pelvic operations are especially risky. The high mortality rate of hysterotomy and hysterectomy as abortion procedures are primarily the result of these complications. The age of the woman is of great significance – thrombo-embolic phenomena are rare in the young.

Anaesthesia

Modern general anaesthesia, for minor short procedures such as early abortion, is very safe. Nevertheless, now that it is known that the risk of death from early abortion is so exceptionally small, anaesthetic dangers must form a significant proportion of the total danger. Preliminary figures from England and Wales suggest that in the first one million legal abortions there were three anaesthetic deaths. Until recently general anaesthesia has been almost universally used in Britain.

LATE COMPLICATIONS
Damage to the uterine cervix

Overstretching of the cervix, preliminary to either curettage or suction aspiration, may result in tearing with haemorrhage, or leave a damaged cervix liable to infection. In this way cervical damage can give rise to an early complication. But, of course, the major importance of overstretching the cervix is the possibility of permanent damage of the internal cervical sphincter, so that *spontaneous* late abortion or premature delivery may occur in subsequent pregnancies.[107–109] Studies from Britain,[107] Hungary[108] and elsewhere[109,110] suggest this possibility but the observations have been disputed. It is an especially difficult topic to study because it is only revealed when such a spontaneous abortion occurs, often years later. For this reason any defect in the woman's recall of her past history is crucial and only careful prospective studies will ever establish the true frequency.[111] It must be remembered that the same overstretching of the cervix with subsequent spontaneous abortion may follow full-term delivery or *D & C* carried out for diagnostic reasons. It is particularly liable to follow a *D & C* performed as a curative measure for painful periods.

One of us has recently analysed eight consecutive cases of abortion due to cervical incompetence, in which the diagnosis has been established by the use of X-ray-opaque media injected into the uterus. In four cases the only relevant history was of a previous *D & C* – three having been done for dysmenorrhoea; in three cases there had been a previous therapeutic abortion – two being mid-trimester vaginal terminations and one abortion being performed at only six weeks' gestation under general anaesthetic and presumably with cervical dilatation. The last woman had, a year previously, delivered her first baby by rapid breech extraction for fetal distress. Usually when a previous abortion is responsible for cervical incompetence then the operator has overdilated the cervix, probably in the course of performing late vaginal abortion, when the use of intra-amniotic urea/prostaglandin would have been safer. If the multiparous cervix is never dilated beyond 14 mm diameter this complication is unlikely to occur. The condition normally responds well to the use of the Shirodkar suture, which prevents the late spontaneous abortion. It may be assumed that early abortions, performed without cervical dilatation, are without risk of long-term cervical damage.

Rhesus immunisation following abortion

The rhesus factor is one aspect of human blood groups (it is also found in monkeys, hence the name), and a baby may have a rhesus-negative mother, but inherit a positive factor from its father. The placenta is a barrier between the maternal and fetal circulation, but at the time of childbirth or abortion, fetal blood can leak into the maternal circulation giving rise to antibodies which will persist and may in turn damage the fetus of a subsequent pregnancy. This possibility has been taken so seriously in Poland that the law has been amended to forbid termination of the pregnancy in rhesus-negative women.

The risk of maternal immunisation in a full-term rhesus-positive pregnancy is about one in eight.[112] The rhesus factor can be demonstrated in fetal blood cells after the thirty-eighth day of pregnancy[113] and the risk of immunisation following spontaneous abortion has been very variously estimated, but recent work suggests that it probably lies at between two and four per cent, depending on the duration of pregnancy when the abortion occurred.[114–116]

Medically induced abortion poses several special features because of the variety of techniques used. Suction curettage in early pregnancy is less likely to cause immunisation than is cervical dilatation and uterine curettage. The concomitant use or non-use of oxytocic drugs at the time of abortion may also be of significance in influencing the passage of fetal cells into the maternal circulation although unfortunately there are no controlled clinical observations.

The most significant work is ably summarised by Queenan and his colleagues.[116] They found that:

First, out of 631 patients admitted for abortion 24 (4 per cent) were found to have fetal blood cells present in blood smears on admission and before operation. For the most part other investigators have not looked for fetal cells prior to abortion.

Secondly, 7.2 per cent of women terminated by suction curettage, and 20.2 per cent of more advanced pregnancies terminated by intra-amniotic injections, were shown to have trans-placental haemorrhage.

Thirdly, incidence and severity of trans-placental haemorrhage were related to the duration of gestation. In all cases of less than 13 weeks' gestation, the trans-placental haemorrhage was always small, as demonstrated by the fact that the ratio of fetal to maternal red cells on blood smear was always less than 10:50000. After 16 weeks of gestation, larger bleeds became more common; and, between 18 and 21 weeks gestation, readings were as high as 40–50 fetal cells per 50000 maternal cells.

There is a great deal of difference between transplacental haemorrhage and true post-abortion rhesus immunisation. In Queenan's series there were 66 rhesus-negative women; three were found to have fetal cells before abortion and were excluded from the trial. Fifteen were given anti-D immunoglobulin (which destroys any fetal cells that have leaked across before they can set up a reaction in the mother) at the time of abortion. Of the remaining 48, only 25 were successfully followed-up four months after abortion. One of these had become immunised to the rhesus factor.

The Ljubljana study did not find a correlation with any specific technique but confirmed that the risks of rhesus immunisation are small in the first month of pregnancy. Trials are needed to confirm or refute the impression that suction curettage is less hazardous than *D & C* and whether transplacental haemorrhage is affected by oxytocic drugs used at the time of abortion. In the absence of more knowledge, the only safe procedure is for all rhesus-negative women who are free of antibodies at the time of abortion to be protected at that time by anti-D immunoglobulin.[117] In all technologically advanced countries this is now routine.

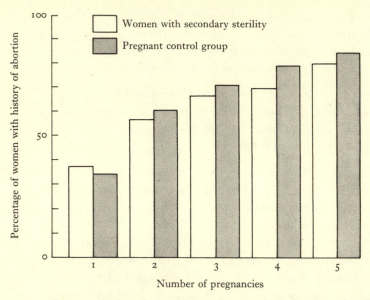

Fig. 35. Induced abortion and secondary sterility. Study of 484 cases of secondary abortion and 3389 control cases of pregnant women (Japan, 1964).

Sterility

Abortion may result in sterility, as may full-term pregnancy. Statistical data are lacking but it seems likely that the two events are approximately equally dangerous from this point of view. In general, sterility is only a remote possibility unless infection occurs with the abortion. The avoidance, and the rapid treatment of, infection are essential features of good abortion care.

The earliest study in this field is that of Gebhard and his co-workers, who were unable to demonstrate any adverse effects following abortion.[118] The study was a retrospective one and had certain obvious limitations. In clinical practice, one frequently encounters the woman seeking investigation of involuntary infertility who admits to a previous criminal abortion, and Gebhard's work is a useful reminder that criminal abortion is common and that it is normally under-reported in obstetric case histories.

In 1959 Lindahl followed up 1132 patients for one to five years after *legal* abortion.[119] Although there were some immediate complications, only 1.6 per cent had radiographic evidence of tubal abnormalities and only five women complained of infertility: this despite the fact that his series contained a high proportion of mid-trimester abortions.

The largest study is that of Hayashi & Momose in Japan.[120] These investigators questioned women complaining of secondary infertility as to whether or not they had had a medically induced abortion; they then asked the same question of women who had just been delivered at full-term. This case-controlled study showed that the incidence of an immediately previous induced abortion was virtually the same in the two groups (Fig. 35).

Future obstetric performance

The length of labour, the blood loss in labour and the incidence of instrumental delivery are all unaffected by previous medically induced abortion.[121]

Ectopic pregnancy – development of the embryo in the fallopian tubes or some other abnormal site – occurs in up to one in 300 pregnancies. The cause of the condition is not understood and guesses based on what appear to be commonsense clinical assumptions can be misleading. However, an induced abortion, by producing infection or the retrograde passage of material along the tube, could theoretically predispose to an ectopic pregnancy in later life. Epidemiological studies are difficult. On the one hand, Japanese hospital records show an increasing number of ectopic pregnancies in the post-war years. On the other hand, the ratio of ectopics to the total number of hospital deliveries has fallen in recent decades.[122] In Novi Sad, Yugoslavia, good records are available from a university obstetric department dealing with the total care of a locality, and here the number of ectopic pregnancies has remained constant while the number of legal terminations has been rising (1960 – 4580 legal abortions, 148 admissions for ectopic pregnancy; 1965 – 5013 legal abortions, 175 admissions for ectopic pregnancy; 1970 – 6445 legal abortions, 121 admissions for ectopic pregnancy.)[123] In Ljubljana women with several induced abortions had a slightly reduced risk of ectopic pregnancy. Perhaps the most useful evidence comes from the one case-controlled retrospective study conducted in Japan. Among 222 case histories of ectopic pregnancy, collected in Nihon University School of Medicine between 1959 and 1964, 117 (52.7 per cent) had a past history of induced abortion, but among normal pregnancies 50.3 per cent also had a history of induced abortion. When controlled for a variety of parameters such as parity, no marked difference was detected between a control group and those with ectopic pregnancies, except in the case of interstitial ectopic pregnancies. The Japanese study concluded that clinical impressions linking ectopic pregnancy and induced abortion were false (except possibly in the case of interstitial pregnancies), although pointing to the need for further study.[124]

Psychological sequelae to abortion

Of all the complications of abortion the psychological are the most difficult to assess. There is a great scarcity of prospective surveys with adequate methodological preparation. Poor sampling techniques, inadequate elimination of possible interviewer bias, failure to assess the psychological status of the woman before her unwanted pregnancy and inadequate follow-up surveillance are features of most reported surveys. Control groups are almost entirely absent.

The interaction between the woman and the doctor is of critical importance in the assessment by the latter of the former's psychological reaction. The woman's emotional response to abortion is influenced by her doctor's reaction on the first occasion when she seeks advice about her unwanted pregnancy, and is further moulded by the responses of all those in whose care she subsequently finds herself. Many doctors feel that the woman has sinned, but that they should extend charitable forgiveness and help her. Such doctors may well perform large numbers of abortions since they are overtly 'sympathetic'. Women under their care tend to feel grateful but ashamed; they might be less damaged by a matter-of-fact non-judgemental approach. The result of this interaction is that it is possible for two sincere and equally honest doctors, each having considerable experience of abortion to report either that shame and regret are common after abortion or that they are almost entirely absent. Only if they were to interview each other's patients would they realise that both reports are true. Those physicians who expect abortion to be associated with guilt may indeed produce guilt in those they terminate and this may account for the fact that Simon & Senturia, surveying the literature in 1966, found the incidence of severe guilt following hospital termination variously reported as between 0 and 43 per cent of all abortions.[124] Henry David has commented,

It is seldom realised that post-abortion psychosis is practically unknown. Since there are some 4,000 documented postpartum psychoses requiring hospitalisation in the United States per year, about one or two per 1000 deliveries, there should be a sizeable number of hospitalised post-abortion psychoses if abortion were as traumatic psychologically for women as term delivery. It would seem unlikely that a significant number of hospitalised psychoses related to abortion could be hidden in the records.[125]

The fact that childbirth is a more psychologically traumatic experience for a woman than abortion is not surprising. After she has had an abortion and has physically recovered, a woman is back in the non-pregnant state that preceded her unwanted pregnancy, and her psychological trauma is basically associated with having been unwantedly pregnant. After childbirth, and most especially if the child is unwanted, the woman has responsibilities and demands thrust upon her by, and on behalf of, the child, which imposes considerable strain.

The most comprehensive data on the psychiatric effects of abortion come from the JPSA study and, out of 73 000 abortions surveyed, a total of 16 major psychiatric complications were found, including two suicides and five depressive reactions associated with major haemorrhage or protracted fever.[51] The JPSA data yield a psychiatric complication rate of 0.2 per 1000 abortions as a minimum estimate and 0.4 per 1000 for local residents with follow-up, which is regarded as a maximum estimate. These figures may be compared with the 1.0–2.0 per 1000 *major* hospitalised psychoses following childbirth.

The traditional expectation that abortion must be mentally injurious runs very deep. Even a liberal writer such as Calderone, highlighting the abortion problem in the USA in 1968 and bringing together a mass of information that was of great value in changing attitudes, claimed that psychiatrists had demonstrated that 'in almost every case, abortion, whether legal or illegal, is a traumatic experience, which may have severe consequences later on'.[126]

When abortion is found to be an emotionally traumatic experience, it is still necessary to distinguish between the various factors which may be at work. Is it a form of stress that gives rise to, or uncovers, emotional instability? Is it possible to isolate the psychological and emotional trauma due to the abortion itself from that due to having unwillingly become pregnant in the first place?

When women seeking abortion are matched against control groups it is found that they exhibit more than usual emotional disturbances. In fact, the unplanned and unwanted pregnancy may itself be a symptom of psychological instability.

Early studies in the field suffered from the paradox that, when terminating pregnancy on psychological grounds, the stronger the psychiatric grounds for termination the more likely the operation was to be followed by emotional disturbance. Until the 1960s in the English-speaking world, only those women who were psychiatrically gravely ill – or pretended to be – obtained abortion,[127,128] and this may explain why so many early writers stressed the perils of unfortunate psychological *sequelae*.

The attitude of society as expressed by its abortion laws will influence the uncertainty and guilt experienced by the woman, as will the moral attitudes, spoken or implied, taken by the medical and nursing personnel through whose hands she passes. A leading Scandinavian psychiatrist has gone so far as to categorise guilt occurring in such circumstances as iatrogenic.

The current position is well summarised by McCoy, who writes, 'women who request abortions for basically social reasons usually reported a few initial or long-term regrets...Patients undergoing abortion for strong medical reasons were often sorry at first but most adjusted well and eventually accepted the necessity for the operation.'[129] Horden comments that 'although it is too soon to pronounce definitely on the psychiatric sequelae of the [British] Abortion Act, what has become apparent so far, is that they have been notable for their absence'.[130]

A fact often overlooked is that long-term psychiatric disturbances after illegal abortions are rare, although the guilt and emotional trauma associated with such an abortion must be far greater than when the operation is done openly and legally. In Gebhard's series, only four per cent of women admitting to criminal abortions reported adverse emotional consequences.[118] Legal abortion, when done on a large scale and for social reasons, is also free of psychological complications. For example, in Hungary, where legal abortions are more frequent than births, it is almost impossible to find an admission to psychiatric inpatient care precipitated by a termination. Of course, like all operations, abortion may be a relevant incident, among a complex of other factors, in the evolution of a woman's psychiatric condition and, like sterilisation or mastectomy, it may be the subject of regret, but it does not seem to carry the emotional penalties imagined of it.[131]

As experience of liberal abortion has spread, there has been an awareness that for many women termination brings genuine relief. The most fulsome rejection of traditional attitudes has come from the USA. Walter epitomises the new viewpoint. 'A whole generation of professional health workers refuses to let the myth die out that abortion will irreparably harm a woman. Extensive review of the literature reveals that this has not been true. In fact, for the healthy woman with a happy marriage, abortion is most often truly therapeutic.'[132]

It would appear that when the women is strongly motivated towards abortion there is little likelihood of guilt reactions. Clinical experience does suggest that age is an important factor in the likelihood of guilt; the very young girl is unlikely to suffer, whereas the older woman, particularly if nulliparous, needs careful assessment.

Benefits

After an abortion the woman usually experiences a sense of relief and an awareness that many of her pressing problems have been solved (Table 24).[133, 134] She can face the future afresh and make new choices. Women, in particular the unmarried, are now able to review their sexual reproductive attitudes and make positive decisions. This represents an important step forward because many may never have truly considered their attitudes on these topics until they found themselves unwantedly pregnant. After abortion many women make new and practical decisions about contraception (p. 491).

No doctor enjoys performing abortions any more than he would enjoy carrying out limb or breast amputations. But it is his appreciation of the improvement in the social and emotional health of the woman that can be expected to follow abortion which encourages him to embark on an intrinsically disagreeable task after weighing the physical risks of the operation against the predicted advantages. The preliminary assessment and counselling of a woman before abortion, as well as supporting her during and after the procedure,

Table 24. *Emotional benefits of legal abortion (360 women having first-trimester abortions in London)*

	Before termination	After termination 3 months–2 years
Psychiatric symptoms requiring treatment	29%	19%
Depression (Hamilton rating scale)	11.67±6.18	4.38±3.95
Interpersonal relationship rated as satisfactory	62%	77%
Sexual adjustment rated as satisfactory	59%	74%

bring the doctor into close contact with the woman and establish the same sort of link between them that is forged by a good obstetrician who cares for his patient throughout pregnancy and delivery.

The decision of a woman, or a couple, to have an abortion is not necessarily made because they dislike children, it is normally an expression of the fact that at this particular time in their life they feel that they cannot offer a child the love, security and physical support which would meet their ideals: the young unmarried girl feels that she cannot give a baby the life she sees as necessary for its proper happy development; the married woman often feels that another child would take away from her existing children too much of the physical and emotional resources available and would mean that in the future all her children would be to some extent deprived. Abortion is usually an altruistic decision.

A new philosophy is arising concerning the possible emotional consequences of induced abortion. Whereas previously the topic was looked at in the same way as some curative procedure in medicine, such as a partial gastrectomy or a hysterectomy, it is now being realised that it may be useful to review the problem from the point of view of decision making. Rather than asking, 'was the operation emotionally traumatic?' it may be more useful to ask, 'did the woman/couple make a healthy choice?' or 'did they have all the relevant information they needed to make their decision, in the context in which they found themselves' or 'do they regret their decision or would they make the same decision again; were they using the decision to hurt themselves or other people; did they learn from the decision?'

From the point of view of society, abortion eliminates unwanted pregnancies and thus frees social resources for the improved care and support of wanted children. In communities with ready access to abortion there will be a highlighting of the positive aspects of wanted pregnancy. It is no accident, but a logical and historical process, that liberal abortion attitudes evolve first in societies that have already shown increasing concern for the welfare of children.

In Britain when abortion was illegal many 'threatened abortions' were in fact the result of deliberate attempts at induced abortion and the humane doctor realised that the woman's genuine desire was certainly not to preserve the pregnancy. Knowing that if she was admitted to hospital every effort would be made to foil the woman's real aims, family doctors often used to treat such cases at home. Nowadays, when most women who are unwantedly pregnant can obtain an abortion if they try hard enough, a doctor faced with a case of threatened abortion will take a much more positive attitude towards preserving the pregnancy and it is a fact that a larger proportion of cases of threatened abortion are now hospitalised.

The benefits to the individual of ensuring that birth shall be by choice rather than by chance also extend to the community at large. We live in a world that is becoming increasingly overcrowded. The overcrowding occurs in rich as well as in poor nations and the birth of an unwanted baby in a rich nation represents a far greater consumption of resources from the common pool. Often, as in the UK, the number of unwanted births happens to be numerically almost the same as the difference between births and deaths. Indeed, most Western nations with liberal abortion laws are also moving towards zero population growth. In developing countries any reduction in births releases capital and resources for the improved social and economic welfare of others. In short, not only do individuals choose abortion with the welfare of existing or potential children in mind, but often it is an essential prerequisite to the health and happiness of the next and subsequent generations.

Contemporary and future developments

Surgical

MENSTRUAL REGULATION

Menstrual regulation, menstrual aspiration, very early abortion, *interception*, and pre-emptive abortion are all terms used to describe the surgical evacuation of the uterine contents shortly after the first missed period. Such terms are usually arbitrarily restricted to 14 days after the first missed period.

The most common technique involves using a hand-held vacuum syringe or vacuum bottle in conjunction with a flexible 4 mm diameter Karman curette, but any source of vacuum can be used.[135-143] The method has been used in three different situations. Certain feminist groups in the USA have used it regularly, each month at, or just before the expected time of menstruation, as a combined fertility regulation and personal hygiene procedure. One underground paper wrote, 'There is available to some women a mechanical form of menstrual insurance that is so simple that any woman can learn to use it at home.' A woman visits feminist groups, asks for a table, and a mirror, lies back, spreads her legs, inserts a speculum and aspirates material from her own uterus. These episodes are some of the more strange in the history of abortion, but no more curious than many of the opposite type of unnecessary restrictions that have been perpetrated by physicians. Unhappily, some of the feminist groups promoting menstrual regulation in the USA are spurred on by an uninformed fear of contraceptives: '. . . the technique offers a method of birth control that will leave her [*the user*] free from dangerous chemicals and devices.'

A second pattern of menstrual regulation is to offer the procedure to all women whose period is late and who might be pregnant. The controversial element in this situation is that some women will not have been pregnant and therefore are exposed to a small but measurable risk of unnecessary complications (Fig. 36).

The third possibility is to restrict the operation to women with a positive pregnancy test. By asking women with negative pregnancy tests to wait as little as one week, the percentage of redundant operations has been cut from 30 to 13.[144]

The use of menstrual regulation is subject to research in many countries. The International Fertility Research Program has over

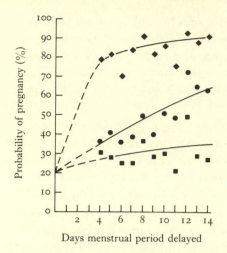

Fig. 36. Incidence of pregnancy by duration of menstrual delay (estimated values). ◆ = woman with positive pregnancy test ($n = 407$); ● = all women ($n = 1440$); ■ = women with negative pregnancy test ($n = 1009$).

8000 cases with follow-up on its computer. Pelvic infection occurred in 1 to 2 per cent of cases. Between 0.6 and 2.8 per cent of cases have required re-aspiration and, as is often the case, the experience of the operator is of key importance in the number of repeat failed operations.[145,146]

Emptying the uterus before the woman knows for certain that she is pregnant profoundly changes the emotional, legal and ethical aspects of early abortion. Gynaecologists investigating involuntary infertility frequently perform a diagnostic curettage of the uterus during the 10 days before the next expected period and they will all recollect having thereby inadvertently performed an early abortion when it was least desired. Indeed very many seemingly normal menstrual periods are in fact early abortions unknown to the woman (p. 60).

Using the name *menstrual regulation* alters the rules of the game which people play in relation to abortion. To describe such an important human problem in terms of a game is not entirely a fantasy. Neither the general public nor the medical profession are logical in their attitudes to abortion. Politicians, lawyers, doctors and women in need all distort reality. It is not practical to write about abortion in a Bangladesh newspaper in a straightforward way, but it has proved acceptable to hold a much-publicised conference on menstrual regulation in Dacca and menstrual regulation is proving popular.[147] It is not prudent to have even a whispered discussion of the role of abortion in family planning in the Philippines; but it generates immediate and widespread interest to discuss menstrual regulation.

Menstrual regulation has become a significant factor in fertility control within the last few years because it meets a need and describes a reality. It is misleading and an affront to language to describe an operation that terminates a 24-week pregnancy by the same noun as a procedure that evacuates the uterus when a woman's period is a few days late. The earlier an abortion is done the safer it is. Menstrual regulation is probably safer than any other pregnancy termination procedure. Emotionally it imposes less of a strain upon the woman than an abortion undertaken when she has already accepted that she is pregnant. Ethically it is the least challenging form of abortion, not only because it may in practice not be abortion at all but because we are here disturbing and destroying an embryo hardly developed from the fertilised ovum and which we know is so frequently lost by natural processes. Recently, the development of highly sensitive pregnancy tests (although not yet in general use) allows pregnancy to be detected before a menstrual period has been delayed. Interestingly, it has been shown that many such tests become positive in the few days preceding an expected period in women using intrauterine contraceptive devices. If this work is confirmed then there would seem to be little difference ethically between using such a device and requesting menstrual extraction.

Legally the option of menstrual regulation has the potential to make a great impact.[148,149] Few women have absolutely regular cycles and a period that is a few days late means no more than that she is *probably* pregnant. Thus, if menstrual regulation is limited to aspiration of the uterus within 14 days of the expected first day of the delayed period then, although both the woman and the doctor may believe that she is pregnant and will mutually agree upon suction aspiration, there will be no proof of pregnancy unless the tissue removed from the uterus is submitted to microscopic examination, which could only be done with the doctor's collaboration. The point is of critical importance in countries where abortion is illegal. In Argentina and several other Latin American countries, a doctor can only be held to have performed an abortion when the woman is first proven to have been pregnant. In the opinion of Latin American lawyers menstrual regulation is not a crime. This is in contrast to the British tradition of law where, under the 1861 statute, it is the 'intent' to commit abortion which is the crime. Therefore menstrual regulation counts as an abortion if the doctor believes the woman is pregnant, but not if he is genuinely investigating a delayed period. This would be true even if the tissue removed during such an investigation actually contained embryonic material.

There are certain cultural aspects of menstrual regulation which are interesting. Both in America and Britain it has already been found that a proportion of woman asking for menstrual regulation prefer not to be told whether or not they had been pregnant. Clearly, even when abortion is legally available some women who seek to be free of pregnancy would prefer not to have to accept the full responsibility for provoking an abortion. It seems likely that, in countries where the religious and legal tenets are against induced abortion, menstrual regulation may be more acceptable than a later procedure. Moral questions relating to abortion at all stages of pregnancy are further discussed in Chapter 15.

There are two main objections to menstrual regulation. First, a woman who believes herself to be pregnant must decide very quickly indeed if she is to avail herself of the procedure. In most cases this will not present a problem but there will be many women, particularly those single girls who have a good and stable relationship with the putative father, where ambivalence is understandable and it would be better to allow adequate time to discuss the situation widely and decide in freedom from haste. Secondly, as many as one-third of the women will be found at operation not to have been pregnant at all (Fig. 36). Although the risks involved are small, it is obvious that unnecessary surgical procedures are undesirable. It should be remembered, however, that there are comparable situations in surgery. Many surgeons will operate on the suspicion of appendicitis and even if they find the appendix is normal they will argue that the risks of operation were far less than those of delay had the organ been diseased. Similarly, some doctors believe that the simplicity and safety of menstrual regulation, bringing instant solution to the woman's worries and problems, completely justify its use.

To some extent menstrual regulation, like marriage, is what the individual chooses to make of it. In certain countries, for example parts of Latin America or the Moslem countries of Asia, it could become, or is already becoming, a politically acceptable reality in situations where routine abortion is unacceptable. Clinical series of several hundred menstrual regulations have been reported from Bolivia, Panama, Indonesia, Malaysia and Chile.[150]

POST-COITAL INSERTION OF AN INTRAUTERINE DEVICE

Lippes has recently reported that, if a woman has unprotected intercourse and seeks action to prevent or possibly to interrupt pregnancy, then the insertion of an intrauterine device within a few days of sex would appear to protect her.[151] He has so far not experienced any failures of this technique but the trial is small and needs to be repeated and assessed.

Medical

THE POST-COITAL PILL

The use of relatively large doses of oestrogens as post-coital contraceptives has already been discussed (p. 204). Other drugs, including anti-oestrogen preparations, have been tried as post-coital contraceptives, but at present the five-day course of oestrogens started within 72 hours of unprotected intercourse would seem to be the most effective. In 2000 cases, Haspels recorded 14 pregnancies, but some of those may have been due to additional coitus after treatment.[152] The side effects of nausea, and subsequently disturbed menstrual pattern, make it a wholly unsatisfactory method of birth control and it is used in 'emergency' situations only. Oestrogens are ineffective after ovo-implantation.[153]

THE ONCE-A-MONTH PILL

In 1968 Ravenholt defined the ideal method of fertility control as a 'non-toxic and completely effective substance which, when self-administered by the woman on a single occasion, will ensure non-pregnancy at the completion of one monthly cycle'.[154] Although the dosage of prostaglandins necessary to induce abortion tends to be larger the earlier they are used in pregnancy, it seems possible that, given at approximately the time of the expected menstrual period, prostaglandins may be capable of inducing either menstruation or very early abortion according to whether the woman had become pregnant or not.[155] Current research with prostaglandin analogues is giving encouraging results.

IMMUNISATION AGAINST PREGNANCY

Immunisation against pregnancy has been sought for many years. Immunisation against sperm, the fetus and against placental extracts have all been tried but so far without any success. However, some of the hormones necessary for pregnancy are antigenic. The three pituitary endocrine-stimulating hormones (thyroid-stimulating hormone, follicle-stimulating hormone and luteinising hormone) carry two antigenic factors the alpha portion of which is common to all of them. The beta factors are specific and, even more important, also different antigenically whether they are produced in the woman's pituitary or by the placenta during pregnancy – although the endocrine actions of the material from these two sources are similar. Careful preparation is necessary to avoid developing cross-immunisation against the pituitary horomones when immunising against chorionic gonadotrophin.[156] This is probably the most hopeful area of fundamental research into a new contraceptive technique.[157,158] It has been successfully used in marmoset monkeys and antibody production that is specific against chorionic gonado-trophin has been achieved in sterile human volunteers.[159] Both active and passive techniques of immunisation are under trial and the problems of reversibility would seem to show promise of ultimate solution. The technique necessarily relies upon very early abortion whenever pregnancy occurs and chorionic gonadotrophin is produced.

Interaction of attitudes and practice

The extent to which abortion is utilised, and the role it plays within the fertility control mechanisms of a community, depend on cultural, ethical and traditional factors. The attitudes of the doctors, legislators and religious leaders are often in sharp contrast to the usage of illegal abortion by the people within the society.

The inhibition of new developments within the field of abortion, which persisted until very recently and which resulted in relatively dangerous techniques being used, particularly in mid-trimester abortion, has been noted. Even more important has been the inhibition of doctors towards using abortion, which resulted in inordinate delays in providing the operation so that frequently, by the time agreement to operate had been made, the procedure was far more dangerous than it need have been. Fortunately, the difficulty recedes as the atmosphere becomes more permissive. The early experience of abortion in Scandinavia and England and Wales illustrates this problem well.

Legislators and administrators are also subject to inhibitions. The British administrative machine, which controls public and private medical practice, effectively (although often without the force of statute) held back the use of outpatient abortions until 1976 by prohibiting it within the private sector even though the private sector has been innovative, has a lower mortality from abortion than the NHS and there was ample statistical evidence of safety and popularity of daycare abortion when available. The main effect of forcing overnight stay upon private patients in Britain was to increase the costs of abortion to those unable to obtain the service from the NHS.

Throughout the abortion debate the real question is 'who has the right to decide?' The woman chooses and requests abortion but the medical profession, at all levels, has been reluctant to diminish its power of decision and veto. Inevitably, those in closest contact with the woman, the family doctors, have been the first to support liberalisation of abortion laws, while doctors in administration or positions of influence – the 'medical establishment' – have in some cases been the most resistant.

Even after the 1967 Abortion Act in Britain and when clinical practice underwent a rapid increase in the utilisation of abortion, the 'establishment' was unwilling to consider statistical evidence of its merits. The low mortality rate of abortion in countries as far apart as Hungary and Japan, and from 1970 onwards in the USA, was disbelieved by leaders of the medical profession. The statistics were called 'unreliable', 'vague' and in some cases 'utopian'. In 1970 Jeffcoate, who was about to become President of the Royal College of Obstetricians and Gynaecologists, wrote:

> Those who repeatedly state that the induction of abortion
> under modern conditions is without hazard generally quote
> figures from behind the Iron Curtain which are politically
> adjusted. Do any of us believe accounts of the invasion of

Czechoslovakia put out by Russia and her satellites? The official reports of their experience with legalised abortion are equally unreliable.[160]

By contrast, in the same year a WHO scientific group wrote, 'Mortality associated with induced abortion performed in hospitals has dropped to exceedingly low values, according to reports from several parts of eastern Europe that have reliable vital statistics.'[161]

Not only have convictions been so strong that they have led to denial of observational data and feelings so passionate that they have defeated experimentation, but social attitudes have interacted with surgical techniques in a destructive way. Some gynaecologists have employed the combination of sterilisation with abortion, not as a rational and mutually accepted option, but as a punitive compulsory addition. A survey of abortion practices in American hospitals in 1967 found that half the teaching hospitals in the sample sometimes made the acceptance of tubal ligation a prerequisite to the granting of abortion. We have already commented upon the very high, and dangerous, rates of sterilisation combined with abortion in the early British statistics of NHS terminations.

The real issues generated by developments in prostaglandins may be more in attitudes than in clinical pharmacology. For the first time a method is evolving that offers the possibility of self-treatment. For the first time a medical (possibly even an oral) method of abortion is on the horizon. Just as the Pill transferred contraception from the lavatory to cocktail party conversation, so prostaglandins may do the same for abortion. The Pill threw out a challenge to the Roman Catholic church that, although formally rejected, sent shock waves through that structure which will continue to knock pinnacles and buttresses off theological constructs for years to come. In the long run, abortion is likely to cause even greater stresses.

While the goal of prostaglandin research, to develop self-administered early abortifacients, is clear, the barriers to its achievement are more obscure. Djerassi has estimated that it could take ten years and cost $18 million to register a new fertility control agent, such as prostaglandin, with the United States Food and Drug Administration.[162] His estimates may be pessimistic, and some countries including the UK are already acting more rapidly than the USA, but, even if a suitable analogue can be developed that has a powerful uterine action but few side effects, it would take several years to bring it into use. Beyond the practical difficulties of developing complex therapeutic agents lies the problem of medical attitudes if their use is oversupervised. Illegal use and use late in pregnancy are bound to present problems and the medical profession is certain to be divided between those who will hope to prevent abuses by very easy access to any possible drug and those who attempt to prevent misuse by close supervision.

To the student of abortion the biggest contrast between countries is in medical attitudes and not in the cultural differences dividing populations. It is hard to find a Russian or a Japanese doctor who can be convinced that the oral contraceptive is as safe a method of birth control as early abortion. In fact, over a reproductive lifetime, control of fertility by the Pill or by repeated early abortion would appear to be about equally safe. Conversely, few American or British doctors would be happy to consider the two techniques solely from the point of view of efficiency and medical hazards.

Where abortion is accepted by the community and its provision by the medical profession is adequate and non-judgemental, some women may consider its repeated usage to be personally more acceptable than other forms of birth control. Moore-Čavar has summarised possible arguments for preferring abortion:

1 Except for sterilization and the IUD no other birth prevention technique is a one-event procedure.
2 As with IUDs and pills, abortion is coitus-independent.
3 Whereas there is always some uncertainty associated with the use of contraception, the woman knows at once and for certain that an abortion has been successful.
4 Abortion is not based on the probabilities of conception (which many women may consider very small given the large number of times they have had unprotected sex without becoming pregnant) but on the certainty of a recognised pregnancy: it requires hindsight, not foresight. Abortion, in this light is 'curative' rather than 'preventive' medicine. We all know that hindsight is a stronger force than foresight and few of us are good at personal preventive care.
5 Abortion is the only method of preventing the birth of a child who may have been desired at the time of conception but which, due to changed circumstances, may no longer be wanted.
6 For the unmarried, separated, widowed or divorced who have

infrequent or unanticipated intercourse, abortion may be
cheaper, less risky and/or more acceptable than other methods.
  7 Abortion need not require the knowledge or consent of the
    male partner.[163]

Paradoxically, those whose cultural taboos regarding sex are
conservative or still developing may find abortion more acceptable
than contraception. The young single girl, who has not yet come
to terms with her own sexuality, may expect to be wooed and won
afresh before every sexual act. Such an attitude can prevent her from
taking preventive contraceptive precautions. It is an attitude often
found amongst contraceptively knowledgeable young nurses requesting abortion. Within Western society more young girls obtaining
abortion are from the groups who fully intended to marry as virgins,
rather than those who planned premarital sexual enjoyment.

From the point of view of the effects of cultural acceptance upon
the type of service provided, wherever the decision to perform an
abortion is regarded as a medical one there will be delays and the
benefits of early abortion are likely to be lost. Wherever abortion
is accepted as a normal part of birth control, then women present
early and the procedure is safer and less traumatic.

Treatment of incomplete abortion

An incomplete abortion may be an extra-legal abortion with
possible infection and/or trauma. The recognition of this possibility
is the paramount factor in its treatment, but whether induced or
spontaneous, the complete emptying of the uterine cavity remains
the most important therapeutic aim, and experience has shown that
the suction curette is superior to the classical method of curettage
in this respect.[164–168]. Since the condition may be spontaneous, and
in countries with liberal abortion laws this will usually be the case,
it is important to try to find the cause so that recurrence may be
avoided. A careful examination under general anaesthesia is often
important in detecting or excluding causes of spontaneous abortion.

Women admitted to hospital following an illegal abortion frequently receive poor-quality treatment, especially in the developing
world. In Latin America alone there are an estimated one million
such admissions per year, and the women usually find themselves
in the oldest and worst-equipped part of the hospital, and may find

themselves two in a bed – or even on the floor. There is an urgent need to up-grade the treatment of such cases, and the provision of equipment for vacuum aspiration curettage would simplify this technically. Once an abortion has taken place, even if illegally induced, the woman deserves and needs dignified and humane treatment. It is essential that she should be afforded realistic contraceptive advice.

Conclusions

Early abortion is a straightforward operation that in series of hundreds of thousands of cases has proved to have a remarkably low mortality and relatively few immediate side effects. As yet there is no evidence of serious long-term side effects, although data are still being accumulated. It is generally concluded that vacuum aspiration is the optimum way to empty the uterus, and where different techniques survive this is because information and awareness of the advantages of vacuum aspiration are still diffusing through the medical community.

First-trimester abortions can be conveniently performed as an outpatient or daycare procedure. The facilities required are simple. A clean room and equipment can cost well under $100 although plans have to be made to deal with possible complications, however rare. For best results a standardised repeatable technique needs to be developed, taught and implemented.

It seems unlikely that there will be any important additional improvements in the surgical technology of early abortion; like appendectomy this particular procedure has arrived at an end-point.

While it is unlikely and undesirable that a doctor would spend the whole of his time performing abortions, the skill which is represented by a single individual doctor is equivalent to a surprisingly large number of early terminations. It is not impossible for a doctor to perform 50 operations in a day, and on a 300-day working year this represents 15000 terminations. Therefore, in a hypothetical situation of a city of one million people with a birth rate of 30 per 1000 of the population, *one doctor's time* devoted to the performance of abortions could halve the birth rate. It would be impossible for the same unit of professional skill to have a similar impact if only contraceptives were being made available. Therefore it is not the technology of abortion or the availability of skills and facilities which limit its use and its potential demographic impact. The use of abortion depends upon the will of the medical community to make it available, upon the legislative context in which they work, and on the desire of the women to terminate unwanted pregnancies. Much of the rest of this book will be concerned with these other variables.

The situation for second trimester abortions is very different. They present a much greater risk to the woman, both of death and of possible complications. There are a number of different ways of emptying the uterus and none is pre-eminently better than any other. It is quite possible that new and much improved ways of doing second-trimester abortions will be introduced, but, however great the improvement, it is very unlikely that second-trimester abortions could ever approach the earlier operation in safety and simplicity.

Second-trimester abortions require a higher degree of surgical skill, specialisation and a greater investment in equipment, operating theatre facilities, professional manpower and nursing care.

Menstrual regulation, or very early abortion, is technically an extension of procedures that are already used and proven. However, it has political, legal, ethical and emotional advantages, which may be of particular value in parts of the developing world, such as South America.

For many decades doctors and scientists took no interest in the possibility of medical methods of terminating pregnancy. Recently some effort has been put into this field. An abortifacient preparation that women could take orally or insert vaginally may, for the first time, be a possibility. However, the surgical methods of early abortion are so successful that a medical method is unlikely to produce equal or better clinical results. The true significance of a self-administered abortifacient is that it places the decision with the woman. Its drawback is that it is likely, for biological reasons, that a medical method would be effective at all stages of pregnancy, and therefore would be open to a form of misuse that would be physically dangerous to the woman and/or could produce an abnormal living baby.

In the case of second-trimester abortions the medical use of prostaglandins is already a real option.

The promising fundamental research into immunisation against pregnancy opens up slightly different horizons. Current research concentrates on immunisation against the conceptus and therefore will act by causing very early abortions – so early that the woman will never know that she was pregnant. Predictably such procedures will raise ethical questions. In practice, the application of the technology on a large scale, especially in developing countries, is likely to be particularly simple and cheap.

But, in the last analysis, from the woman's point of view current and future changes in abortion are likely to lie not so much in new technical developments as in the more ready and sympathetic availability of services based on those techniques which we already possess.

References

The literature on various methods of inducing abortion is larger than that on any other aspect. Potts & Diggory have reviewed the clinical literature (Termination of pregnancy. In *Human Reproduction* (1973), eds. E. S. E. Hafez & T. N. Evans, p. 405. Harper & Row, New York). Tietze & Murstein provide the most comprehensive summary of mortality and morbidity statistics in the Population Council 'Induced Abortion: 1975 Factbook'. (Tietze, C. & Murstein, M. C. *Reports on Population/Family Planning*, **14** (second edition).) The publications of the International Fertility Research Program, Chapel Hill, North Carolina, analyse many aspects of the treatment of incomplete abortion, menstrual regulation, induced abortion and the use of prostaglandins. The *Population Reports* of the George Washington University Medical Center (Series F and G) provide up-to-date reviews of abortion techniques.

Specialist bibliographies exist on *Post-Implantation Antifertility Substances* (A. L. Walpole, 1970), *Effects of Prostaglandins on the Reproductive System* (V. Pickles, 1971) and *Outpatient Abortion* (D. M. Potts, 1972), from the Reproductive Research Information Service, Cambridge, England, and on the *Psychosocial Aspects of Fertility Regulation*, from the International Reference Center for Abortion Research, Bethesda, Maryland.

1 Pearsall, R. (1969). *The Worm in the Bud*. Weidenfeld & Nicolson, London.
2 Ricci, J. V. (1949). *The Development of Gynecological Surgery and Instruments*. Blakiston, Philadelphia.
3 Edelstein, L. (1942). *The Hippocratic Oath*. Columbia University Press, New York.
4 *Nux Elegia*, lines 23–34.
5 Lair, S. (1828). *Nouvelle méthode de traitment des ulcères, ulcérations et engorgemens de l'utérus*. Paris.
6 Nelson, M. R. (1945). History of the uterine curette. *Contributions from the Department of Gynecology of the City of New York*, **8**, 72.

7 von Braun-Fernwald (1904). Instrumental termination of abortion. *Zentralblatt für Gynäkologie*, 17 September.

8 Pritchard, E. W. (1864). Abortion procured by tents of common sea tangle (*Laminaria digitata*). *Obstetrical Transactions*, **5**, 198.

9 Simpson, J. Y. (1863). *Clinical Lectures on Diseases of Women.* Blanchard & Lea, Philadelphia.

10 Barnes, R. (1873). *Clinical History of the Medical and Surgical Diseases of Woman.* Churchill, London.

11 Bykov, S. G. (1927). A method of preventing pregnancy. *Vrachebnoe Delo*, **9**, 21.

12 Wu, Y. T. & Wu, H. C. (1958). Suction in artificial abortion: report of 300 cases. *Zhong Fuchanke*, **2**, (6), 447.

13 Wu, Y. T. & Wu, H. C. (1958). Suction curettage for artificial abortion: preliminary report of 300 cases. *Chinese Journal of Obstetrics*, **6**, 26.

14 Kerslake, D. & Casey, D. (1967). Abortion induced by means of uterine aspiration. *Obstetrics and Gynecology, N.Y.*, **30**, 35.

15 Nilsson, C. A. (1967). Vacuum aspiration of uterine contents in legal abortion and allied conditions. *Acta obstetricia et gynecologica scandinavica*, **46**, 501.

16 Beric, M. B. (1937). *National Congress on Health and Treatment of Village Women.* (In Serbocroat.)

17 Beric, B. M. & Kupresanin, M. (1971). Vacuum aspiration, using paracervical block for legal abortions as an outpatient procedure up to the twelfth week of pregnancy. *Lancet*, **ii**, 619.

18 Karman, H. (1972). The paramedical abortionist. *Clinical Obstetrics and Gynecology*, **15**, 379.

19 Mullick, B., Brenner, W. E. & Berger, G. (1973). *Termination of Pregnancy with Intrauterine Devices.* International Fertility Research Program, Chapel Hill, North Carolina.

20 Barns, H. H. F. (1947). Therapeutic abortion by means of soft soap pastes. *Lancet*, **ii**, 825.

21 Diggory, P. L. C. (1969). Some experiences of therapeutic abortion, *Lancet*, **i**, 873.

22 Boero, E. A. (1935). Avortement par formaldéhyde. *Gynécologie et Obstétrique*, **32**, 502.

23 Watteville, H. & de'Ernst, J-P. (1950). L'avortement thérapeutique par hydramnios artificiel. *Gynaecologia*, **130**, 425.

24 Brosset, A. (1958). The induction of therapeutic abortion by means of a hypertonic glucose solution injection into the amniotic sac. *Acta obstetricia et gynecologica scandinavica*, **37**, 519.

25 Bengtsson, L. P. & Stormby, L. (1962). The effect of intra-amniotic injection of hypertonic sodium chloride in human midpregnancy. *Acta obstetricia et gynecologica scandinavica*, **41**, 115.

26 Greenhalf, L. J. O. & Diggory, P. L. C. (1971). Induction of therapeutic abortion by intra-amniotic injection of urea. *British Medical Journal*, **1**, 28.

27 Bonney, V. (1918). Abdominal hysterectomy. *Lancet*, **ii**, 518.
28 Jorgensen, P. I. (1969). Paracervical block use in curettage for diagnostic purposes and for abortion. *Acta obstetricia et gynecologica scandinavica*, **48**, 446.
29 Penfield, A. J. (1972). Abortion under paracervical block. *New York State Journal of Medicine*, **71**, 1185.
30 Ganesh, K. & Hingorani, V. (1973). Paracervical block anaesthesia for gynaecological operations. *Journal of Obstetrics and Gynaecology of India*, **23**, 600.
31 Chatfield, W. R., Suter, P. E. N. & Kotonya, A. O. (1970). Paracervical block anaesthesia for the evacuation of incomplete abortion – a controlled trial. *Journal of Obstetrics and Gynaecology of the British Commonwealth*, **77**, 462.
32 Hulka, J. F., Lefler, H. T., Angelere, H., & Lachenbrack, P. A. (1972). 'A new electric force monitor to remove factors influencing cervical dilation for vacuum curettage.' IFRP. (Duplicated document.)
33 Stewart, G. K., Margolis, A. J., Murr, W. & Kerner, J. A. (1970). Cervical dilation by vibration. *Obstetrics and Gynecology, N.Y.*, **35**, 949.
34 Dingfelder, J. R., Brenner, W. E., Hendricks, C. H. & Staurivsky, L. G. (1974). Reduction of cervical resistance induced by prostaglandin suppositories prior to dilation for induced abortion.' IV Congress of Obstetrics and Gynaecology, Kuala Lumpur, Malaysia. (Duplicated document.)
35 Potts, D. M. (1970). Termination of pregnancy. *British Medical Bulletin*, **26**, 65.
36 Olsen, C. E., Borch, N. H. & Ostergaard, E. (1967). Legal induced abortion: an analysis of 21,730 notifications to the Danish Health Department (1961–1965). *Ugeskrift for Laeger*, **129**, 1341.
37 Bluett, D. G. (1973). A review of one thousand uncomplicated vaginal operations for abortion. *Contraception*, **7**, 11.
38 Fang Liu (1966). A comparison of the three methods of artificial abortion: suction with an injection instrument, electrical suction and uterine curettage. *Chinese Journal of Obstetrics and Gynaecology*, **12**, 287.
39 Williford, J. F. & Wheeler, R. G. (1975). Advances in non-electrical vacuum equipment for uterine aspiration. *Advances in Planned Parenthood*, **9**, 3.
40 Lewis, S. C. (1971). Vacuum termination of pregnancy. *British Medical Journal*, **4**, 365.
41 Filshie, G. M., Alhluwalia, J. & Beard, R. W. (1973). Portable Karman curette equipment in management of incomplete abortions. *Lancet*, **ii**, 1114.
42 Wu Pao-chen (1966). The use of vacuum bottle in therapeutic abortion. *Chinese Medical Journal*, **85**, 245.
43 Branch, B. M. & Bridgman, M. (1973). The use of pre-evacuated reservoirs for uterine aspirations. *Lancet*, **i**, 520.

44 Dvořák, Z., Tonka, V. & Vašíček, R. (1967). Termination of pregnancy by vacuum aspiration. *Lancet*, **ii**, 997.

45 Vojta, M. (1967). Therapeutic abortion by vacuum aspiration. *Journal of Obstetrics and Gynaecology of the British Commonwealth*, **74**, 768.

46 Nathanson, B. M. (1971). Suction curettage for early abortion: experience with 645 cases. *Clinical Obstetrics and Gynecology*, **14**, 19.

47 Lewis, S. C. (1972). Some trends in the management of early induced abortion. *Journal of Obstetrics and Gynaecology of India*, **22**, 411.

48 Tietze, C. & Lewit, S. (1972). Joint program for the study of abortion (JPSA); early medical complications of legal abortion. *Studies in Family Planning*, **3**, 97.

49 Novak, F. & Andolšek, L. (ed.) (1974). *Comparison of the Medical Effects of Induced Abortion by Two Methods: Curettage and Vacuum Aspiration. Final Report.* National Institutes of Health, Center for Population Research, Bethesda Maryland.

50 Menget, W. F. & Slate, W. G. (1963). Diagnostic dilatation and curettage as an outpatient procedure. *American Journal of Obstetrics and Gynecology*, **70**, 727.

51 Margolis, A. J. & Overstreet, E. W. (1970). Legal abortion without hospitalization. *Obstetrics and Gynecology*, N.Y., **36**, 479.

52 Margolis, A. J., Stewart, G. K., Easter, M., Lee, G. F., Galen, D. I., Fisk, D. & Ostermann, F. K. (1971). Therapeutic abortion without hospitalization. *Advances in Planned Parenthood*, **6**, 165.

53 Strausz, I. K. & Schulman, H. (1971). 500 outpatient abortions performed under local anesthesia. *Obstetrics and Gynecology*, N.Y., **38**, 199.

54 Fairchild, E. & Penfield, A. J. (1971). Should family planning clinics perform abortions? *Perspectives in Family Planning*, **3**, 15.

55 Nathanson, B. M. (1972). Ambulatory abortion, experience with 26,000 cases. *New England Journal of Medicine*, **286**, 403.

56 Goldsmith, S. (1974). Early abortion in a family planning clinic. *Family Planning Perspectives*, **6**, 119.

57 Nathanson, B. M. (1974). Deeper into abortion. *New England Journal of Medicine*, **291**, 1189.

58 Branch, B. N. (1972). Outpatient termination of pregnancy. In *New Concepts in Contraception*, ed. M. Potts & C. Wood, p. 175. Medical & Technical Press, Lancaster & Oxford.

59 Hull, M. G. R., Gordon, C. & Beard, R. W. (1974). The organisation and results of a pregnancy termination service in a National Health Service hospital. *Journal of Obstetrics and Gynaecology of the British Commonwealth*, **81**, 577.

60 Manabe, Y. (1971). Laminaria tests for gradual and safe cervical dilatation. *American Journal of Obstetrics and Gynecology*, **110**, 743.

61 Newton, B. W. (1972). Laminaria tent: relic of the past or modern medical device? *American Journal of Obstetrics and Gynecology*, **113**, 442.

62 Laufe, L. E. & Kreutner, K. (1971). Vaginal hysterectomy: a

modality for therapeutic abortion and sterilization. *American Journal of Obstetrics and Gynecology*, **3**, 1096.

63 Ward, C., Booth, R. & Pinkerton, J. H. (1962). Induction of labour by intra-amniotic injection of hypertonic glucose solution. *British Medical Journal*, **2**, 706.

64 Wagner, G., Karker, H., Fuchs, F. L. & Bengtsson, L. P. (1962). Induction of abortion by intra-amniotic installation of hypertonic saline. *Danish Medical Bulletin*, **9**, 137.

65 Cameron, J. M. & Dayan, A. D. (1966). Association of brain damage with therapeutic abortion induced by amniotic fluid replacement. *British Medical Journal*, **1**, 1010.

66 Manabe, Y. (1969). Danger of hypertonic saline-induced abortion. *Journal of the Americn Medical Association*, **210**, 22.

67 Kovacs, L., Resh, B., Szöllósi, P. & Herczeg, J. (1970). The role of foetal death in the process of therapeutic abortion induced by intra-amniotic injection of hypertonic saline. *Journal of Obstetrics and Gynaecology of the British Commonwealth*, **77**, 1132.

68 Jakobovits, A., Traub, A., Farkas, M. & Morvay, J. (1970). The effect of intra-amniotic injection of hypertonic saline on the structure and endocrine function of the human placenta. *International Journal of of Obstetrics and Gynaecology*, **8**, 499.

69 Csapo, A. I., Sauvage, J. P. & Wiest, W. G. (1970). The relationship between progesterone, uterine volume, intrauterine pressure and clinical progress in hypertonic saline-induced abortion. *American Journal of Obstetrics and Gynecology*, **108**, 950.

70 Karim, S. M. M. & Sharma, S. D. (1971). Second trimester abortion with sjngle intra-amniotic injection of prostaglandin E_2 or $F_{2\alpha}$. *Lancet*, **ii**, 47.

71 Roberts, G., Gomersall, R., Adams, M. & Turnbull, A. C. (1972). Therapeutic abortion by intra-amniotic injection of prostaglandins. *British Medical Journal*, **4**, 12.

72 Mehta, A., Talati, R., Mirchandani, S. & Katrak, J. (1974). Mid-trimester pregnancy termination.' India Fertility Research Programme Conference. IPPF, London. (Duplicated paper.)

73 Weilerstein, R. W. (1944). Intrauterine pastes. *Journal of the American Medical Association*, **125**, 205.

74 Williams, G. F., Domino, E. A. & Davies, V. J. (1955). Intrauterine pastes for therapeutic abortion. *Journal of Obstetrics and Gynaecology of the British Empire*, **62**, 585.

75 Bach-Nielsen, P., Wilkjehn, A. & Wilhjelm, B. J. (1958). Abortus provocatus. *Ugeskr for Laeger*, **120**, 1009.

76 Sood, S. V. (1971). Termination of pregnancy by the intrauterine insertion of Utus paste. *British Medical Journal*, **ii**, 315.

77 Anonymous (1947). Abortifacient pastes. *British Medical Journal*, **2**, 317.

78 Nabriksi, S. A., Kalmanovitch, K., Lebel, R. & Brodman, V. (1971).

Extraovular transcervical injection of Rivanol for interruption of pregnancy. *American Journal of Obstetrics and Gynecology,* **110**, 54.

79 Manabe, Y. (1969). Abortion in midpregnancy by extraovular installation of Rivanol solution correlated with placental function. *American Journal of Obstetrics and Gynecology,* **103**, 232.

80 Ingermanson, C. A. (1973). Legal abortion by extra-amniotic installation of Rivanol in combination with rubber catheter insertion into the uterus after the twelfth week of pregnancy. *American Journal of Obstetrics and Gynecology,* **115**, 211.

81 Manabe, Y. (1967). Metreurynter-induced abortions at midpregnancy. *American Journal of Obstetrics and Gynecology,* **99**, 557.

82 Ganzoni, M. & Widmer, H. (1930). Uber die therapeutische Schwangerschaftsunterbrechung durch Röntgenstrahlen. *Strahlentherapie,* **38**, 754.

83 Stern, S. (1928). *American Journal of Radiology,* **19**, 133.

84 Thiersch, J. B. (1958). Effect of *N*-desacetyl-thio-colchine (TC) and *N*-desacetyl-methyl-colchine (MC) on the rat fetus and litter *in utero.* *Proceedings of the Society for Experimental Biology and Medicine,* **98**, 479.

85 Emmens, C. W. (1970). Postcoital contraception. *British Medical Bulletin,* **26**, 45.

86 Nathanson, B. M. (1970). Drugs for the production of abortion: a review. *Obstetrical and Gynecological Survey,* **25**, 727.

87 Kar, A. B. (1969). Non-steroidal antifertility agents interfering with different phases of reproduction in the female. *Journal of Scientific and Industrial Research,* **28**, 45.

88 Vojta, M. & Jirasek, J. (1966). 6-Azauridine-induced changes of the trophoblast in early human pregnancy. *Clinical Pharmacology and Therapeutics,* **7**, 162.

89 Morris, J., McLean, C., van Wagenen, G., McCann, T. & Jacob, B. (1967). Compounds interfering with ovum implantation and development. *Fertility and Sterility,* **18**, 7 and 18.

90 Nicholson, J. O. (1968). Cytotoxic drugs in pregnancy. Review of reported cases. *Journal of Obstetrics and Gynaecology of the British Commonwealth,* **75**, 307.

91 Thiersch, J. B. (1952). Therapeutic abortion with a folic acid antagonist 4-aminopteroylglutamic acid (4 amino P.G.A.) administered by the oral route. *American Journal of Obstetrics and Gynecology,* **63**, 1298.

92 Meltzer, H. J. (1956). Congenital anomalies due to attempted abortion with 4-aminopteroylglutamic acid. *Journal of the American Medical Association,* **161**, 1253.

93 Bourne, F. M., Friedman, S. O. & Jordan, G. E. (1957). Intoxication by aminopterin used as an abortifacient. *Canadian Medical Association Journal,* **76**, 473.

94 Goetsch, C. (1962). An evaluation of aminopterin as an abortifacient. *American Journal of Obstetrics and Gynecology,* **83**, 1474.

95 Vengadasalam, D., Lean, T. H., Kessel, E., Berger, G. S. & Miller, E. R. (1975). 'Estrogen-progesterone Withdrawal Bleeding in Diagnosis of Early Pregnancy.' XIX All India Congress in Obstetrics and Gynaecology, Jamshedpur, India. (Duplicated document.)

96 von Euler, U. S. (1935). Uber die spezifische blutdrecksenkende Substanz des menschlichen Prostata und Samenblasensekretes. *Klinische Wochenschrift*, **14**, 1.

97 Karim, S. M. M. (ed.) (1972). *The Prostaglandins*. Medical & Technical Press, Oxford & Lancaster.

98 *Population Reports*. Series G.

99 Beazley, J. M., Dewhurst, C. J. & Gillespie, A. (1970). Induction of labour with prostaglandin E_2. *Journal of Obstetrics and Gynaecology of the British Commonwealth*, **77**, 193.

100 Karim, S. M. M. & Filshie, G. M. (1970). Therapeutic abortion using prostaglandin $F_{2\alpha}$. *Lancet*, **i**, 157.

101 Roth-Brandel, U., Bygdeman, M., Wiqvist, N. & Bergström, S. (1970). Prostaglandins for induction of therapeutic abortion. *Lancet*, **i**, 190.

102 Simms, M. (1973). *Report on Non-Medical Abortion Counselling*. Birth Control Trust, London.

103 UK Statistics are reviewed regularly in *The State of the Public Health: The Annual Report of the Chief Medical Officer of Health; The Registrar General's Statistical Review of England and Wales Supplement(s) on Abortion; Report(s) on Confidential Enquiries into Maternal Deaths in England and Wales*; and *The Registrar General's Statistical Review of England and Wales*, which are all publications of HMSO, London.

104 US abortion statistics are reviewed in a series of publications and articles. (1) United States Center for Disease Control, Atlanta, *Abortion Surveillance*. (2) The National Academy of Sciences (review of extant data up to 1974–75) *Legalized Abortion and the Public Health: Report of a Study by the Committee of the Institute of Medicine* (1975), Washington D.C. (3) 'Legal abortion in the United States: its effect on the health of women' (1976). New Developments in Fertility Regulation, Pathfinder Conference, Airlie House, New York. (Duplicated document.)

105 Buckle, A. E. R., Anderson, M. M. & Loung, K. C. (1970). Vacuum aspiration of the uterus in therapeutic abortion. *British Medical Journal*, **2**, 456.

106 Hodgson, J. E., Major, B., Portmann, K. & Quattlebaum, F. W. (1975). 'The prophylactic use of antibiotic tetracyclines for patients undergoing first trimester abortions.' Meeting of the American Association of Planned Parenthood Physicians, 1975. (Duplicated document.)

107 Wright, C. S. W., Campbell, S. & Beazley, J. (1972). Second trimester abortion after vaginal termination of pregnancy. *Lancet*, **i**, 1278.

108 Central Statistical Office (1972). *Perinatalis Halalozas.* Budapest, Hungary.

109 Kralj, B. & Lavrič, V. (1974). Cervico-isthmic incompetence. In *Comparison of Medical Effects of Induced Abortion by Two Methods, Curettage and Vacuum Aspiration,* ed. F. Novak & L. Andolšek, National Institutes of Health, Bethesda, Maryland.

110 Stefanos, N., Pantelakis, G. C. & Doxiadis, S. A. (1973). Influence of induced and spontaneous abortion on the outcome of subsequent pregnancies, *American Journal of Obstetrics and Gynecology,* **116**, 799.

111 Hogue, C. J. (1977). Low birth weight subsequent to induced abortion: an historical prospective study of 948 women in Skopje, Yugoslavia. (In preparation.)

112 Morrison, J. (1967). The effect of some obstetrical factors on rhesus iso-immunisation. *Journal of Obstetrics and Gynaecology of the British Commonwealth,* **74**, 419.

113 Bergström, H., Nilsson, L. A. & Ryttinger, L. (1967). Demonstration of Rh antigens in a 38 day old fetus. *American Journal of Obstetrics and Gynecology,* **99**, 130.

114 Gelleń, J., Kovács, Z., Szontágh, F. E. & Boda, D. (1965). Surgical termination of pregnancy as a cause of rhesus sensitization. *British Medical Journal,* **2**, 1471.

115 Matthews, C. D. & Matthews, A. E. B. (1969). Transplacental haemorrhage in spontaneous and induced abortion. *Lancet,* **i**, 694.

116 Queenan, J. T., Shah, S., Kubarych, S. F. & Holland, B. (1971). Role of induced abortion in rhesus immunisation. *Lancet,* **i**, 815.

117 Judelsohn, R. G., Townsend, A. M. & Branch, B. M. (1973). Optional utilization of Rh. immunoglobulin in induced abortion. *Obstetrics and Gynecology, NY,* **42**, 827.

118 Gebhard, P. H., Pomeroy, W. B., Martin, C. E. & Christenson, C. V. (1959). *Pregnancy, Birth and Abortion.* Heinemann, London.

119 Lindahl, J. (1959). *Somatic Complications Following Legal Abortion.* Scandinavian University Books. Stockholm.

120 Hayashi, M. & Momose, K. (1966). Statistical observation on artificial abortion and secondary sterility. In *Harmful Effects of Induced Abortion,* ed. Y. Koya, p. 36. Family Planning Federation of Japan, Tokyo.

121 Furusawa, Y. & Koya, T. (1966). The influence of artificial abortion on delivery. In *Harmful Effects of Induced Abortion,* ed. Y. Koya, p. 74. Family Planning Federation of Japan, Tokyo.

122 Sawazaki, C. & Tanaku, S. (1966). The relationship between artificial abortion and extrauterine pregnancy. In *Harmful Effects of Induced Abortion,* ed. Y. Koya, p. 49. Family Planning Federation of Japan, Tokyo.

123 Beric, B. M. (1972). Personal communication.

124 Simon, N. & Senturia, A. (1966). Psychiatric sequelae of abortion. *Archives of General Psychiatry,* **15**, 378.

125 David, H. P. (1972). Psychological studies in abortion. *American Journal of Orthopsychiatry*, **42**, 61. See also, David, H. P. (1974). Abortion is psychosocial perspective. In *Abortion Research: International Experience*, ed. H. David, p. 109. Lexington Books, Lexington, Mass.

126 Calderone, M. S. (1968). *Abortion in the United States*. Harper & Row, New York.

127 Bolter, S. (1962). The psychiatrist's role in therapeutic abortion: the unwitting accomplice. *American Journal of Psychiatry*, **119**, 312.

128 Ford, C. U., Atkinson, R. M. & Bragonier, R. (1971). Therapeutic abortion: who needs a psychiatrist? *Obstetrics and Gynecology, NY*, **38**, 206.

129 McCoy, D. R. (1968). Emotional health after abortion. *Journal of Obstetrics and Gynaecology of the British Commonwealth*, **75**, 1054.

130 Horden, A. (1971). *Legal Abortion: the English Experience*. Pergamon, London.

131 Ekblad, M. (1955). Induced abortion on psychiatric grounds. A follow-up study of 479 women. *Acta Psychiatrica et Neurologica Scandinavica, Suppl.* **99**, 238.

132 Walter, G. S. (1970). Psychologic and emotional consequences of elective abortion. *Obstetrics and Gynecology, NY*, **36**, 483.

133 Pare, C. M. B. & Raven, H. (1970). Follow-up of patients referred for termination of pregnancy. *Lancet*, **i**, 635.

134 Greer, H. S., Lal, S., Lewis, S. C., Belsey, E. M. & Beard, R. W. (1976). Psychosocial consequences of therapeutic abortion. King's termination study III. *British Journal of Psychiatry*, **128**, 74.

135 Karman, H. & Potts, M. (1972). Very early abortion using syringe as vacuum source. *Lancet*, **i**, 1051.

136 Davis, G. & Potts, D. M. (1974). Menstrual regulation: a potential breakthrough in fertility control. *Journal of Reproduction and Fertility*, **37**, 467.

137 Potts, M. (1974). Early ambulatory termination of pregnancy; techniques and results. In *Avortement et Parturition Provoqués*, ed. M. J. Bosc, R. Palmer & C. Sureau, p. 409. Masson et Cie, Paris.

138 Davis, G. (1974). *Interception of Pregnancy*. Angus & Robertson, Sydney.

139 Beric, B. M. & Kupresanin, M. (1975). Regulation des menstruations. *Journal de Gynécologie, Obstétrique et Biologie de la Réproduction*, **4**, 873.

140 Dawn, C. S. (1975). *Menstrual Regulation. A New Procedure for Fertility Control*. Dawn Books, Calcutta.

141 Hodgson, J. E., Smith, R. & Milstein, D. (1974). Menstrual extraction: putting it and its synonyms into proper perspective as pseudonyms. *Journal of the American Medical Association*, **228**, 849.

142 Van der Vlugt, T. H. & Piotrow, P. T. (1973–74). *Population Reports*, Series F: vol. **1**, *Menstrual Regulation – what is it?*; vol. **3**, *Uterine Aspirations Techniques*; vol. **4**, *Menstrual Regulation Update*.

143 Goldsmith, S. & Margolis, A. (1974). Menstrual induction. *Advances in Planned Parenthood*, **9**, 7.

144 Miller, E., Fortney, J. A. & Kessel, E. (1976). Early vacuum aspiration: minimizing procedures to non-pregnant women. *Family Planning Perspectives*, **8**, 33.

145 Kessel, E., Brenner, W. E. & Stathes, G. H. (1973). Menstrual regulation in family planning services. 101st meeting of the American Public Health Association. (Duplicated paper.)

146 Pachauri, S. (1973). 'Menstrual regulation study of the International Fertility Research Program.' Conference on Menstrual Regulaton, University of Hawaii. (Duplicated document.)

147 Khan, A. R., D'Souza, S. M. & Hanum, H. (1975). 'A preliminary experience with menstrual regulation in Bangladesh.' Johns Hopkins Fertility Research Program. (Duplicated document.)

148 Lee, L. T. & Paxman, J. M. (1974). *Legal Aspects of Menstrual Regulation*. Law and Population Monographs Series, no. 19.

149 Dourlen-Rollier, A. M. (1974). Legal problems related to abortion and menstrual regulation. *Symposium on Law and Population, Tunis*, p. 120. United Nations Fund for Population Activities, New York.

150 Editorial (1976). *Lancet*, **i**, 947.

151 Lippes, J., Malik, T. & Tatum, H. J. (1977). The postcoital copper IUD. (In preparation.)

152 Haspels, A. A. (1972). Postcoital oestrogen in large doses. *IPPF Medical Bulletin*, **6**(2), 3.

153 Bačič, M., Wesselius de Casparis, A. & Diczfalusy, E. (1970). Failure of large doses of ethinyl estradiol to interfere with early embryonic development in the human species. *American Journal of Obstetrics and Gynecology*, **107**, 53.

154 Ravenholt, R. T. (1968). In *Abortion in a Changing World*, ed. R. E. Hall, vol. **2**, pp. 49–52. Columbia University Press, New York.

155 Karim, S. M. M. (1971). Once-a-month vaginal administration of prostaglandins E_2 and $F_{2\alpha}$ for fertility control. *Contraception*, **3**, 173.

156 Mitchison, N. A. (1974). Long-term hazards in immunological methods of fertility control. In *Research Methods in Reproductive Endocrinology*, Karolinska Symposium, vol. **7**, ed. E. Diczfalusy, p. 405. Karolinska Institute, Stockholm.

157 Stevers, V. C. (1974). Fertility control active immunisation using placental proteins. In *Research Methods in Reproductive Endocrinology*, Karolinska Symposium, vol. **7**, ed. E. Diczfalusy, p. 357. Karolinska Institute, Stockholm.

158 Moudgal, N. R., Jagannadha Rao, A. & Prahalada, S. (1974). Can hormone antibodies be used as a tool in fertility control? *Journal of Reproduction and Fertility, Supplement*, **21**, 105.

159 Hearn, J. P., Short, R. V. & Lunn, S. F. (1975). The effects of immunizing marmoset monkeys against the β-subunit of HCG. In *Physiological Effects of Immunity Against Hormones*, ed. R. G. Edwards and M. H. Johnson, p. 229. Cambridge University Press, London.

160 Jeffcoate, T. N. A. & Foot, P. (1970). Abortion. In *Morals and Medicine*, p. 29. BBC, London.

161 World Health Organisation (1970). *Spontaneous and Induced Abortion. Technical Report Series*, **461**, WHO, Geneva.

162 Djerassi, C. (1969). Prognosis for development of new chemical birth control agents. *Science, Washington*, **155**, 468.

163 Moore-Čavar, E. (1974). *International Inventory of Information on Induced Abortion*. International Institute for the Study of Human Reproduction & Columbia University Press, New York.

164 Marik, J. J. & Langlois, P. L. (1968). Clinical and pathological evaluation of uterine vacuum curettage for incomplete abortion. *Journal of Reproductive Medicine*, **1**, 187,

165 Eaton, C. J. & Doil, K. L. (1969). Uterine aspiration in the management of incomplete abortion. *Surgery, Gynecology and Obstetrics*, **129**, 588.

166 Tan, P. M., Ratnam, S. S. & Quek, S. P. (1969). Vacuum aspiration in the treatment of incomplete abortion. *Journal of Obstetrics and Gynaecology of the British Commonwealth*, **76**, 834.

167 Rashid, S. & Smith, P. (1970). Suction evacuation of uterus for incomplete abortion. *Journal of Obstetrics and Gynaecology of the British Commonwealth*, **77**, 1047.

168 Solish, G. I. (1970). Aspiration curettage in the treatment of incomplete abortion. *Advances in Planned Parenthood* **5**, 213.

7

The illegal abortionist

Induced abortion is one of the most common procedures in the spectrum of medical provision yet, until recently, the majority of cases were handled by untrained, unqualified personnel whose activities were explicitly illegal and who were open to criminal charges. In much of the world this situation still obtains. Therefore, in historical and in contemporary geographical terms, the illegal abortionist is one of the most unusual of public servants.

While illegal abortionists are a less homogeneous group than most other medical specialists, certain patterns of recruitment, in the gaining of experience and in the practice, financing and motivation of their activities, can be discerned.

Recruitment

Abortionists are recruited both from those who have had first-hand experience of the need for abortion, and from those who take up the career from choice. Nurses, midwives, medical students, doctors and pharmacists are obvious recruits, because they are already partly trained and likely to be subject to numerous requests for help.

Self-induced abortion is known in nearly all societies. For reasons of fear or shame, some women attempt to induce their own abortion even in a situation where there is a liberal law. In Britain in 1971 among 16000 women coming to the British Pregnancy Advisory Service, 2070 (12 per cent) had themselves attempted to induce an abortion before seeking help from the Service.[1] The great majority (1920) used self-medication, but 106 had used a syringe or some instrument. Twenty-four had sought help from a second person. In

Australia 30 per cent of women coming to the Fertility Control Clinic in Melbourne had attempted to terminate the pregnancy.[2] Women who succeed in aborting themselves may subsequently help others. A woman who has obtained help from another person – a husband, boyfriend, sister, neighbour or a more experienced abortionist – may also learn the technique by observation.

A large number of illegal abortions are probably performed by abortionists who do relatively few procedures, mainly helping their family, friends and local community. Very few people choose to take up criminal abortion as a lifetime career, but this small number do a very large number of operations.

In North America, the medically qualified practitioner probably accounted for the majority of the country's illegal operations prior to the reform and repeal of US abortion laws. Self-induced abortions appear to have been rare in the USA during most of the twentieth century. Six per cent of 686 illegal abortion cases collected by Stix from the poor quarter of New York were of the self-induced type.[3] Whittemore interviewed five abortionists in an American town of less than 300 000 inhabitants. One was a practising doctor, two had had partial training in medical school, one was a black practical midwife and one a garage mechanic. In total, they were performing about 1000 abortions a year, although these were unequally divided between one who was doing approximately one operation a month, one approximately one a week, and one practitioner who was doing two or more a day.[4]

In many parts of Latin America the physician is one of the most important illegal operators. Paradoxically, it is also true to say that Latin American physicians as a group have been even more reluctant than their colleagues in other countries to consider the problem of abortion objectively. One survey in Mexico established that 34 per cent of reported illegal abortions were performed by physicians, 28 per cent by trained or untrained midwives and 19 per cent by the woman herself.[5] In Argentina it is believed that 50 per cent of abortions are performed by medical doctors, 30 per cent by graduate midwives and only 20 per cent by unskilled operators.[6]

In many developing countries, traditional healers take on that role which is undertaken by the qualified doctor in the Western world. For example, in Awan's study in Pakistan, doctors were responsible for four cases of illegal abortion while non-qualified healers and *dais* (traditional midwives) had carried out 18. Six abortions were self-

induced.[7] In another small series of illegal abortions from the
Lebanon, five were self-induced, six were undertaken by a 'madame'
(traditional midwife), two by qualified midwives and one by a
trained doctor.[8] But, in further study, 67 per cent were performed
by doctors and only 1 in 10 by midwives.[9] In this last case, the
social background of the hospital (the American University, Beirut)
from which the survey was conducted was probably the unusual
factor. In Thailand 13 out of 28 serious cases of illegal abortion were
induced by lay people, 13 by qualified or traditional paramedical
personnel, but none was by a doctor.[10]

Italy is an example of a country falling between the USA and
developing countries with respect to the balance between medically
qualified and non-medically qualified operators. Of 61 women with
illegal abortions, studied in great detail by Rene Figa-Talamanca,
36 were performed by doctors and 16 by qualified nurses or
midwives.[11]

In the absence of changes in the law, patterns of illegal abortion
probably only change slowly. For example, in Europe in the nineteenth century, midwives seem to have provided many of the illegal
abortionists. In 1881 Tardieu found midwives to be responsible for
21 out of 32 cases of criminal abortion.[12]

Qualifications and training

The training of the illegal abortionist will vary according to
his or her background and experience. The woman who aborts
herself or is aborted by someone else, and who then later goes on
to abort others, is almost certain to repeat the technique that was
used upon her. The husband or boyfriend, desperately driven to
attempt a novel surgical procedure, often seeks advice from someone
in the medical or nursing professions. The pharmacist, nurse,
medical student and doctor all possess at least some access to
reliable medical information. A recently convicted abortionist in
England, a chiropodist by profession, performed his first abortion
on a girlfriend after telephoned advice from an old friend, then
medically qualified. By the time he was convicted he had virtually
abandoned chiropody for his new profession.

An important feature in the training of the illegal abortionist is
that, because of the need for secrecy, information on techniques and
problems is not discussed between different practitioners. Illegal

abortionists do not have national or international conferences, nor do they publish a journal. They tend to be individualists, convinced of their own high ability. Moreover, illegal abortionists, even if medically qualified, rarely keep records. An exception was one licensed physician in the USA who allowed his records of over 30 000 abortions, personally performed, to be reported anonymously.[13]

While it is not surprising that the totally unqualified illegal abortionist should remain secretive and hidebound to his particular technique, it is noteworthy that, until recently, even in those countries where the laws are such that many doctors were able to perform 'pseudo-legal' abortions, a stigma remained and publication and discussion of clinical results was virtually impossible. Until the late 1960s the medical journals of the Western world gave few references to therapeutic abortion techniques. The situation has changed radically since the laws were liberalised, but much of the world, such as Latin America or southern Europe, remains in the old situation.

The perception of those who seek the help of illegal abortionists is somewhat different from those who review the scene from without. Although illegal abortionists have no systematic training and no recognised qualifications, within the community in which they work they become recognised and their ability and status tend to be artifically inflated by their clients. Figa-Talamanca[11] points out that the majority of women who had abortions were quite convinced about the high qualifications of the 'doctor' who performed the operation. Confidence in the professional qualifications and the ability of the abortionists may be a part of the phenomenon of 'optimism' found in the pre-operative stages among many women. One woman aborted by a midwife is quoted as saying, 'She must have been competent. She had all kinds of diplomas on the wall. There were always many women waiting when I went and I used to wait for many hours.'

Techniques

'Abortifacient' drugs

Often a woman who attempts to abort herself will start by using drugs and medicaments. The efficacy of such self-medication has probably been described to her by some friend or relative who believes herself to have achieved an abortion by its use.

There is a widespread trade in so-called abortifacient drugs throughout the world. In developed countries they are sold by pharmacists and druggists, and in developing countries by herbalists and by traditional medicine men. These suppliers, qualified or unqualified, have a perfect market. If, having taken their medicament, the women menstruates following a delayed period, or aborts spontaneously, the salesman will be given credit. If the medicament fails, the woman is in no position to complain, though she may return to the person who sold the item, who may gain further rewards by acting as a referral point for a surgical abortion.

Epidemics of poisoning have frequently occurred because of the popularity of a particular abortifacient. Sometimes the first realisation of the effectiveness of a compound as an abortifacient appears to have resulted from poorly regulated hazards facing female factory workers early in this century. In 1901 Hedrén wrote a doctoral thesis on criminal abortion in Sweden for the Karolinska Institute.[14, 15] He traced 1553 cases from 1851 onwards and in 1410 cases the women died and a *post mortem* was performed. Only eight cases involved mechanical trauma but a spectacular 1408 involved phosphorus matches. Sweden was the home of this industry until it was banned in 1901. Hedrén commented, 'Other substances, more or less injurious to women's health, will take the place of phosphorus until public opinion has reached the stage, "by enlightenment", where all these unreliable and, for the woman herself, often perilous agents...are replaced by the mechanical agent that will certainly, in all civilized countries, become the fetus-expelling agent of the future.'[14]

In Britain, workers in paint factories were exposed to the risks of lead poisoning and women sometimes aborted. A localised and slowly spreading epidemic of lead poisoning caused by abortifacients occurred in the Midlands, beginning with the first recorded case in Leicester in 1893. Further cases were reported in Birmingham in 1898, Nottingham one year later and in south Yorkshire by the turn of the century. Hall & Ransom polled 200 medical practitioners living within 30 miles of Sheffield in 1906 and 50 replied reporting 100–200 cases of lead poisoning a year among women in that part of the country.[16] Six deaths were recorded. Hall remarked, 'For my part I believe it is *not* any particular pill or medicine, either advertised or not, but rather the secret information...which every woman knows.'

The problem still existed in 1913,[17] and today, in contemporary

Malaysia, pills made from olive oil and lead oxide (diachylon paste) remain in use.[18]

In 1937 the Midwives' Institute collected evidence for presentation to the Birkett Committee (see Chapter 8) which was studying abortion.[19] They received 1200 replies to 7500 questionnaires. The price of abortifacients ranged from a few shillings to many pounds. 'It is a common thing when patients come to book' remarked one midwife, 'for them to say they are booking as they could not get rid of it.' Another midwife thought that the reason women so frequently asked if the baby was 'all right' at birth was because they had so often taken abortifacient drugs. Among the medicines quoted were ergot (12 oz bottles, 12s 6d ($1.25)) 'silver coated quinine pills' (7s 6d (75 cents) for 50) and Dr Reynolds' Lightening pills. Vaginal douches in use in the 1930s included iodine, turpentine and water, carbolic soap and Lysol. Intrauterine foreign bodies included bark, wax tapers, crochet hooks, goose quills, meat skewers and hair pins. In the same decade, Janet Chance, one of the founders of the Abortion Law Reform Association in Britain, surveyed abortion practices amongst women attending a London birth control clinic. Of 21 women who had had at least one pregnancy, 16 had 'taken pills or drugs, or in some way attempted to terminate, without a doctor's advice, an unwanted pregnancy'. Chance also quoted a woman shopkeeper who claimed a lively trade in abortifacients saying, 'It's the only talk among women, they're very loyal together, and what one knows goes all up the street.'

Immediately before the 1967 reform of the British abortion laws, an interesting survey of the sale of abortifacient drugs was carried out in Birmingham. Volunteers visited chemists, herbalists and rubber goods stores carrying concealed taperecorders.[20] The male investigators stated that their girlfriend's period was overdue, the women merely stated that they thought they might be pregnant. Most shops had something to offer (see also Chapter 5).

At the turn of the century the *Lancet* ran a number of articles on the sale of abortifacients. The trade was apparently similar to that found in the Birmingham survey of 1966. The drugs were advertised under 'advice to females' and for women who had suffered 'any unusual delay'. One was labelled 'my remedies are the most powerful and strongest on earth; effectual after all others have failed. May be taken by the most delicate... price 4/6d.' In one case a manufacturer brought an action against a newspaper for refusing an advertisement. The judge asked the jury to decide whether the advertisement was intended to advertise a medicine that would procure an abortion. The advertisement was found to be immoral and judgement given to the defendant. In 1905 the British Medical Association, after consultation with the Pharmaceutical Society and the Council for Public Morality, suggested that parliamentary action should be taken to control the sale of abortifacients. In 1908 a joint committee of both Houses introduced at least two Bills but neither became law.[21] But, in parts of the USA and the state of Queensland, Australia, legislation did progress to the statute book.

The same pattern, though modified to suit the local environment, can be found all over the world; basically it consists of the sale of a large number of harmless but inefficient drugs at grossly inflated prices, mixed with a small number of medicaments that are potentially dangerous to the woman, the fetus, or to both and may cause abortion in extreme cases.

In developing countries, many herbal remedies that supposedly act as abortifacients are available. For example, in the Philippines an infusion of banana and *kalachulchi* leaves is drunk. Aqueous and alcoholic infusions of barks rich in turpinols are also used. One of the most curious sites for the sale of abortifacients is in central Manila, next to the Quiapo. The Quiapo is the busiest and most loved church in Manila. Mass is celebrated in relays from 6.30 a.m. on Sundays and the church is crowded for many hours, with hundreds standing in the aisles. Immediately outside the church – in physical contact with its walls – are rows of booths. They sell three things: religious pictures (of a tinsel, folk art variety), candles (poorly cast in the shape of saints) and herbal remedies (of which those for late periods are the most important). A bottle of abortifacient medicine (always sold in the local San Miguel beer bottle) costs 1.50 pesos (25 cents). An average stall sells about 20 bottles on a Sunday to women going to, or leaving mass. There are 40–50 stalls clinging to the walls of the Quiapo. The whole is a vivid demonstration that neither the congregation nor priests perceive the intent to terminate a very early pregnancy as a sin. Indeed, the Quiapo on Sunday morning may well represent the busiest family planning clinic in the Philippines – it is illegal, may be ineffective and is contrary to the teachings of the formal religion, but culturally it is more acceptable than the programmes for family planning erected on the basis of millions of dollars of foreign aid and national investment.[22] In the Cameroons 13 fatalities occurred among 1165 abortion admissions, and in two cases death was believed to have been associated with the toxic effects of herbal abortifacients.[23]

Self-medication by the medically qualified, or partly qualified, is more than usually likely to involve the use of active, dangerous drugs. At one London teaching hospital, during the mid-1960s, a series of illegal abortions were attempted by medical students using anti-metabolite drugs. In three cases the abortion was successful, though in one case incomplete, and in the fourth case the drug was administered with resultant sickness but without apparently interfering with the pregnancy. At this stage the situation was disclosed, and it was decided that therapeutic abortion was strongly indicated because of the danger of fetal abnormality. Subsequently the regulations covering the ward storage of anti-metabolite drugs were drastically up-graded!

External trauma

Deliberate or accidental violence is a commonly quoted cause of abortion. However, careful study has shown accidental trauma to have no demonstrable effect on the possibility of abortion.[24] The woman who claims she fell down a flight of stairs or from a chair before the vaginal bleeding began is acting out a fictitious role in a well-rehearsed drama and, in reality, is either telling the doctor that she had an induced abortion or she is a statistical oddity.

The only possible exception concerns the practice of 'massage' by traditional midwives in the developing world. Most traditional birth attendants (and the majority of the deliveries taking place each year in the world as a whole are not attended by a trained person) are familiar with requests to terminate unwanted pregnancy. Among the techniques they use is heavy abdominal pressure, exerted with the full weight of the midwife's body and continued, if necessary, for up to an hour and until vaginal bleeding begins. A bimanual technique, with one hand in the vagina, does not seem common. The pregnant woman usually keeps her clothes on. The process is very painful for the woman. Here, then, is an important method of fertility regulation, widely known and accessible to tens of millions of women, yet it has never been studied scientifically and has rarely or never been observed by Western-trained medical practitioners. Our limited insight comes from histories given by women who have suffered the procedure – both successfully and unsuccessfully.

Simple instrumentation

The passage of a foreign body through the cervical canal into the pregnant uterus has been practised as a means of producing abortion throughout recorded time. In Hawaii a special instrument made of wood, over 20 cm long, slightly tapered and the same diameter as the average index finger, has been described. The handle was carved with a grotesque head and the instrument, called a *Kapo*, regarded as an idol.[25] The use of boiled twigs from thorn bushes remains common in India and in much of the developing world. One variant of the method involves the use of a straight twig or stick, usually about 20 cm long. The woman is assisted by two friends and, after placing stones on the ground and the twig upright above them, she is lowered so that the end of the twig enters the vagina when her friends, instead of supporting her, abruptly drop her upon the projecting stick, which with fortune will enter the cervical canal and the uterus. However, needless to say, perforation of the uterus or vaginal vault is common and mortality and morbidity high. In some communities the need to prevent infection is crudely understood and procedures such as boiling or peeling the bark off a twig before use are routinely applied, whereas in other areas no sterile precautions of any kind are attempted. In Victorian England steel instruments were often used – the ubiquitous crochet hook, umbrella ribs, hairpins, bicycle spokes and, of course, knitting needles. Some of these instruments remain in vogue. Feathers are used in the Middle East and parts of Asia. In Western Australia in the years of the Depression, when farmers and their families were said to exist solely on 'wheat and rabbits', many women carried out abortions using fencing wire.[26] The aim of all such instrumental methods is either to rupture the membranes or so disturb the placental attachment that an abortion occurs some time later, being either complete or incomplete.

Cervical dilatation

In China, where necessity has so often been the mother of invention, dried asparagus lucides soaked in alcohol have been used as cervical dilators and this has also been a traditional method in eastern Europe. In Japan, dried seaweed is used. Karman experimented with compressed balsa wood. Slippery elm is another organic cervical dilator. In Parish's study of illegal abortion in Camberwell, London, in 1935, slippery elm accounted for 16 out of

1000 cases of incomplete abortion.[27] Two women entered hospital with 6 in. (15 cm) slivers embedded in the uterus. At one time, dried slippery elm was available at most British chemists and it is difficult to see for what other use it could have been intended. In the 1930s a regulation was made insisting that all slippery elm available for sale by a chemist should be broken into short lengths not exceeding 2 inches (5 cm).

When tightly compressed dried organic material is introduced into the cervical canal and left *in situ* for many hours, it absorbs water from the cervical secretions, swells and dilates the cervix. Abortion usually follows after a day or so. Reference has already been made to the method in Chapter 6, describing the modern use of laminaria tents. Clearly, the danger facing the illegal abortionist is one of infection.

Objects introduced into the uterine cavity

Soft pliable objects that can be pushed through the cervical canal and will then lie within the uterine cavity irritate the uterus and cause abortion. They may also cause placental separation with fetal death prior to the actual onset of abortion. The method is particularly useful in later pregnancies and tends to be the domain of the more experienced illegal abortionist.

Both in the Western world and in the developing countries, the urinary catheter or other suitable small-bore rubber tubing is popular. In general, the abortionist inserts the catheter, leaving a short projecting end at the cervix, sends the woman home with instructions to remove it herself once the pains have become strong and it is usually understood that she may require physical assistance from trained personnel later. In many communities the whole procedure is well understood and the hospital doctors are well aware of what has preceded the admission for abortion, even though the woman will generally deny any criminal interference.

The symbiotic relationship between the illegal abortionist and the hospital doctor can become a parasitic one. In Hong Kong, some doctors draw a sample of intravenous blood from a woman seeking an abortion and then squirt it straight into her vagina. She is told to report to hospital and complain of uterine bleeding, where she is admitted and a *D & C* is performed for threatened abortion. Sometimes they refer to a colleague, sometimes to themselves, travelling from their private rooms to the hospital outpatients to treat the woman for a contrived complaint. Women are charged heavily for their part in the game and fees as high as 1000 Hong Kong dollars (US $250) are demanded.

In Iran the midwife, or lay abortionist, tapes the end of the catheter to the woman's thigh, and tells her to remove it after 24 hours and to go to hospital when bleeding commences. Typically, the hospital is overworked and makes no effort to investigate the woman's history in depth and proceeds to an immediate curettage. In Thailand, among 652 cases of illegal abortion, over 80 per cent involved rubber catheters or the infusion of liquids. In Paraguay, in one closely studied series, 94 out of 249 illegal abortions involved the catheter or *sonda*.[28] The catheter is also familiar outside Latin America. A doctor approached to perform an abortion in the Philippines often says 'See my nurse'. The nurse then inserts a catheter, telling the woman to return next day when the doctor (for a fee) completes what he diagnoses as an 'incomplete' abortion.

One illustrative case from England, prior to abortion reform, provides a scenario that could be replicated in most countries where abortion is illegal. A woman was admitted with uterine bleeding, a high temperature and septicaemia. Her condition became extremely serious and, being a Roman Catholic, she was given the last rites, still denying criminal interference. Shortly after she aborted and her condition improved. The expelled fetus was accompanied by a rubber catheter.

Intrauterine injections and pastes

Intrauterine injections with syringes of various fluids to induce abortion are used worldwide. The method may have been particularly widely used in England. The Higginson syringe, nominally manufactured as an enema, was long marketed through outlets dealing with abortifacients. A wide variety of fluids was used to procure abortions, the commonest types being strong solutions of soapy water or Dettol solutions. In the Caribbean and some other areas, the preferred fluid was Coco-Cola – which in fact has quite good antiseptic properties. In Parish's study of illegal abortion in Camberwell in the 1930s, the syringe was the major method, accounting for 336 out of 1000 hospital admissions. Ten of these 336 women died.[27]

The dangers of intrauterine injections, apart from those of infection, are that the syringe can inject either fluid or air under pressure. Invariably some air is injected with the fluid unless a very careful technique is adopted and this air can enter the placental sinuses and therefore pass on to the maternal circulation causing air emboli and possible death. Additionally, many fluids used, if introduced into the maternal circulation, will cause haemolytic destruction of the red cells. A further danger is that the fluid under pressure can encircle the conceptus, travel along the fallopian tubes and into the peritoneal cavity, causing chemical or bacterial peritonitis.

The use of pastes, legitimate use of which as a medical technique has already been reviewed (see p. 202), started in the illegal sector in Germany. The flow of information from the illegal and extra-legal operator into the acknowledged body of licit medical practice is a unique interaction in the evolution of medical techniques. The German chemist, Heiser, in the 1920s used various oils as vehicles, mixed with codeine as an antiseptic and an irritant. He claimed to have treated 11 000 women. He acted outside the law and his invention eventually gained him a three-year prison sentence. His methods were taken up by a physician, Leunbach, in Denmark – who also spent three years in jail as well as five years' disqualification from medical practice.[29,30]

One of the consequences of illegal invention is that re-invention – sometimes of a less satisfactory method – can take place several times as society can only learn slowly. In the 1950s various tooth-pastes were used in Britain to induce abortion because their consistency, osmolarity and the presence of antiseptics made them particularly suitable. One specific brand was marketed with a cone-shaped nozzle resembling a cake-icing nozzle and its appropriateness for illegal abortion was immediately recognised. Its use for this purpose became so widespread that the manufacturer was induced to change its presentation. The dangers of paste methods have already been mentioned in the previous chapter (p. 202); in the illegal field some highly unsuitable substances have been used. In particular, unsaturated fatty acids may be used and these are rapidly withdrawn from the placental walls through the placental sinuses and not infrequently result in fat emboli.

Corrosive materials

The fact that the medical profession has always been sympathetic and lenient towards the woman admitted with a potentially illegal abortion has been capitalised upon by the consumer to the extent that the induction of a threatened abortion or even of a 'false' abortion often leads, once the woman is admitted to hospital, to the emptying of the uterus. The use of tablets of potassium permanganate inserted into the vagina was particularly common in England at one stage. Their action was to cause vaginal bleeding, which, in early pregnancy, was then accepted as evidence of an abortion by the medical profession who generally acceded to the woman's obvious desire for a termination. The method, in fact, never really damaged the pregnancy, although it could lead to serious local damage and even to bladder or rectal perforation.

Dilatation and curettage

In Britain, this procedure belongs to the realm of the experienced illegal abortionist, such as the disqualified doctor, the one-time nurse or theatre attendant. Before the 1967 Abortion Act it was common for the operation to be performed without anaesthesia, except for alcohol, aspirin or other mild analgesic. In other countries medically qualified practitioners simply work illegally in their own clinics. This is true of much of Latin America. Sometimes the work is performed quite openly. The most extreme example is Korea, where in Hong's study 1390 out of 1484 (94 per cent) of illegal abortions were curettages performed by qualified doctors.[31] In the experience of one of the authors, full aseptic precautions and adequate anaesthesia were used.

The major aim of the illegal operator is to have a conscious patient fit to leave his clinic as rapidly as possible. This pressure can stimulate some aspects of good medical practice. Harvey Karman benefited from observing the techniques of illegal abortionists in California and went on to develop the no-anaesthetic flexible plastic cannula for terminating early pregnancies. Another American physician pioneered some of the most efficient and humane ways of handling large numbers of patients, while working for the Clergy Referral Service in Louisiana prior to major law reform in the USA. After the repeal of the New York State law in July 1970, he was able to build on experience gained outside the law and was soon performing 50–60 legal terminations a day. Several factors contributed to his success: the strict limitation of all but the most exceptional doctors to operating before 12 weeks of gestation; the use of paracervical block and vacuum aspiration; and the assignment of every woman to a counsellor, who stayed with her throughout the procedure. All the counsellors had had abortions themselves. They helped the woman to talk about any possible guilt feeling, advised on future contraceptive practice, detailed the operative procedure to be followed and reassured the woman during the course of the operation. The surgeon was then able to rotate between patients, spending just sufficient time with each to check the details of the medical and social history and perform the operation.

Advertising

Most abortionists, like most doctors, are recommended by grateful patients. Like doctors, they are not allowed to advertise, but often develop effective ways of recruiting new customers. Fee-splitting, which is also a practice in sections of the medical profession, occurs, with some criminal abortionists. Again there is probably a clear division between the small number of people who do a large number of operations and go to considerable lengths to set up a network of referrals and the casual operator who helps friends and neighbours two or three times a year. Unlike doctors, illegal abortionists have to beware of the *agent provocateur*. Where the tradition of the police force is one of healthy benevolence they will often overlook the activities of the criminal abortionist, unless he or she appears to be acting unwisely. However, in other situations the intention of the police may not be so much to stop the abortionists, as to get a slice of the turnover. The illegal abortionist may enter into a corrupt relationship with the police, both groups ultimately taking their strength from unwilling pregnant women. Australia had a long tradition of medically qualified abortionists, often functioning with a fair degree of visibility and performing outpatient abortions with moderate competence. (Unfortunately, as in other countries, a few appear to have passed on their own uncertain position in society to the women they aborted by a punitive omission of local or general anaesthesia during dilatation and curettage.) The police, especially in Melbourne and Sydney, tolerated the situation as long as the market would carry the doctors' fees (US $150–$2400) and pay the police bribes.[32] When oral contraceptives entered Australia they were adopted with unusual rapidity and the number of married women seeking abortions fell, increasing the competition between abortionists. Some doctor/police units then began to engineer the exposure and arrest of others. In Melbourne, Victoria, in the late 1960s this disturbance of the traditional equilibrium was particularly acute. Wainer reports that in 1969 Inspector Ford of Victoria State Homicide Squad was willing to enter into a verbal agreement to protect certain grateful abortionists from arrest for 10 per cent of their fees. Eventually an enquiry into police corruption cited nine members of the force of whom four were convicted and the remainder disciplined under police regulations.[32] These events, like the originally budgeted costs of the Sydney Opera House, reflected only a small portion of the total situation in Australian cities. The illegal unqualified abortionist is usually less able to bribe those who choose to prosecute him. One Turkish abortionist in Melbourne, whose patient died in the 1960s, was convicted of homicide and sentenced to death, although the execution was subsequently commuted to imprisonment.

Elsewhere, a more tolerant attitude towards abortion exists or has existed. Early twentieth-century Britain was such a case. An example of open advertising, that could be multiplied a thousand times, comes from a Hull newspaper at the outbreak of World War I:

> *Mrs Stafford Brookes, the Eminent Lady Specialist*
> *in all Female Complaints, has much pleasure in*
> *announcing that her remedy for restoring regularity*
> *WITHOUT MEDICINE is the only positive, safe,*
> *certain and speedy one known. It acts almost*
> *immediately, and does not interfere with household*
> *duties. I guarantee every case. Send at once*
> *stamped addressed envelope for full particulars*
> *and most convincing testimonials (guaranteed*
> *genuine under penalty of £5,000) to Mrs Brookes*
> *(664 Dept) Ardgowan Road, Catford, London*[33]

It is not clear how much of an element of confidence trickery there was in Mrs Brookes' advertisement. Perhaps copy from Korean newspapers of the 1950s and 60s is even more direct,

> *We offer quick family planning services with*
> *new electronic device.*

Here the implication is that the doctor has a vacuum aspirator. Where advertising is very open, as in Korea, services, are often cheap but good. The charge to the Korean middle classes for a doctor-induced abortion often ran at $7–8, falling to as low as $3 for the very poor woman. In the Philippines abortion is one stage more concealed – and therefore less well done and more expensive. Yet for those who can afford to attend physicians the Filipino newspapers carry moderately direct advertisements,

> *VD check up – rapid XR: Circumcision – painless,*
> *bloodless, German cut: Pregnancy test – 3 mins.*
> *WOMEN'S DISEASES.*

Prior to law reform in the USA, many women travelled to Puerto Rico, where, although abortion was illegal, the laws were applied with a looseness typical of developing countries. Nevertheless, some camouflage was deemed necessary and one abortion mill used a Catholic priest as the point of first contact. The woman was then collected from the church in a taxi and taken for operation at a secret address.[34]

Fees and motivation

Moya Woodside interviewed 44 women serving sentences for criminal abortion in Holloway Prison, London, in the 1960s.[35,36] Most were married and had children of their own. Thirteen were grandmothers and the group as a whole ranged in age from 28 to 80 years, but most were between 50 and 70. They did not regard themselves as criminals and within their own community had usually been hailed as public benefactors. Some had produced testimonials of their respectability at their trials. Most did not deny that they took money or gifts, but financial gain does not appear to have been their main motivation. One woman accepted a bunch of flowers from her client as the only payment. Their aim was to help their fellow women. 'I am not ashamed of what I have done,' said one woman, 'even though it's against the law. It's human nature, and women have to help each other.' A study in Italy in 1970 showed a similar lack of guilt amongst abortionists in a country where the law remains restrictive.

Maurice Hinton was a Birmingham illegal abortionist of the 1950s who died while serving a six-year prison sentence. The judge described him as 'a clever abortionist'; 'You were never slovenly in the attention you bestowed on those who foolishly sought your help,' he declared. Ferris interviewed a woman who knew him well. He had used an intrauterine injection of *Dettol* or *Ibcol* and normally charged a hundred guineas ($210), splitting fees with whoever referred the woman. In 1960 he had seen 135 women. Among his patients were two policemen's wives and a lady doctor.[37]

Obeng[38] in a study of women admitted with the consequences of illegal abortion to a London hospital in 1960 found they had paid £5–£80 ($10–$160), although a minority had the operation for nothing from sympathetic friends. Even allowing for inflation these rates are lower than those found in private practice immediately after the 1967 Abortion Act. Obeng also interviewed three illegal abortionists in active practice; none expressed any guilt and each had drifted into the profession after an initial attempt to help someone in desperate circumstances. Tietze, in the USA in the 1940s, reported on the work of two physicians who performed abortions. They charged $300–$500, which was much higher than charges were to become in legal practice 30 years later.[39]

Abortion prices have always been flexible. The casual operator sometimes charges little and may be content with a small gift, which in many developing countries will come as food or clothes. The more professional operator, with a large turnover, will charge higher fees, although he may adapt them to the demands of the market. In the Philippines the abortion rate for the bar girls in Manila is 10 pesos ($1.50) for each week of pregnancy. In Nigeria a doctor-performed illegal abortion in Lagos costs 50–80 naira ($155–$248) but in Karno only 15 ($46.5), while a lay abortionist charges 'a few naira'.

Undoubtedly some illegal abortionists make a large sum of money, but the image of the criminal abortionist as a money-grasping butcher can be a misleading simplification. Some have been motivated by humanitarian concerns. Some have been men or women of culture. One art gallery in a provincial city in a southern European country was built up by the city's illegal abortionist, who was a man of taste, and when he died he gave his collection to the city. In this way the city acquired a low birth rate and an art collection including a Rembrandt and a Rubens.

Mortality and morbidity

One of the few things that conservatives (in terms of abortion attitudes) and liberals have been able to agree about is that illegal abortion presents serious dangers to life and health. Like many aspects of abortion it is a conclusion based on impressions arising from isolated, often dramatic, experiences.

Mortality due to illegal abortion is perhaps the most difficult of all abortion statistics to review both because the denominator (the number of deaths) is open to falsification and the numerator (the number of abortions) is uncertain. In addition, any answer may be expected to be subject to wide variation depending upon the background of the operator. Current estimates have a wide range, part of which is probably genuine and part of which reflects uncertainty in the measurements themselves. In Chile it is thought that there is a death rate of between 150 and 200 per 100000 illegal operations. About one-third of the illegally induced abortions are believed to be associated with complications that are sufficiently serious to take the woman to hospital. (Approximately 50 per cent of the self-induced abortions end up in hospital but fewer than a quarter of the doctor- or midwife-performed operations do.) Although medical facilities are inadequate for the health needs of the country, an estimated 184000 'bed-days' were taken up with the complications of abortion even as early as 1960, and 42 per cent of all emergency admissions were the consequences of abortion.[40,41] Even here it is difficult to know how much the figures reflect poor surgery and how much a 'symbiosis' in which the illegal operator initiates vaginal bleeding and the hospital doctor, albeit reluctantly, completes the procedure. Certainly the latter relationship is common in many countries, although it does not entirely prevent the inexperienced causing a great deal of suffering, ill health and occasional deaths. A comparison between hospital admissions for septic abortion and hospital-induced abortions in Accra, Ghana, established that the mean hospitalisation time was 2.17 and 1.54 days, respectively.[42]

In general, the risks of abortion are highest where the risks of childbirth are also high. For example, in Jordan over 2000 abortion cases (illegal and spontaneous) were admitted to one hospital over a period of three years and there was one death, but death due to childbirth over the same interval ran at 2.5 per 1000 deliveries. In

Thailand there were nine deaths in 779 hospital admissions for illegal abortion. Even in developing countries antibiotics and the availability of blood transfusion, which is not universal but is increasingly available for really serious cases, allow lives to be saved that would previously have been lost.[43] Taussig,[44] in the inter-war years, estimated death rates from abortion to be at a level slightly above one in 100 (he believed 25–30 per cent of all abortion deaths were registered under a false diagnosis) and Freudenberg made a similar estimate in Germany.[45]

One complication which remains difficult to deal with is that of tetanus. Among 27 cases of tetanus associated with pregnancy admitted to Lagos University Teaching Hospital (1963–67), 22 followed illegal abortions and half of these died. Even this mortality rate is lower than in many other series.[46]

Some countries have remarkably low death rates from illegal abortion. For example, Hong Kong has a population of 4.5 million, medical attitudes are very conservative and only about 100 legal abortions are performed each year. Many thousands of illegal operations occur, and it is believed that many are performed by non-medical personnel. However, only three or four women a year die as a result of illegal abortion. It is thought that some women return to the Chinese mainland for legal operations, but even so the community appears to have established not only an effective, but a relatively safe, illegal network. In Seoul, South Korea, an attempt was made to trace all the deaths attributable to illegal abortion. Hospitals were contacted and about 200 relatives of women who died in their fertile years were questioned. Of the 68 maternal deaths taking place in 1967, 18 were believed to be due to infection following induced abortion and four to haemorrhage.[47] As the number of illegally induced abortions in Seoul is approximately 50 per cent of the number of legal abortions in the UK, it seems reasonable to assume that the death rate in the two situations is of the same order of magnitude. In Korea, as noted elsewhere, most illegal abortions are performed by experienced doctors.

But whether the risks of illegal abortion are high or low, the woman seeking an illegal abortion, like the soldier on the battlefield, makes life and death decisions from a different point of view from that of the academic analyst. Even if she believes the risk of death to be one in a hundred, she still identifies with the ninety and nine who will survive.

Conclusion

The illegal abortionist has played an essential role in the evolution of modern industrial urban living, with its low birth rates, intensive education and nuclear family system. Isolated, working outside the law and in many cases handling a low volume of work, the illegal abortionist nearly always performed at a lower level than the existing technology would have allowed in a more open, systematised situation.

The illegal abortion was, and is, rarely prosecuted, yet the private nature of the work and conventional social attitudes invariably make it easy, for any who wish, to exploit their clients financially and in other ways (when a woman is attractive, intercourse may be demanded).

It is argued elsewhere in this book that the incidence of induced abortion depends more on socio-economic factors and the maturity of contraceptive practice within society than on whether the operation is legal or not. A vast toll of human suffering would have been avoided in nineteenth- and twentieth-century Christendom if abortion laws had been otherwise. But unlike war, the abortion casualties are never concentrated at one point and rarely talked about publicly.

Very occasionally the famous are caught by historical analysis or publicity, exposed to self-induced or second-person illegal abortions in the same way as hundreds of thousands of their contemporaries have been, but whose private tragedies remain unrecorded. Arthur James Balfour had an aristocratic background, was educated at Eton and Cambridge and became Prime Minister of Britain between 1903 and 1905. Later, at the end of World War I he was Foreign Secretary, representing Britain at the Paris Peace Conference and, among other things, committing Britain to a role in finding a home for the Jews in Palestine. He had a number of love affairs including a long liaison with Lady Mary Elcho, and his biographer,[48] recounts how she wrote to him of a self-induced abortion which took place in 1898. Turning from Queen Victoria's Britain to twentieth-century Hollywood, the private wounds which Marilyn Monroe sustained in her personal war against unwanted fertility became public knowledge under the journalistic scrutiny that characterised the years of her later marriages and death: '. . . she had many abortions, perhaps as many as twelve! And in cheap places – for a number of these abortions were in the years [*1950s*] when she was modelling or a bit player on seven year contracts – thus her gynaecological insides were unspeakably scarred.'[49]

But for the bulk of women having abortions, the event was likely to have been the most private and secret thing that ever happened to them.

Some image of the scale of human experience involved in the illegal abortion practices of developed countries during the first half of the twentieth century can be formed by comparing it with a well-described male endeavour of similar proportions. Within one month of the invasion of Normandy in World War II, a million Allied troops had been landed; 60000 were casualties and 9000 dead – a death rate of approximately one in 100. If we bring together the epidemiological evidence concerning illegal abortion in Europe, reviewed earlier, and the insights into illegal abortion practices covered in this chapter, we can see that for every year, decade in and decade out, in Europe alone well over a million women must have had illegal abortions and they often faced an ordeal as frightening and sometimes as potentially dangerous as one of the epic battles of World War II. Their motives, in risking so much in the battle against excess fertility, were identical to those found in most wars – they wanted to give their children a better world. Women seek abortion because they feel unable to fulfil their own ideals for the welfare of their offspring. The graves of women who died from illegal abortions are not concentrated in cemetries where flags fly and inscriptions are carved in granite, but the demographic, economic and social changes which have occurred in Western civilisation as the result of the prevalence of illegal abortion are as great as those resulting from any battle fought by men.

In the war against fertility, the developing world is recapitulating the evolution of the developed countries, but on a more massive scale and within a different time frame: legal and medical attitudes are changing relatively earlier in the demographic transition. The optimum role that abortion could play in global fertility regulation is discussed in Chapter 13. The way in which attitudes towards abortion have changed and are changing in the developed and developing worlds are discussed in the intervening chapters.

References

1 British Pregnancy Advisory Service (1972). *Client Statistics for 1971 with Commentary*. British Pregnancy Advisory Service, Birmingham.
2 Wainer, B. (1974). Personal communication.
3 Stix, R. K. (1935). Effectiveness of birth control. *Milbank Memorial Fund Quarterly*, **13**, 347.
4 Whittemore, K. R. (1970). The availability of nonhospital abortions. In *Abortions in a Changing World*, ed. R. E. Hall, vol. **1**, p. 212. Columbia University Press, New York.
5 Aldama, A. (1963). 'El aborto provocado problem de salud pública, Mexico 1963.' Population Council, New York. (Duplicated document.)
6 Viel, B. (1974). Personal communication.
7 Awan, A. K. (1967). *Provoked Abortion amongst 1,447 Married Women*. Maternal and Child Health Association of Pakistan, Lahore.
8 Ghosn, G. (1972). Report on abortion from the French University Hospital, Beirut. In *Induced Abortion: A Hazard to Public Health?* ed. I. R. Nazer, p. 233. IPPF, Beirut.
9 Harfouche, J. K. (1972). Abortion in Lebanon. In *Induced Abortion: A Hazard to Public Health?* ed. I. R. Nazer, p. 239. IPPF, Beirut.
10 Suporn Koetsawang (1973). Investigation of illegal abortion cases admitted to Siriraj Hospital (Bangkok). In *Sterilization and Abortion Procedures*, Proceedings of the first meeting of the IGCC Expert Group Working Committee on Sterilization and Abortion, ed. R. A. Esmundo & K. C. Arun, p. 45. Penang, Malaysia.
11 Figa-Talamanca, R. (1971). Social and psychological factors in the practice of induced abortion as a means of fertility control in an Italian population. *Genus*, **27**, 99.
12 Tardieu, A. (1868). *Etude médico-légale sur l'infanticide*. Baillière & Son, Paris.
13 Spencer, R. D. (1970). The performance of nonhospital abortions. In *Abortion in a Changing World*, ed. R. E. Hall, vol. **1**, p. 218. Columbia University Press, New York.
14 Hedrén, G. (1901). Om fosterfördrivning från rattsmedicinsk synpunkt. Doctoral thesis, Karolinska Institute, Stockholm.
15 Sjövall, H. (1972). Abortion and contraception. *Zeitschrift für Rechtsmedizin*, **70**, 197.
16 Hall, A. & Ransom, W. B. (1906). Plumbism from the ingestion of diachylon as an abortifacient. *British Medical Journal*, **1**, 428.
17 Oliver, S. T. (1913). Diachylon or duty: a call to action. *British Medical Journal*, **1**, 1199.
18 Thambu, J. A. M. & Marzuki, A. (1974). Personal communication.
19 Simms, M. (1974). Midwives and abortion in the 1930s. *Midwife and Health Visitor*, **10**, 114.
20 Cole, M. (1966). 'Abortifacients' for sale. In *Abortion in Britain*, Proceedings of a conference held by the Family Planning Association,

p. 43. Pitman Medical, London. Also distributed as a duplicated paper in a more detailed presentation.

21 Parry, L. A. (1932). *Criminal Abortion.* John Bale, Sons & Dannielsson Ltd, London.

22 Potts, M. (1976). Abortion: 1871–1975. (In preparation.)

23 Lantum, D. M. (1973). 'Some characteristics of women dying from Abortion in Cameroon'. IPPF Conference on the Medical and Social Aspects of Abortion, Accra. (Duplicated paper.)

24 Fort, A. T. & Marlin, R. S. (1970). Pregnancy outcome after noncatastrophic maternal trauma during pregnancy. *Obstetrics and Gynecology, NY,* **35**, 912.

25 Devereux, G. (1960). *A Study of Abortion in Primitive Societies.* Thomas Yoseloff, London.

26 Greenwood, I. Personal communication.

27 Parish, T. M. (1935). A thousand cases of abortion. *Journal of Obstetrics and Gynaecology of the British Empire,* **42**, 1107.

28 Castagnino, D. (1968). *Aborto Provocado.* Centro Paraguaya de Estudios de población. Asunción, Paraguay.

29 Levy-Lenz, L. (1931). A non-operative method for the interruption of pregnancy. In *The Practice of Contraception,* ed. M. Sanger & H. H. Stone, p. 180. Baillière, Tindall & Co., London.

30 Leunbach, J. H. (1931). A new abortus provacatus method. In *The Practice of Contraception,* ed. M. Sanger & H. H. Stone, p. 92. Baillière, Tindall & Co., London.

31 Hong, S. B. (1966). *Induced Abortion in Seoul, Korea.* Dong-A Publishing Co., Seoul.

32 Wainer, B. (1972). *It Isn't Nice.* Alpha Books, Sydney.

33 *Hull Times,* 27 June 1914.

34 Interview with former client (New York, March 1975).

35 Woodside, M. (1963). Attitudes of women abortionists. *Howard Journal,* **2**, 93.

36 Woodside, M. (1966). The woman abortionist. In *Abortion in Britain,* Proceedings of a conference held by the Family Planning Association, p. 35. Pitman Medical, London.

37 Ferris, P. (1967). *The Nameless.* Pelican Books, London.

38 Obeng, B. (1967). 500 Consecutive cases of abortion. Ph.D. thesis, University of London.

39 Tietze, C. (1949). Report on a series of abortions induced by physicians. *Human Biology,* **21**, 60.

40 Armijo, R. & Monreal, T. (1963). Factores asociados a los complicaciones del aborto provocado. *Revista Chilena de Obstetricia y Ginecología,* **91**, 4.

41 Plaza, S. & Briones, H. (1962). 'Demanda de recursos de Atención médica del aborto complicado.' Congreso Medico Social Panamericano, Santiago, Chile. (Duplicated paper.)

42 Chi, I-cheng, Bernard, R. P., Ampofo, D. A. & Suporn Koetsawang (1973). 'Incomplete abortions in Accra and *Bangkok University*

Hospitals, 1972–73. IFRP, Chapel Hill, North Carolina. (Duplicated document.)

43 Ampofo, D. A. (1970). 330 cases of abortion treated at Korle Bu Hospital: the epidemiological and medical characteristics. *Ghana Medical Journal,* **9,** 166.

44 Taussig, F. J. (1936). *Abortion, Spontaneous and Induced: Medical and Social Aspects.* Kimpton, London.

45 Freudenberg, K. (1932). Frequency of abortion deaths. *Münchener Medizinische Wochenschrift,* **79,** 758.

46 Adadevoh, B. K. & Akinla, O. (1970). Postabortal and postpartum tetanus. *Journal of Obstetrics and Gynaecology of the British Commonwealth,* **77,** 1019.

47 Hong, S. B. (1972). Personal communication.

48 Young, K. (1963). *Arthur James Balfour* Bell, London.

49 Mailer, N. (1973). *Marilyn.* Grosset, New York.

8
Abortion and the law in Britain

British legal practice has influenced not only the Commonwealth but the USA. British legal tradition itself is an amalgam of the tradition of the Roman legal system and the influence of Christianity. The Romans, like the ancient Greeks, tolerated abortion and in the later Empire it was an *extraordinarium crimen*, not classified as homicide but as a crime against the husband. (Plato wrote in the *Republic*, 'When both sexes have passed the age assigned to procreating children to the state, no child is brought to light.') Canon law followed the same pattern and St Augustine drew a distinction between the *embryo informatus* and *formatus*, abortion of the former only meriting a fine.[1] English Common Law, likewise, made a distinction between early and late abortion, drawing the dividing line at quickening. Bracton, in the thirteenth century, only considered abortion to be homicide after animation, or entry of the soul. Prior to 1803, abortion before quickening was not regarded as a crime and even abortion later in pregnancy was not severely punished. The great Elizabethan lawyer Coke believed abortion after quickening was a 'great misprision' or misdemeanour, not a murder.[2]

However, in other places and at other times a stricter interpretation of abortion was to be found. 'It is believed beyond doubt' wrote St Fulgentius in the sixth century, 'that not only men who come to the use of reason, but infants, whether they die in their mother's womb, or after they are born, without baptism...are punished with everlasting punishment in eternal fire, because though they have no actual sin of their own, yet they carry along with them the condemnation of original sin from their first conception and birth.'[3]

It was in the spirit of this type of theology that in sixteenth-century Germany a man attempting to induce an abortion after quickening was put to death by the sword, while the woman was drowned. In France, those who 'get rid of the fruit of their womb in a hidden manner' were 'punished by death and the last penalty with such rigour as the particular nature of the case deems and as to be an example to all'.[4,5] Up until the Socialist Revolution, Tsarist Russia made abortion punishable by solitary confinement. In medieval England abortion was regarded as an ecclesiastical crime and ecclesiastical courts may have followed the continental trend, treating the denial of eternal life to an unbaptised soul with increasing severity. However, first with the Reformation and even more so after the Civil War, the power of Ecclesiastical Courts was greatly diminished and England trod a more moderate path, with regard to abortion, than many other nations.

Early nineteenth-century legislation

The modern history of abortion legislation in Britain begins in 1803. But the statute that was passed in that year does not appear to have been motivated by any strict theology or new puritanism, but rather to have been a piece of legal tidying up. Lord Ellenborough's Act[6] included, as set out in the title, clauses related to 'attempting to discharge loaded fire arms, stabbing, cutting, wounding, poisoning and the malicious using of Means to procure Miscarriage of Women and also the malicious setting Fire to Buildings'. This unlikely juxtaposition reappears in the text where abortion is one of many in a long list of felonies that qualify for the death penalty. '. . . or thereby to cause and procure the miscarriage of any woman then being quick with child: or shall wilfully, maliciously, and unlawfully set fire to any house, barn, granary, hop oast, malthouse, stable, coach house, outhouse, mill. . .'

The attempt to procure an abortion where the woman may not be 'quick with Child at the Time' was not classified as a capital offence but warranted the pillory or transportation. The Act repealed several earlier statutes including one of 1623[7] that had sought to convict those mothers of illegitimate children who waited until birth, killed the baby and then declared that a still-birth had occurred. (The Scots law was also rewritten in 1803, but there the 1623 Act was amended to become a capital offence.) There appears to have been no debate or contemporary comment concerning the 1803 legislation and it is uncertain whether, as Noonan claims, the law was continuing the ecclesiastical tradition of distinguishing between the *embryo informatus* and *formatus*, or merely following a pragmatic and common sense approach to a difficult topic. The fact that the law does not refer to the woman who attempts to procure her own miscarriage suggests the possibility of the latter explanation.

The 1803 Act did not signify any legal or social revolution towards abortion and it was fully eight years before the first indictment under the Act was made and when this did happen the drafting of the Bill was torn to shreds by an alert defence. Hannah Mary Goldsmith was unmarried and four months pregnant when one Mr Phillips gave her 'divers large quantities, that is to say six ounces, of the decoction of a certain shrub called savin' (*Rex* v. *Phillips* (1811)). The defence argued that the medicine was an infusion not a decoction, then they claimed the accused did not know the woman was pregnant but the judge ruled that 'if the prisoner believed at the time it [*the decoction*] would procure abortion and administered it with intent, the case is within the Stature'. Finally Miss Goldsmith swore she had never felt the fetus move and the Judge directed an acquittal. In a later case (*Rex* v. *Soudder*), mere proof that the woman was not pregnant at the time of the attempted abortion was held as a valid defence.

Unlike France, where the *Code Napoléon* replaced Roman law and attempted to be an all-embracing legal system, in Britain only modest efforts at codifying and reorganising laws were made in the nineteenth century. Much of the material covered in the 1803 Act was redrafted by Lord Lansdowne in 1828.[8] The wording is more careful, and the oasthouses and stables have disappeared, while murder manslaughter and maim are listed in a rational order. In the case of abortion, not only the abortionist but 'every Person counselling, aiding or abetting such Offender' was included, although the status of the woman herself remained ambiguous. The division between before and after quickening, made in 1803, continued.

Further recodification took place in 1837 with An Act to Amend the Laws relating to Offences against the Person.[9] In the context of early nineteenth-century law-making, the 1803 and 1828 Acts made the penalties for abortion relatively mild, equating abortion after quickening with the arson of farm buildings and before quickening as a lesser offence than the 'abominable crime of buggery' – which in the 1838 Act met with 'the Death of a Felon'. The 1837 Act saw some moderation in the use of the death penalty under the humane influence of Lord John Russell and abortion was one of the several crimes that ceased to be a capital offence. However, the distinction between abortion before and after quickening was lost. The reason is uncertain. Perhaps it was little more than a simplification of drafting. Certainly it was not viewed as of any great significance because early abortion was not yet a real technical possibility. The Act read,

> And be it enacted That whosoever, with Intent to procure the Miscarriage of any woman, shall unlawfully administer to her or cause to be taken by her any Poison or other Noxious thing, or shall unlawfully use any Instrument or other means whatsoever with the like Intent, shall be guilty of Felony, and being convicted thereof shall be liable at the Discretion of the Court, to be transported beyond the Seas for the Term of his or her natural life, or for any Term not less than Fifteen Years, or be imprisoned for any Term not exceeding Three Years.

Again prosecutions were relatively few and acquittals on flimsy grounds occurred. In 1853 a young woman was aborted by a quack doctor using a syringe. The defence claimed the treatment was an attempt to cure gonorrhoea and the abortionist was acquitted. In the case of *Rex* v. *Dale*, it was claimed that a feather quill could be inserted into the uterus for an 'innocent purpose' and again an acquittal resulted.

In 1846 the Criminal Law Commissioners[10] commented on the 1837 Act and suggested, 'Provided that no act specified in the last proceeding Article shall be punished when such act is done in good faith with the intention of saving the life of the mother where miscarriage is intended to be procured.' The suggestion was not put into practice but foreshadowed a theme that has recurred over the succeeding one and a quarter centuries.

The law of 1861

The 1861 Offences against the Person Act covered a wide range of legal problems. Section 58 deals with abortion, in the following terms:

> Every Woman, being with Child, who, with Intent to procure her own Miscarriage, shall unlawfully administer to herself any Poison or other noxious Thing, or shall unlawfully use any Instrument or Other Means whatsoever with like Intent, and whosoever, with Intent to procure the Miscarriage and any Woman whether she be or not be with Child shall unlawfully administer to her or cause to be taken by her any Poison or other noxious Thing, or shall unlawfully use any Instrument or other Means whatsoever with Intent, shall be. . .liable at the Discretion of the Court to be kept in Penal Servitude for Life or any Term not less than Three years. . .with or without Hard Labour, and with or without Solitary Confinement.[11]

Section 59 deals with the supply of 'noxious Things' and 'Instruments' to second parties.

The Act was one 'to consolidate and amend the Statute Law of England and Ireland'. A draft Bill was published on 14 February 1861 and then passed to a Select Committee of 16 members, under the Lord Advocate. The records of the Committee are unenlightening: on 7 May 1861 'clauses 54, 55, 56, 57, 58, 59 and 60 severally read, and agreed to'. (At this stage clauses 59 and 60 corresponded to 58 and 59 mentioned above.) The Bill became law on 6 August 1861. Inspection of *Hansard* shows that the Act, which was to determine English abortion practice for over a century, which is still in force (although amended) in England and Wales, which remains unamended in Eire and Ulster, and which has been the basis of legislation for much of the British Commonwealth, passed without debate in the chamber of the Mother of Parliaments. Inspection of *The Times* shows that no mid-Victorian clergymen wrote letters about the moral aspects of the problems and the correspondence and editorial columns of the *Lancet* and *British Medical Journal* are equally silent. In short, the Act only contained minor modifications of that drafted in the first year of Victoria's reign, and it appears to have engendered no public or professional comment. The only legal change was to include the woman herself as a possible felon.

Society in 1861 had not developed the machinery to discuss any aspect of sex openly or objectively. *The Times* was able to publish one exceptional letter from a prostitute and to pass editorial comment on that topic, but abortion never even penetrated as far as the underground literature of Victorian England.[12] Menstruation and masturbation were also topics where ability to intellectualise about the problem had not yet evolved. Prior to the sort of vocabulary and insight which Darwin and Freud gave to the world, some problems were just not open to analysis – and abortion was one of them.

It is also important to remember that the problem of abortion did not present itself in the terms in which we see it today. Medically, the procedure was sufficiently dangerous, in the years before antiseptics and anaesthesia, to be limited to only the most pressing of cases. The biology of human reproduction was very imperfectly understood. Conception was thought to occur at the time of menstruation, the human embryo (and even the embryo of other mammals) had not been studied in any detail and the techniques of preserving and sectioning material for microscopic study had not been invented. In both the Anglican and Catholic Churches some of the most restrictive of theological attitudes were still to develop.[13]

The last reason for the lack of public interest was that abortion was of little significance as a problem. The Act was passed before the late-Victorian upsurge in absolute abortion numbers, which accompanied the changing fertility practices of the 1870s. A great many other more immediate and more demanding problems were available to prick the middle-class conscience – child and female labour in factories, chimney boys, flogging in the armed services, and all the degrading cruelty that goes with poverty and the exploitation that arises when there is a great gulf between rich and poor.

The only groups who could not totally escape the reality of abortion were the medical and legal professions. Although they had provided no immediate exegesis on the passing of the 1861 Act, the possibility of therapeutic abortion sometimes arose. The word 'unlawful' was coupled with the adjective 'malicious' in the early nineteenth-century legislation, but in 1837 it stood by itself. What nuances of meaning was it meant to convey?

Twenty years after the 1861 Act, William Priestly, consulting physician at King's College Hospital, discussed induced abortion as a therapeutic measure.[14] He gave an assessment of the dangers of abortion and compared them with the dangers of allowing pregnancies complicated by disease to continue to term. The dangers of Caesarean section in the 1880s hardly need emphasis. 'It is true', writes Priestly, 'that the law makes no exception in favour of medical men who adopt this practice [*abortion*], nor does it in the statute of wounding make any exception in favour of surgical operations, but what is performed without evil intention would not be held unlawful.' He concludes that 'Members of the medical profession are so far trusted by Members of the public and even by those of Authority, that upon them devolves a special responsibility of resisting any attempts to destroy immature foetal life which are *not* absolutely necessary, but to be able to speak confidently as to when such an operation is necessary.' He proposes as a general rule that 'the induction of abortion is only a legitimate operation *when the life of the mother is so imperiled by the continuance of pregnancy that emptying the uterus presents itself as the only alternative to save the patient*' (his italics). In the 'animated' debate which followed the presentation, his lines of reasoning appear to have been well accepted. If Priestly's paper and ensuing discussion are representative of medical thinking of the second half of the nineteenth century, then it would appear that the 1861 Act was liberally interpreted. The need for strong indications to perform abortion, and the suggestion that it should only be considered when the woman's life was at stake, seem to have been as much the result of the dangers of surgical procedures as of any moral concern.

In 1896 the Royal College of Physicians sought Counsel's opinion on the legality of abortion performed by a doctor to save the life of the mother. The opinion was given that *bona fide* efforts to save the life of the mother provided a reasonable defence. Edgar's *The Practice of Obstetrics* (1911) confirms this attitude: 'For the conscientious physicians the interruption of pregnancy naturally involves great responsibility, but when it is the only method of saving the life of the mother, or when without it her life is placed in imminent danger, it is usually regarded as not only justifiable but imperative.'[15]

Health and rights (1929–39)

Although a trend towards pragmatism is apparent in nineteenth-century legislation and thought, induced abortion entered the twentieth century as a medical enigma wrapped in legal antiquities. In 1929 parliament passed the Infant Life (Preservation) Act.[16] This piece of legislation specified that 'the destruction of children at or before birth' would not be regarded as a felony, when it was carried out in good faith in order to preserve the life of the mother. The medical profession now found itself in an illogical position. It had clear guidance on the rare and dramatic cases when a mother's life was endangered during delivery of a full-term fetus, but remained in a no-man's land concerning the possibility of destroying a fetus early in pregnancy.

Therapeutic abortions were performed in moderate numbers in the 1920s and 30s, particularly in the case of women with tuberculosis, where it was considered dangerous to allow the pregnancy to continue. (Prior to World War II, tuberculosis was still a very common disease.)

The pragmatism of British medical practice may have been slightly more liberal than that in some other countries, but it was of the same quality. Almost all medical communities will perform therapeutic abortion when the woman's life is demonstrably at risk, whatever the letter of the law. This would be the practice in contemporary France or Italy, and in Latin America. The sticking point for the medical profession has been, and in many places remains, the problem of dealing with cases of abortion performed for social reasons.

The prevalence of illegal abortion in the 1930s (see Chapter 3) must have continually brought the problem before doctors (Fig. 37). Efforts were made to involve the British Medical Association (BMA) and somewhat reluctantly a Committee on Abortion was set up in 1935 under Professor James Young of Edinburgh. It reported in 1936 and stated, 'while the Committee has no doubt that the legalisation of abortion for social and economic reasons would go far to solve the problem of the secret operation it realises that this is a matter for consideration by the community as a whole and not by the medical profession alone'.[17] This comment was a good deal more liberal than many of the things which the BMA was to say in the succeeding generation. The Committee was in no doubt that the existing law was undesirably vague and it was clear that abortion should be legalised on the grounds of physical and mental health. They also felt that abortion should be legal in cases of rape and where there was 'reasonable certainty that serious disease would be transmitted to the child'. The report was not kindly received by the BMA Conference, but at least it got as far as publication.

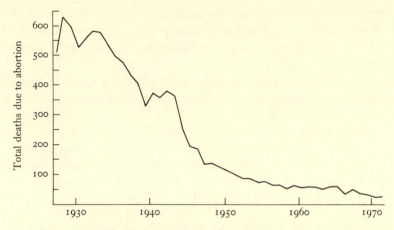

Fig. 37. Total deaths due to abortion (all causes). England and Wales, 1928–1970.

ALRA

The judiciary and a minority of far-sighted lay people were ahead of the medical profession. In 1936 the Abortion Law Reform Association (ALRA) was founded.[18] Janet Chance, a wealthy woman with influential friends, was its first chairman. The Association was feminist and no men and no doctors were involved at its foundation, but it received support from the whole political spectrum, although heavily weighted towards the left. A few courageous doctors, including Joan Malleson and Aleck Bourne later became involved in activities of the organisation. The subscription was 2s 6d (25 cents) per year. The philosophy of the founders was radical, even by the standards of the 1970s, hoping to remove all restrictions on abortion other than that limiting the procedure to doctors. Stella Browne, the vice-chairman, considered illegal abortion a relic of the middle ages like 'burning, branding, mutilation and stoning'. She proclaimed:

> The woman's right to abortion is an absolute right, up to the viability of her child, in other words until the time when the child could survive if born. Abortion must be the key to a new world for women. It should be available for any woman, without insolent inquisitions or numerous financial charges, or tangles of red tape. For our bodies are our own.[19]

Stella Browne often embarrassed her own supporters. She was a Communist, she quoted the experience of the USSR, although her own belief in repealing the law against abortion pre-dated the Russian experiment, being first made public in 1915. She asked scientists to invent a 'perfectly reliable and otherwise tolerable abortifacient'.

But even before the founding of ALRA, back in 1931 Mr Justice McCardie, when trying a series of criminal abortionists in Leeds, said,

> This accused was only trying to help. The last thing she
> wanted to do was cause the death of the mother, and so I can
> only describe the charge against her as brutal. I express the
> view clearly that in my opinion the law of abortion as it exists
> ought to be substantially modified. It is out of keeping with the
> conditions that prevail in the world around us. The law as it
> stands does more harm than good...In my view the time has
> come when the nation should be warned. I warn it today. I
> cannot think it right that a woman should be forced to bear a
> child against her will.[18]

McCardie's philosophy was strikingly different from that of the medical profession, when he said, 'I cannot think it right that a woman should be forced to bear a child against her will'. Indeed it was McCardie who influenced Alice Jenkins to take up the abortion cause. He appears to have been motivated partly by humanitarian concern and partly by a fashionable belief in eugenics. He was ostracised by his colleagues and committed suicide within two years. Nevertheless, whatever the reasons, the leadership of the legal profession, traditionally conservative and chauvinistic, was not just a flash in the pan – within a lifetime the American Supreme Court was to fire the greatest broadside in abortion repeal the world has ever seen.

The Birkett Committee and the Bourne Case

McCardie, ALRA, the BMA and growing public concern eventually brought Stanley Baldwin's government to adopt the traditional temporising measure of appointing a Government Interdepartmental Committee (Health and Home Office) on Abortion. It was chaired by Sir Norman, later Lord, Birkett. The main body of the evidence presented to the Committee, and the discussions that took place, were identical to the debate that was to occur in the 1960s in the press and parliament. The ALRA evidence had acid moments,[19]

Birkett [Chairman]: Have you considered how frequently a 14th or 15th child in a family has become a very great man?

Chance [ALRA]: Have you considered how rapidly maternal death rises after the fifth child?

Birkett: If a distinguished gynaecologist were to assert that from his knowledge and experience any form of abortion may be injurious to the human system, you would have no medical knowledge to put against that?

Browne [ALRA]: No trained medical knowledge...but other gynaecologists of equal experience I know take another view. I have also – and I say this as a matter of public duty – the knowledge in my own person that if abortion were necessarily fatal or injurious I should not now be before you.

The evidence of the British (later to become Royal) College of Obstetricians and Gynaecologists mingled morality and epidemiology, a tradition which persists in some quarters.

Thurtle [Member of the Committee]: Your memorandum, Sir Beckwith, stresses your view that abortions are medically very risky.

Whitehouse [British College of Obstetricians]: Do you mean that to have an abortion is not any detriment to a woman? Haven't we made that point clear?

Thurtle: I'm not really satisfied on this point. I know it's almost *lèse-majesté* to say so, but I'm still not too happy about the alleged ill effects on women of an abortion carried out under proper conditions. We don't seem to have much information or statistics. Can I ask directly...do you want to stop abortions being carried out because you are satisfied they have a bad effect on maternal mortality and maternal health?

Whitehouse: Yes, yes, but you'll remember that there's a fundamental oath on our part not to perform these operations. We've taken an oath when qualifying against the induction of these illegal operations.

The College of Obstetricians and Gynaecologists did get as far as supporting a law that would permit abortion in cases where a girl had been raped *and* was under the age of consent.[20] This went beyond the recommendations of the League of National Life, which stated, 'Where the shock of rape has already been experienced it is highly undesirable and inexpedient to add the further shock of abortion'.

This was indeed an era when strong Fascist opinions had a public following. Dr Halliday Sutherland, a Roman Catholic, who had been involved in a libel action over birth control with Marie Stopes and was an active member of the League of National Life (a between-the-wars right-to-life organisation), praised the Nazi Penal code of 1936 (see also p. 381) which made the 'public ridicule of marriage and maternity, and all propaganda in favour of birth control' into criminal offences. Even as late as 1947, Sutherland classified contraceptive manufacturers with traitors – 'if saboteurs deserve to hang so do they'.[21] Measured against opinions of this type, the Birkett Committee made considerable strides.

The Committee finally reported in 1938, recommending a change in the statute law to allow abortion in cases where the mother's life was imperilled. Dorothy Thurtle pleaded for much wider grounds for legalised abortion. It is interesting that a similar report, at a similar time, to the Swedish government led to the first change in the Swedish law and to that country's tradition of liberal abortion. England, meanwhile was on the brink of war, and attempts at abortion law reform were set aside for well over a decade.

While the Birkett Committee was sitting, the 1861 law was tested in the courts by the actions of Mr Aleck Bourne. Bourne was a gynaecologist of great integrity, a brilliant teacher, much loved by his students, but in no way a radical reformer. He was a man of compassion acting in a strictly traditional medical framework. In 1938 he was asked to see a girl of 14, pregnant after rape by two guardsmen. Dr Joan Malleson said in the referral letter, 'the girl's parents are so respectable that they do not know the address of an [illegal] abortionist'.

'After getting the consent of her parents', wrote Bourne many years later, 'I admitted her on June 6th 1938. I kept her in bed in the ward for eight days to be sure of the type of girl I was dealing with; many of the prostitute type or those of low intelligence are completely undisturbed by pregnancy, except that for the first of these groups it is an obvious nuisance but nothing more'.[23] Bourne operated on the morning of 14 June and was interviewed by the police in the evening. He went for trial at the Old Bailey a month later.

Among Bourne's mail was a letter hoping he would receive 20 years' hard labour and a telegram from the police wishing him well. The defence argued that the health of the girl was in danger. The judge, Mr Justice Macnaghten, summing up, said,

> it [the 1861 Act] does not permit of the termination of
> pregnancy except for the purposes of preserving the life of the

mother. But I think myself that these words ought to be construed in a reasonable sense: if the doctor is of the opinion, on reasonable grounds and on adequate knowledge, that the probable consequences of the continuation of the pregnancy would indeed make the woman a physical or mental wreck, then he operates, in that honest belief, for the purpose of preserving the life of the mother.[22]

Macnaghten also argued that the application of the adjective 'unlawful' to abortion in the 1861 statute implied that some abortions must be lawful.

The jury returned a verdict of not guilty, the speculations of the nineteenth-century doctors such as Priestly were vindicated, the discussions of the Birkett committee had a nucleus around which ideas and recommendations could crystallise and a case precedent (which was never to be seriously challenged) was created.

Bourne escaped to a yachting holiday. He 'returned to a crowd I had not imagined. Not the press this time but women who, because of the wide publicity of the trial, thought that I would be easy on abortion and ready to relieve them of their unwanted pregnancies.'[23] Bourne, however, remained 'very strict in the interpretation of the law' and, at the time of the 1967 Act, was to join SPUC (Society for the Protection of the Unborn Child). He believed it might 'be a counterweight against the growing propaganda for "abortion on demand" which would be a disaster for our womanhood'.[24]

Reform

Politically, it is interesting and fortunate that in Britain, no one party ever espoused the cause of abortion reform. In parliament, legislation outside party politics is either moved by a private member, or introduced by the government in power but permitting a free vote. At the begining of each parliamentary session, all members of parliament who wish to sponsor new legislation take part in a ballot and those who appear within the first 10 or 15 may be able to gain parliamentary time to introduce their measures. In cases where the proposed Act is highly controversial it is essential to be very high on the list, since opposition is certain and procedural delaying tactics to be expected. The time allocated for debating Private Members' Bills is limited, though where the House of Commons itself and the public at large show considerable interest, the government of the day may agree to provide extra time to ensure adequate debate and a final vote.

Early attempts at parliamentary legislation

The reform of the British law has been adequately chronicled by Simms and Hindell.[25,26,27] The campaign was a long one, with several false starts, and medical attitudes, public opinion and political issues all altered as the movement progressed.

In the 1952/53 session of parliament, Joseph Reeves introduced a Bill to permit abortion 'done in good faith for the purpose of preventing injury to the mother in body or health'. Cardinal Griffin of Westminster led the opposition to the Bill, declaring it was 'against the whole tradition of English law, of natural law and of divine law'. The House of Commons devoted *one minute* of its debating time to the Bill. Among the other sponsors of the Reeves Bill were Douglas Houghton and Kenneth Robinson, who were both to figure prominently in later debates.

Reform flagged until the thalidomide tragedy of 1961 brought the question of therapeutic abortion to public attention. ALRA met again in 1945 after the war, but then entered a long political pause before being invigorated by a dramatic change of leadership in 1963. Vera Houghton, wife of Douglas Houghton (later to become a member of the Labour Cabinet at the time of the 1967 Act) became the new chairman and brought determination and enormous attention to detail. Previously Mrs Houghton had been the vigorous executive secretary of the newly formed International Planned Parenthood Federation. With a handful of hardworking, dedicated and well-informed committee members she launched a highly influential campaign upon the members of parliament (Commons and Lords) and the public at large. Not only was ALRA tiny in numbers, its budget was minute. In the 1950s and early 60s the total expenditure fluctuated between £50 ($100) and £600 ($1200) per year. From 1961 onwards over half of ALRA's financial support came from the Hopkins Donation Fund of Santa Barbara, California, which gave by 1967 a total of $24 500 (over £8500). The remainder of the budget was provided by UK sympathisers. Membership of ALRA only passed 1000 in 1966, women were in a majority and one in three had sought an abortion. Of the membership, 74 per cent were non-believers, 51 per cent Labour supporters, 21 per cent Conservative and 13 per cent Liberal. There was a 31 per cent overlap with membership of the National Trust, a conservation organisation.

In 1954 Lord Amulree, a Liberal Peer and a distinguished physician, introduced a Private Member's Bill in the House of Lords along similar lines to that proposed by Joseph Reeves, but withdrew it after disagreement with his supporters.

In 1961, Kenneth Robinson, a doctor's son who later became Minister of Health, introduced another Commons Bill. He included clauses concerning pregnancy following rape or cases where there was a risk of a grossly deformed child being born. Like the Reeves Bill it was talked out by the Catholic opposition, i.e. a filibuster was used to exhaust the allocated time and the Government of the day refused to provide extra time for further debate and for a vote to be taken. In 1963 a further Bill was introduced by Mrs Renee Short (later to be a sponsor of the successful 1967 Bill), but again it was talked out.

Throughout this time the majority of the medical profession remained comparatively uncommitted and silent; virtually all the initiative for reform came from lay quarters, primarily ALRA. Writing about his own Bill, Mr Robinson made the preceptive judgement, 'it's perhaps no exaggeration to say that most doctors prefer to have nothing to do with termination of pregnancy in any circumstances and that those who are prepared to exercise their professional judgement in what is nearly always a difficult problem constitute a small minority'.

The 1967 Act

In 1967 an Act was finally passed by both Houses of the British parliament reforming the abortion law. The passage followed nearly two years of intense parliamentary and public debate. This debate, of itself, was almost as important as the actual change in the law. The issue of abortion was brought into the open and for the first time its magnitude was widely appreciated. Opinion began to polarise and independent ballots taken by reputable opinion pollsters established that there already existed widespread support for liberalisation of the law, not only among the lay public but also among the general practitioners. The number of hospital and private practice abortions performed rose rapidly, even before the change in the law occurred (Fig. 38, p. 300). Perhaps most important of all, the English debate had repercussions abroad, especially in America (where up to that time the legal position and indeed public opinion had been much more conservative than in the UK).

Events in the House of Lords helped to prepare the way for the Commons legislation of 1967. The British House of Lords no longer has any executive function, but has been in the forefront of social reform including the fields of homosexuality, abortion and free contraception. The debating power of the Upper House had been strengthened by the establishment of life peerages in the 1950s. Amongst the first generation of life peers was Lord Silkin, a former Minister in a Labour government. He introduced a Bill in September 1965 to permit abortion where (1) 'if the pregnancy were allowed to continue there would be grave risk of the patient's death or serious injury to her physical and mental health', (2) 'there would be a grave risk of the child being born grossly deformed or with other serious physical or mental abnormality', (3) 'in the belief that the health of the patient or social condition in which she is living (including the social condition of her existing children) make her unsuitable to assume the legal and moral responsibility for caring for a child, or another child, as the case may be', and (4) where the woman became pregnant as the result of a sexual offence. This far-sighted piece of legislation was probably a more lucid statement of the aims of those attempting to reform the law than the Bill that eventually came out of the Commons in 1967, which was partly the result of political compromise. In contrast to the Commons, there was no time limit to debate in the Lords and many issues were thoroughly discussed. The Lords debate was also important in stimulating discussion within such bodies as the BMA, the Medical Protection Society and the Church of England.

The so-called social clause within the Bill was severely criticised and a somewhat mangled version received a third reading and therefore passed the House of Lords early in 1966. Normally it would then have proceeded to the Commons for their debate, but a general election took place at this time and all unfinished legislation lapsed.

The new government had a strong Labour majority. Among the tiny minority of Liberal members of the new parliament was David Steel, a 28-year-old lawyer, a Christian, whose father was a Minister of the Church of Scotland. He came third in the ballot for Private

Members' Bills. He was approached by a number of groups who wanted legislation to be carried but initially he was uncertain as to whether to handle an Abortion Bill and it seemed as if Edwin Brooks (Labour), who had come seventh in the ballot, would take this Bill. Finally, Steel accepted the advice of a senior civil servant in the Home Office who suggested he espouse the cause of either homosexuality or abortion. He chose the latter. The Bill which David Steel introduced to the House of Commons (June 1966) was based very much on that which had been successfully carried through the House of Lords by Lord Silkin. It allowed abortion to be performed where (1) pregnancy involved serious risk to the life or health, physical or mental, of the woman, (2) there was a 'substantial risk' of a congenital abnormality, (3) it was held that 'the pregnant woman's capacity as a mother will be severely overstrained by the care of a child, or another child as the case may be', and (4) the pregnant woman was a mental defective, became pregnant while under the age of 16, or became pregnant as a result of a sexual crime.

The important features of this proposed Bill, already accepted by the House of Lords, were that two doctors were required to certify that indications for abortion existed and that the operation itself was to be performed only within a National Health Service Hospital, or in a registered nursing home or some other place officially approved.

From 1965, when Lord Silkin first introduced his Bill in the House of Lords, the abortion issue caught the public interest and became, and remained, front-page news. From then until the final enactment of the Abortion Act in the Autumn of 1967 the moral debate raged fiercely. The problem of fetal abnormality was central to the debate and the rarest of indications received the strongest support. Later the medico-social clause became the sticking point and now medical organisations, such as the BMA, joined with religious groups in resisting reform, although most subsequently yielded to public pressure and the common experience of their members. At the height of the Commons debate, the President of the Royal College of Obstetricians and Gynaecologists, Sir John Peel, and E. A. Gerrard, chairman of the BMA Committee on therapeutic abortion, wrote in *The Times*, 'all factors affecting health should be considered, including age, social problems and the circumstances under which the pregnancy started.'

One of the major factors focusing public attention on abortion was the formation of SPUC in January 1967, a political body set up to oppose ALRA. Unlike Planned Parenthood/World Population in the USA, the Family Planning Association stood apart from the debate. ALRA and SPUC, each small but intensely dedicated, fought each other in the press, radio, television and in public meetings up and down the country. Books, pamphlets and letters were showered upon the members of the House of Commons and the House of Lords, and the public was treated to the spectacle of learned professors demonstrating bottled fetuses at public meetings, playing taperecorded fetal heartbeats or discussing the pain felt by the unborn fetus at its termination. The emotional level ran high.

SPUC had much Roman Catholic support, but members of Moral Rearmament were more to the front. In reality many Catholics followed a moderate line and of the 32 Catholic members of parliament only 14 were present at the second reading of Mr Steel's Bill.

One significant factor of the debate was the demonstration by national opinion polls that the public strongly supported liberalisation of the abortion law. There is no doubt that these polls (which were financed by ALRA) had considerable effect upon the voting of many parliamentary members. It was also demonstrated that the family doctors (but not gynaecologists) were supportive of abortion law reform.

The parliamentary debate was long and tortuous in the chamber of the Commons, in Committee stage, and in the Lords. It involved all-night sittings and extra sessions. Alastair Service, a publisher, educated at Eton and Balliol College, Oxford, and a member of the ALRA Executive Committee, and Vera Houghton worked endlessly, lobbying members of parliament and coming to know more about them than they knew of themselves. Although the Bill divided all three Parties along non-political lines and the government was officially neutral, the legislation would not have proceeded had the Cabinet not decided to grant extra parliamentary time for debate. Roy Jenkins, the Home Secretary, played a crucial part in the granting of this time.

The Bill was modified in a number of ways as it progressed. There was a fierce debate on the so-called social clause and the original draft was eliminated.

Outside parliament the Churches had much to say. An Anglican report *Abortion: An Ethical Discussion*[28] (which was commended by the Church Assembly) helped to advance public thinking. It regarded abortion as justified in those cases where 'it could be reasonably established that there was threat to the mother's life or wellbeing' and suggested that 'health and wellbeing must be seen as integrally connected with the life and wellbeing of her family'. Similar views have been expressed by other denominations. In a survey of nearly 500 London clergymen, over 80 per cent of the Protestant clergy were in favour of abortion to preserve the mother's health and a majority felt it was right to take social grounds into consideration. (Almost half the Catholic priests, but less than a quarter of the Anglicans, had been consulted by women on the problem of abortion.) In 1966 the Methodist Conference had expressed the perceptive view that 'the most important fact about a woman seeking an abortion is not that she is about to commit a crime, but that she is a human being in need'.[29]

The Commons accepted that the operation was to be agreed by two registered medical practitioners, but efforts to specify one of these as a consultant obstetrician and gynaecologist were finally defeated, although it had been urged by the Royal College of Obstetricians and Gynaecologists. During the Commons debate requirements about notification of the operation were added, becoming the basis of the British statistics which now exist.

The debate in parliament, as in the country and in the medical profession, was very bitter at times. But one constructive element which came out of these debates was the addition of a conscience clause. This clause, which has subsequently been adopted in other countries, stated that 'no persons shall be under any duty, whether by contract, or by any statutory or other legal requirements, to participate in any treatment authorised by this Act to which he has a conscientious objection'. It is interpreted as applying not only to doctors, but to nurses and other personnel. The onus is on the person maintaining the conscientious objection to establish that his objection is on conscientious grounds. The clause was jointly drafted by Norman St John-Stevas, a Roman Catholic Conservative member of parliament and David Steel. Mr St John-Stevas is a lawyer, a leading lay Catholic thinker who is critical of the Papal Encyclical on family planning,[30] but remains implacably opposed to abortion. He led, and continues to lead, much of the parliamentary opposition to abortion. Nevertheless, in commenting upon the conscience clause in the *Catholic Herald*, St John-Stevas pointed out that a doctor with conscientious objections to abortion is morally and legally obliged to refer a woman to another doctor, adding, 'The decision whether or not to have an abortion is ultimately one for the patient to make. It is not the doctor's moral duty to make that decision for her.' The conscience clause does not permit anyone to refuse to take part in an abortion where the woman's life is at stake. It is interesting that, even in the minutiae of the 1967 Act, the nineteenth-century tradition of approving abortion where the woman's life is at stake persists.

Legislation for the future?

There were, therefore, two streams of thought in the 1967 Acts: one was to codify what had always been accepted, the other broke new ground as social indications for abortion were discussed. The idea of abortion on request and the problem of the woman's right to choose very rarely broke through and when it did was positively rejected by ALRA, as well as by SPUC. With hindsight and nearly ten years' experience of the implementation of the 1967 Act, the question must now be asked: 'Were these debates valid?'

References

The book *Abortion Law Reformed* (1971), by M. Simms & K. Hindell (Peter Owen, London), presents a detailed account of the political and social pressures and counter pressures leading up to the 1967 Act. *Legal Abortion: the English Experience* (1971), by A. Horden (Pergamon Press, London), covers some of the same ground more briefly and reviews early experience of the Act.

1 Noonan, J. (ed.) (1970). *The Morality of Abortion: Legal and Historical Perspectives*. Havard University Press, Cambridge, Mass.
2 Williams, G. (1958). *The Sanctity of Life and the Criminal Law*. Faber & Faber, London.
3 *De Fide*. Quoted in Noonan (1970); see note 1.
4 Henry I (1556). Quoted in Parry (1932); see note 5.
5 Parry, L. A. (1932). *Criminal Abortion*. John Bale, Sons & Danielsson, London.
6 43 Geo. III c. 58 (1803).
7 21 Jas. I c. 27 (1623).
8 9 Geo. IV c. 31 (1828).
9 1 Vic. c. 85 (1837).
10 British Parliamentary Papers – Reports of the Commissioners, 1846. 24.42 (Art. 16). Quoted in Dickens, B. M. (1966). *Abortion and the Law*. McGibbon & Kee, London.

11 24 & 25 Vic. c. 100 (1861).

12 Marcus, S. (1966). *The Other Victorians*. Weidenfeld & Nicolson, London.

13 O'Mahony, P. J. & Potts, M. (1967). Abortion and the soul. *Month*, **38**, 45.

14 Priestly, W. (1881). On the introduction of abortion as a therapeutic measure. *Obstetrical Transactions*, **22**, 271.

15 Edgar, J. C. (1911). *The Practice of Obstetrics*. Rebman, London.

16 20 Geo. V c. 34 (1929).

17 British Medical Association (1936). *Report of Committee on Medical Aspects of Abortion*. BMA, London.

18 Jenkins, A. (1960). *Law for the Rich*. Gollancz, London.

19 Hindell, K. (1973). Personal communications. See also Browne, S. (1930). The right to abortion. In *Sexual Reform Congress*, ed. N. Haire, p. 178. Kegan Paul, London.

20 Simms, M. (1974). Gynaecologists, contraception and abortion – from Birkett to Lane. *World Medicine*, **10**, 49.

21 Simms, M. (1975). The compulsory pregnancy lobby – then and now. *Journal of the Royal College of General Practitioners*, **25**, 709.

22 Report by the BMA Special Committee on Therapeutic Abortion (1966). *British Medical Journal*, **2**, 40.

23 Bourne, A. (1962). *A Doctor's Creed*. Gollancz, London.

24 Bourne, A. (1967). Personal communication.

25 Simms, M. (1970). Abortion law reform: how the controversy changed. *Criminal Law Review*, October, 567.

26 Hindell K. & Simms M. (1968). How the abortion lobby worked. *Political Quarterly*, **39**, 269.

27 Hindell, K. & Simms, M. (1971). *Abortion Law Reformed*. Peter Owen, London.

28 Church of England Assembly, Board for Social Responsibility (1965). *Abortion: an Ethical Discussion*. Church Information Office, London.

29 Methodist Church Report on Resolution (1966). *Methodist Recorder*, 14 July.

30 St John-Stevas, N. (1971). *The Agonising Choice*. Eyre & Spottiswoode, London.

9

The working of the 1967 Abortion Act in Britain

In 1974 a Committee chaired by Mrs Justice Lane reported on the first four years' experience of the working of the 1967 Abortion Act. This chapter draws on the Lane Report[1] to a great extent. In addition, it outlines the political and administrative consequences of the Act, the sociological effect on its beneficiaries and on the medical profession, and provides some additional data that have become available since the Lane Report went to press.

'Antenatal' influence of the Act

The Abortion Bill, in one form or another, was under discussion in Parliament from November 1965 to October 1967 and a further interval of six months elapsed between the passage of the Act and its implementation. Throughout the whole of this period, a fierce debate by and between the public and the medical profession produced enormous changes in public and professional attitudes. The number of hospital abortions increased steadily (Fig. 38) and public opinion became more liberal, as demonstrated by a systematic series of opinion polls over this period.

An immediate and constructive effect was to encourage family planning legislation. Mr Edwin Brooks (Labour, Bebington) had achieved a high position in the 1966 poll for Private Members' Bills. Initially he had considered promoting a Bill to amend the abortion law but, when this was taken over by David Steel, he turned his attention to contraceptive legislation. What would normally have been a controversial measure was passed with remarkable ease. 'The intensity of the lobbying against the alleged "murder" of the fetus,' wrote Brooks later, 'was itself sufficient to absorb the energies of those involved, but there was also the difficulty of denouncing abortion yet at the same time appearing to be hindering the extension of contraceptive services which would help reduce the need for terminations.'[2] During the debate on the 1967 Family Planning Bill, the Speaker of the House of Commons was forced actually to solicit opposition speeches, although no major disagreement arose on the measure.

While the Abortion Act was being discussed, individual members of the Abortion Law Reform Association, and a few other concerned individuals, foresaw that the National Health Service (NHS) would be unable to meet potential national needs, and began planning to set up charitable bodies to help women seeking abortions. The Birmingham Pregnancy Advisory Service, under the leadership of Dr Martin Cole and Mrs Nan Smith, came into operation on the first day of the new Act in April 1968. A non-profit-making organisaton, charging only a small fee to cover the cost of its professional services, it counselled and referred women seeking abortions to carefully selected private gynaecologists who agreed to restrict their fees to a relatively modest level. Before the end of 1968, they acquired a nursing home, the Calthorpe, and employed their own surgeons to perform first-trimester abortions, for an inclusive fee of £65 ($130). In London, a similar pregnancy service arose under the leadership of Mr Alan Golding, and later established an exclusive relationship with the Fairfield Nursing Home, London, where surgeons were employed on a salaried basis, instead of receiving payment case-by-case. Two businessmen, Mr T. Heathcote and Mr R. Reynolds, advanced the initial capital involved in both nursing homes. The two pregnancy advisory services have performed an increasing share of the non-NHS abortions in England and Wales.

Implementation

In tracing the workings of the Act, it is appropriate to distinguish three types of service: (i) the private sector, (ii) the charitable pregnancy advisory services and (iii) the NHS.

Private sector

The initial effect of the 1967 Act on the private sector was to reduce the total number of operations and possibly the total

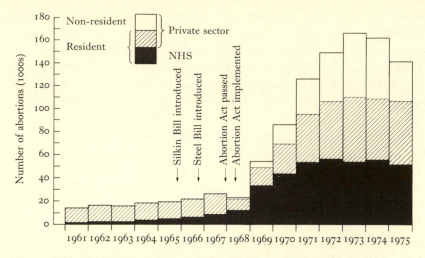

Fig. 38. Legal abortions in England and Wales (1961–75).
(Virtually all non-resident women are treated in the private sector.)

number of surgeons operating. The Act required that operations were only to be performed in licensed nursing homes, which had been inspected and approved by the Ministry of Health (later to become the Department of Health and Social Security – DHSS). The process was a slow one and the Ministry was strict in the application of its criteria. Prior to the Act, a number of abortions had taken place in doctors' surgeries and in small specialised units, neither of which were approved after April 1968.

Despite the slow beginning, there was a rapid recovery in private-sector abortions. In non-charity private nursing homes approved for termination, the beds were intensively used and sometimes women were discharged within a few hours of the operation. A new group of rather inexperienced surgeons entered the field, and while the 1967 Act cast out some devils in the form of backstreet abortionists, it also allowed in a few medically qualified goblins. Some individual abuses were well publicised and caught the attention of the public. SPUC and ALRA (see Chapter 8) remained in existence, following up on conflicting stories of successes and abuses in the Act. As summarised in the Lane Report, adverse criticisms fell into three main categories. It was claimed that the Abortion Act was interpreted too liberally, that women seeking abortion in the private sector were financially exploited, and that the standard of service was sometimes low.

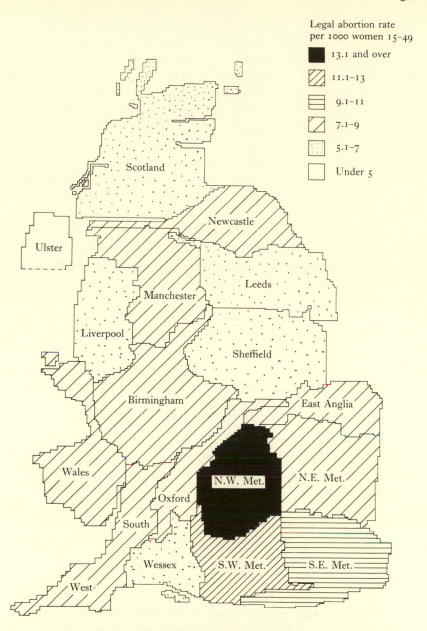

Legal abortion rate
per 1000 women 15–49

- 13.1 and over
- 11.1–13
- 9.1–11
- 7.1–9
- 5.1–7
- Under 5

Fig. 39. Legal abortion rate per 1000 women (15–49) by residence in 1971. (The map of Britain is drawn so that the area of each NHS region is proportional to the population of that region. N.W. Met. etc. = London and adjacent counties, as far as the coast.)

It was predictable that important differences of philosophy would arise between the private sector and the NHS. In the UK, the NHS, both at hospital and general-practitioner level, is financed out of taxes. Hospital consultants receive a basic salary, general practitioners are paid a fee for every patient on their list, whether sick or well. Doctors are often poorly informed about the detailed costing of any therapy. NHS consultants are allotted a fixed number of inpatient beds with relevant nursing care and ancilliary services, but no particular annual budget. In the private sector, the motivation for work and the appreciation of cost of the individual procedures are similar to those in private practice throughout the world. Obviously there is an interest in the fee, although in practice there is virtually always a commitment to the underlying needs of the patient and fees may be reduced or waived in cases of hardship. The abuses that did arise in the private sector probably involved very few doctors. The Lane Committee commented, 'in consequence of the Abortion Act a situation has arisen in which a very small number, of perhaps about 20 or 30 members, of the medical profession and those associated with them, have brought considerable reproach upon this country, both at home and abroad.'

Those opposed to the operation created a doubly complex image: by emphasising the dangers, they turned a simple operation, appropriate for a properly supervised general practitioner to perform, into one that only the most experienced gynaecologist was supposed to conduct, and then they criticised the level of fees paid. Abortion has inflamed emotions to the extent that it seems almost as if, unlike delivering a baby or performing routine surgery, no professional fee or reward should be asked.

Pregnancy advisory services

Both services have grown since their founding. The Birmingham Pregnancy Advisory Service opened several referral centres in other towns, purchased a number of clinical facilities, and changed its name to the British Pregnancy Advisory Service (BPAS). By the end of 1974, it had completed over 100 000 abortions, whilst the PAS in London had counselled 50 000 women. Both services reduce fees, waive them altogether, or make loans to women who are too poor to pay the £65–£67 ($130–$134) requested. Unfortunately, both services have been inhibited by the DHSS from providing daycare facilities, which would enable them approximately to halve their fees.

By 1970 the two PASs were performing 15 per cent of all registered abortions, or 33 per cent of all private cases. However, whereas a quarter of private abortions in that year involved women from overseas, the PASs dealt almost exclusively with British residents, amongst whom they have come to perform over four out of every ten non-NHS terminations. In fact, by the 1970s, the total number of abortion beds available in hospitals and clinics was probably equal to, or slightly in excess of, needs. As a consequence, some clinics in the private sector began to draw in more and more women from continental Europe.

The London-based private sector has always dealt with the majority of overseas patients (Fig. 38). The volume of European women seeking abortion in Britain has grown with time and the profile of country of origin has also altered. France has supplied many women; even in the first quarter of 1975 (after the change of the French law (Chapter 11)) over 7000 women travelled to Britain. However, while West Germany supplied over 13000 cases in 1971 its contribution had fallen to one-third of that figure by 1975. Conversely the number from Italy and Spain has risen steadily (1001 and 949, respectively, in the first-quarter of 1975).

The National Health Service

A woman seeking an NHS abortion has two hurdles to clear. First, she must convince her general practitioner that her case falls within the provisions of the law. It is unlikely that she will have canvassed his opinion on abortion before she accidentally became pregnant. Originally, she may have selected and registered with him as the nearest doctor when she moved house or when her children first had measles. Should she discover that her doctor is hostile to abortion, she has the right to transfer to another general practitioner, but such a process is time-consuming and requires considerable determination, in practice the option is rarely exercised.

Wherever the woman seeking abortion lives, her general practitioner is likely to refer her to the local hospital, where there may be from one to four consultant gynaecologists. Her general practitioner will know the attitudes of these local gynaecologists towards abortion and this enables a sympathetic doctor to select a sympathetic gynaecologist and conversely a hostile general practitioner to play at sending his patient for abortion whilst actually referring her to a gynaecologist he well knows will not agree to perform the operation. Apart from the possibilities of much chicanery, it may well be that, in a given district, the only available gynaecologist, or all the gynaecologists, are basically hostile to abortion. In such districts, few NHS abortions will be performed and we shall show later that the most important factor in the situation is the attitude of the gynaecologist. Unfortunately, although gynaecologists are in general willing to see women from outside their normal catchment area, this rarely applies to women referred for consideration of abortion. All NHS gynaecologists have a waiting list of patients requiring less urgent operations. Any woman accepted for abortion, must be given priority over this list and in addition, if a given gynaecologist who is liberally inclined toward abortion works alongside one who is hostile, it will rapidly follow that the liberal gynaecologist finds himself performing large numbers of abortions and providing a delayed service to his other patients – because of which delays, the routine and possibly also the fascinating gynaecological cases are referred to his illiberal colleague who is refusing to share the abortion load.

Unfortunately, the problem of varying medical attitudes is aggravated by wide variations in gynaecological facilities within the NHS. The Lane Committee called attention to the fact that in 1971, the number of gynaecological beds per 100000 women varied from 52 in East Anglia to 91 in the South-West Metropolitan area. Strangely, such wide variations in available facilities are not in any way correlated with the number of abortions performed; in the instance given above, there were 72.4 abortions per 1000 women aged 15–44 years in East Anglia and only 58.3 in the South-West Metropolitan area. To show even more clearly that medical attitudes are more important than facilities, one may contrast the Newcastle and Liverpool areas, which have almost identical facilities but were performing respectively 79.6 and 41.6 abortions per 1000 women of reproductive age (Fig. 40). To complete the contrast it should be noted that the *total* number of hospital bed-days per million of the population, devoted to therapeutic and 'other' abortions, was greater in Liverpool (31.3 per million) than in, say, East Anglia (24.1).

Ultimately the actual numbers of beds available may be virtually irrelevant. Buckle & Anderson[3] in Lewisham first showed, almost as soon as the Abortion Act came into force, that more than three-quarters of women could be aborted safely on an outpatient or daycare basis. King's College and St Mary's,[4] both London teaching

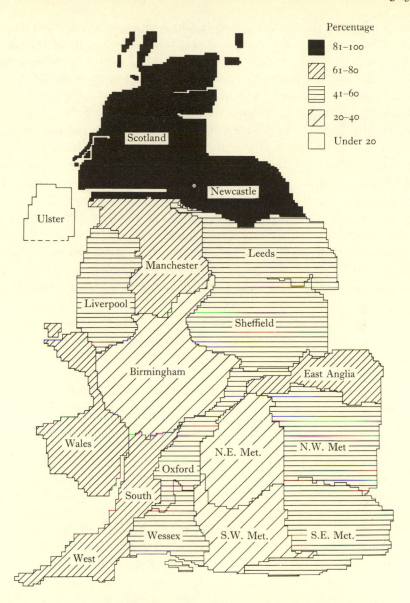

Fig. 40. Percentage of resident women in each NHS region who obtained an abortion in NHS hospitals of their home region in 1971. (See also Fig. 39.)

hospitals, and the teaching hospital in Nottingham also went on to establish very successful daycare abortion facilities.[5] It is probable that many general, provincial NHS hospitals would have followed this lead but for financial starvation.[6] Daycare abortion facilities were only established at Kingston Hospital on the outskirts of London when the Pregnancy Advisory Service made the hospital a grant of £2000, which was sufficient to buy essential equipment to start a unit capable of performing up to 600 operations per year (working only two days per week). This was the first unit where assessment and outpatient abortion is performed by trained general practitioners working within the NHS.

As a result of differing interpretations of the 1967 Act by general practitioners and consultant gynaecologists, the NHS abortion rate varies two-to-three-fold in different parts of England and Wales (Fig. 40).

The range of variation has remained roughly constant since 1968. After four or five years the so-called 'conservative areas' came to perform NHS abortions at the rate which the 'liberal areas' had first adopted, although by that time, the latter had moved on to permit even higher rates. Few facts illustrate the arbitrary nature of medical decisions so clearly.

The pattern of general practitioner, consultant gynaecologist and consultant psychiatrist decision-making has been analysed in depth in Aberdeen and is partially understood in other parts of Britain. In Aberdeen[7-9] there was a 10-fold variation between individual consultants in the number of women they 'approved' for abortion. Refusal was more likely in the case of single than married women. In various parts of Britain, consultants tend to refuse a fifth to a third of women referred for abortion by general practitioners,[10-12] although many of those refused on the NHS seek, and obtain, non-NHS abortions. Todd,[13] reviewing experience in Glasgow, commented, 'it is likely that restriction of the criteria for termination in general would simply lead to patients "shopping around"'.

Ingram[14] has described the treatment of women seeking abortion under the 1967 Act as *abortion games*. He describes what he terms 'Pontius Pilate' and 'Bounced Cheque' manoeuvres by uncertain or antagonistic referring doctors (the 'Bounced Cheque' involves delaying the woman's referral until it is too late for the surgeon to operate). The 'Big White Chief' and 'Little Indian' games revolve around dominating senior gynaecologists who impose their views on a whole hospital, town or even region. The 'Plumber' game is played by a doctor who asks others to tell him what to do and is the reverse of 'Amateur Psychiatrist' or 'Young Dr Kildare'. Ingram concluded 'the concealed function of all abortion games is to abolish or minimise personal responsibility for decisions made for or against termination, whether by patient, doctor or society'. In ethical terms it is hard to decide if this is a serious condemnation of the British Abortion Act, or merely a reflection upon those who operate it at all levels.

Northern Ireland

The 1967 Abortion Act specifically excludes Ulster, which continues to operate the 1861 Act in its unamended form. The Criminal Justice Act (Northern Ireland) 1945 does permit infant destruction in the third trimester when it is necessary to save the woman's life. That is, Ulster perpetuates the paradox that the baby may be legally killed at seven months, but that it is illegal to destroy the embryo seven days after the missed period. This same anomaly applied in England between 1929 and 1967 (see p. 279).

Women from Ulster and the Republic of Ireland are allowed to travel to England for a legal abortion if they can find the money and make the contacts. An Ulster Pregnancy Advisory Association was founded in 1971.[15] Through this and other channels, in 1974 1100 women a year travelled from Ulster (1968 – 36; 1969 – 96; 1970 – 199; 1971 – 649; 1972 – 775; 1973 – 1093). The age and marital status of women seeking to have a legal abortion performed in England are identical to those of English residents. Among those referred by the Pregnancy Advisory Association, 20.7 per cent were Roman Catholic. Thirty-five per cent of the Ulster population are Catholic, but the proportion of Catholic women seeking legal abortion is rising year by year. More Catholics were unmarried (72.2 per cent as compared with 65.1 per cent of Protestants), were somewhat younger, and came slightly later in pregnancy. Middle-class urban women appear to be setting the pace for those from across the Irish Sea who seek legal abortion. In 1973 1200 women from Eire obtained abortions in England and in the first nine months of 1974 about 1450 had already availed themselves of the same facilities.

The medical response

The volume of medical opposition to induced abortion lessened as more and more doctors came to face the visible reality of the problem of unwanted pregnancy among their patients.[16] As the Lane Committee was to comment in 1974. 'From the evidence we have received it appears to us that there has been some change of opinion within the medical profession towards a readier acceptance of abortion as a means of preserving health.' While recognising the need for abortion for mixed medico-social reasons, doctors contrived to rationalise their actions within the traditional framework of curative medicine. In the first year of the new Act, 72 per cent of abortions were registered as being performed on grounds of 'risk of injury to the physical or mental health of the woman' while only 4 per cent of cases were registered under the much-contested medico-social indications.

By 1970, the chairman of the British Medical Association, Dr H. Gibson, and Professor Sir Norman Jeffcoate,[17] soon to become president of the Royal College of Obstetricians and Gynaecologists, felt able to express their support for all the main clauses of the Act. They still believed that the operation is best performed under the supervision of a consultant in the NHS, or by a doctor of equivalent status. But an amendment to this effect attracted insignificant support in a parliamentary debate in February 1970, and was talked out by its own supporters. Addressing a meeting of the Royal College of Obstetricians and Gynaecologists in 1969, Dr T. L. T. Lewis, Secretary of the College, said, 'We thought there would be a slightly more liberal attitude towards the problem for that, after all, was the purpose of the new law. How wrong we were. I am afraid we did not allow for the attitude of, firstly, the general public and, secondly, the general practitioners'.[18] Three months later, a *Lancet* editorial commented,

> 'Things were certainly easier for the gynaecologists before the public and Parliament made their wishes known in the Act – but they were much harder for women. There is a minority of gynaecologists who, though making no claim to religious or conscientious objections, unhappily retreat from an awkward situation behind a barrier of moral disapproval and take little part in the operation of the Act. They thus deprive patients of emergency treatment to which they are entitled and increase the strain on their NHS colleagues.[19]

The grounds for sustaining continued opposition are mixed, and range from a reasoned concern for the ethical problems posed by abortion to peevish arguments about overloaded departments, lack of government assistance and reducing doctors to the 'role of technicians'. The ethical consideration of the problems reached their nadir in a BBC discussion on *Morals and Medicine* in 1970, when Professor Jeffcoate laid bare the muddled motivation of, at least some, doctors who opposed the Act.

> One can understand some women, with their new emancipation, taking the view that they themselves should decide whether their pregnancy should be terminated or not; that they should have the right to demand its removal. If there were an acceptable method of inducing abortion which they themselves could employ I can see no reason why they should not be free to do so, providing they appreciated the risks. There may come a time when an efficient oral abortifacient is discovered. A woman might then choose to take this, just as she can now elect to take oral contraceptives or to smoke cigarettes, despite any hazard involved. Meanwhile, however, abortion necessitates an operation, carried out by a skilled team, consisting of a surgeon, anaesthetist and nurses. These are all motivated by a strong ethical code and are dedicated to protect life and health. Only they can form a detached and professional opinion as to what are the best interests of the patient.[20]

The members of the British Medical Association continued to resist the Act after it was passed, as they had during its passage. They set up their own enquiry into the working of the Act in 1971 and appointed Professor Ian Donald as Chairman. (A few months earlier, Professor Donald had stated that, as a result of the liberal abortion law, it was becoming difficult to find enough doctors to act as 'executioners' in the NHS.)

The Royal College of Obstetricians and Gynaecologists remained cool. The evidence it presented to the Lane Committee was vague and often biased.

The attitude of surgeons in private practice has frequently been pilloried, but observations by consumers, women attending NHS hospitals, can also be harrowing. The history of a woman aged 41 years with four children and a recent episode of tuberculosis was passed on to the Lane Committee. She reported being 'submitted to the most humiliating interview in which the NHS gynaecologist expressed his personal distaste for carrying out terminations and succeeded in making me feel both irresponsible and immoral, so that I came out in tears – as had the patient ahead of me'.[21]

The high percentage of sterilisations accompanying abortions within the NHS (over 50 per cent of married woman having NHS abortions in 1968–69 were sterilised)[22] may reflect a punitive attitude among some NHS gynaecologists as well as a genuine answer to the need for fertility control.

The response of the nursing profession shadowed that of doctors. Some welcomed, most accepted, but a few protested bitterly. For some young nurses the operation can present a particular challenge and a wise surgeon will be careful both to listen and explain. When young nurses care for women seeking abortion, and have the opportunity to talk at length with them, they commonly come to take a sympathetic view. The Lane Committee concluded that the Abortion Act had little or no effect on nursing recruitment. It also commented that morale was often very high in clinics doing only abortions, because the nurses employed clearly believed in the value of the work they were doing. In 1969, the Board of Social Responsibility of the Anglican Church gave it as its view 'that it would be wrong and useless for matrons and nurses to attempt to interfere to delay cooperation in a case actually under treatment. Responsibility must be allowed to rest where it is placed by the Act' (i.e. with the certifying doctors).

In December 1970 the Catholic Nurses' Guild of Scotland issued guidelines to its members. 'Nurses who object to abortion,' they pointed out, 'should always demonstrate their charity to patients having abortions.' Concerning cases in the wards, the guidelines suggested that Catholic nurses 'should be prepared to look after these [i.e. abortion] patients in all neutral matters, giving pain-relief and comfort, and post-operative care'. It was suggested that in the theatre 'Catholic nurses may not give essential assistance, such as handing over instruments or sutures. Standard sets of sterilised instruments and towels may be provided on a trolley, as these are equipment for gynaecological operations and are morally "neutral"'.

Whatever nurses and their spokesmen say about the Abortion Act there is no doubt that, as a group, they are heavy users of its facilities. Diggory[23] and Ingham & Simms[24] as well as others have shown that, when women seeking abortion are analysed according to occupation, nurses are over-represented.

Political pressure groups

The membership of the Abortion Law Reform Association diminished once it had achieved its objectives. Even its name became a misnomer. Money was difficult to raise. Nevertheless, a clear niche remained for a propagandist organisation to meet criticisms which were made about the implementation of the Act in the media, parliament and elsewhere. The Women's Right to Choose campaign was launched jointly by the Abortion Law Reform Association (ALRA) and the National Council for Civil Liberties on 1 January 1975 to meet this need.

In contrast, the Society for the Protection of the Unborn Child (SPUC) still had clearly defined political goals and grew both in membership and financial strength. It sought explicitly to restrict the Act in a number of ways, although it came to recognise the role of abortion in cases where the woman's life was genuinely at risk. SPUC suggested the Act had been pushed hastily through parliament (although it followed one of the longest debates known), sought the setting up of a Royal Commission and suggested referees to review each case before termination.

Life, a charity to give advice to girls unwillingly pregnant, was created as a political alternative to the PASs, emphasising ways in which girls could keep their babies or obtain an adoption. This new option was useful, although the PAS had always been willing to assist in providing adoption advice to those requesting it. Some people regretted the fact that Life had not been founded prior to the Abortion Act, when the need was as great, or greater.

Some of those who had been involved in ALRA, together with some new activists, set up the Birth Control Campaign in 1970. The aim of this group was mainly to lobby parliamentarians to produce rational, total family planning services. In 1971/72, Mr Philip Whitehead steered the National Health Service (Family Planning) Amendment Bill through parliament, permitting Local Authorities, which had previously been in an anomalous administrative position, to pay for vasectomy operations. Edwin Brooks' Family Planning Act of 1967 began to succeed and a number of Local Authorities set up entirely free contraceptive services. The public response to these free services was gratifying.

In 1973, there were debates in the House of Commons and the House of Lords, concerning making contraceptive advice available nationwide without cost to the user. When the NHS was reorganised in April 1974, family planning was included as an intrinsic part of the responsibilities of the new Area Health Authorities. And in 1974 the Secretary of State for Social Services abolished prescription charges for contraceptives within the NHS or Area Health Authorities' clinics.

It is instructive to recollect that all the legislative advances in birth control provisions followed rapidly on the protracted debate and passage of the 1967 Abortion Act.

Backlash

The opinion of those who remained opposed to the 1967 Act was summarised in 1970 by Goodhart, a founder member of SPUC.

> Until a few years ago abortion presented few problems to the ordinary respectable man or woman in the street. It was either regarded as a criminal offence, common enough perhaps, but the less said about it the better, or else it was a matter for the professional judgment of obstetricians: and they had better be sure that there were really good medical reasons for an abortion, if they wanted to keep out of trouble.[25]

The backlash which occurred expressed the elements of Goodhart's summary with varying degrees of emphasis. The 'keep out of trouble' attitude – more suitable perhaps as an admonition to a Cambridge college rowing club after the May races, than a statement of deep concern – sometimes found expression in more hysterical terms of condemnation. The implication that the serious social problem of induced abortion could not only be flushed away like sewage – 'the less said the better' – but that it could be eliminated without any kind of visible drainage system is implicit in most of the criticisms of the Act. Those opposed behaved as if abortion were a new phenomenon and as if embryos had not been deliberately destroyed before 1967. Few had the straightforwardness of Goodhart's comment 'common enough perhaps'.

In May 1970 the Roman Catholic member of parliament Norman St John-Stevas, speaking in the privileged confines of the House of Commons, where the laws of slander do not apply, claimed that live fetuses were being sold for medical experiments.[26] One newspaper, reporting this speech, carried the headline, 'Clinic Sells Abortion Babies for Research'. A Committee was set up to 'consider the

ethical, medical, social and legal implications' of using fetal material
for research. The report of this Committee has never been published. In a parliamentary written answer, Sir Keith Joseph wrote,
'The investigation resulted in a decision to take no further action
beyond the setting up of the inquiry'. No public accusation has ever
been made.[27]

Opinion concerning the 1967 Act has been studied in a number
of surveys and was tested in a direct way in early 1971, when Mr
Peter Mahon stood as the Labour and Against Abortion candidate
at a by-election in a strongly Catholic area of Liverpool. Peter
Mahon and his brother Simon talked out the 1965 Abortion Bill
and contributed at great, and frequently irrelevant, length to the
1967 debates. He gained less than 1000 votes and lost his deposit.

A number of attempts have been made in parliament to alter the
1967 Act. Mr John Hunt presented a reasonable Medical Services
(Referral) Bill to parliament in 1970/71 but it failed to progress.
Another attempt to regulate referral agencies was made by Mr
Michael Grylls, who introduced an Abortion (Amendment) Bill in
May 1974, but this lapsed because of the refusal of anti-abortion
members of parliament to provide a quorum. They wanted a more
restrictive measure. The first attempt to amend the law during
the life of the October 1974 parliament was moved by Mr James
White, supported by several of those who had opposed the 1967
Act, including Leo Abse, Simon Mahon and Jill Knight.

The Lane Committee

In June 1971 the then Secretary of State for Social Services,
Sir Keith Joseph, appointed a committee 'to review the operation
of the Abortion Act 1967'. The committee took nearly three years
to report. It is a convention of British parliamentary procedure that
no major alteration to the legislation should be made prior to such
a report being received. These three years were exceptionally
important for the 1967 Act. The total number of abortions rose,
mortality rates fell and the public and medical profession became
more used to, and more inclined to accept, legal abortion. It is
reasonable to postulate that, if the Lane Committee had not been
set up, some restrictions of the Act might have been taken through
parliament during the earlier days of its history, when facts were
less certain and the hostile lobby was well organised.

The establishment of a special committee empowered to examine and report on the working of the established part of the law is a fundamental device used by the British parliament to obtain authoritative, unbiased advice and analysis. The committee to review the Abortion Act was chaired by the first British woman High Court Judge, the Honourable Mrs Justice Lane, and comprised a cross-section of professional and lay groups (obstetricians, a general practitioner and a social worker, a headmistress and others).

Members of such a committee are chosen by the responsible Minister and his advisers. It is axiomatic that the persons chosen should not only be experienced but, up to the time of their serving on the committee, should have refrained from overtly partisan activities concerning the subject under review.

The Lane Committee used its powers to employ the services of two well-known sociologists from the Institute of Social Studies in Medical Care to carry out a survey of abortion patients.[28] The Committee had full access to government statistical departments and requested and obtained a range of data not previously recorded. Most fundamental, confidential notifications of abortions, containing data on such features as social class and previous obstetric history, became available for the first time. The Committee had 54 days of meetings; its members individually, and in groups, visited a large number of hospitals, abortion clinics, referral agencies and individual practitioners and they received memoranda from nearly 200 organisations and over 500 individuals. The final Report is the most comprehensive official document on legal abortion and its effects ever published in any country.[1]

It is surprising, but a considerable tribute to Mrs Justice Lane, that the final report on this highly controversial subject was unanimous. Previously, there had been two government commissions on abortion (Chapter 8) and neither achieved unanimity. Fair-minded and responsible people had been selected to sit on the Lane Committee and it is clear that, initially, all shades of opinion on abortion were represented. It is significant that as evidence was received, a genuine liberal consensus arose.

The Justices of the US Supreme Court, discussing the same issues at the same time, decided to support abortion on request early in pregnancy. It is said they found a compromise impossible and Mr Justice Blackmun, who drafted most of the judgement, is reported to have said that they had 'no choice' but to reach such a radical conclusion. Perhaps the US Constitution encourages absolute decisions. The Lane Committee was not asked to establish a new philosophy; it was charged with commenting on the working of existing legislation. The Report gives a great many reasons why abortion might be available on request in the first-trimester of pregnancy, and no strong reasons why it should not . It continues to squeeze abortion into the therapeutic, medical mould: 'We regard it as a matter of principle that the care of the woman who seeks an abortion should remain within the mainstream of general medicine and gynaecological practice.'

The Committee ingeniously bracketed the basically conservative approach in the 1967 Act with a liberal view to medical practice. The 'patient should be treated as a whole person' and the amelioration of social problems is rated as important as the cure of disease. Some of the more strident claims of the feminist movement are translated into softer, but nevertheless meaningful, terms and the contemporary woman is said to be less submissive, less resigned and less willing 'to suffer unhappiness or pain which are deemed avoidable: what is desired is sought more actively. Many women are no longer prepared to accept the burden of often repeated, unwelcome and debilitating child-bearing: they see a far wider spectrum of choice open to them and the possibility of a greatly enhanced quality of life for themselves and their children'.

Daycare abortion services

Several of those who gave evidence to the Committee spoke of the need and opportunity to set up daycare services, and some of the Committee's secretariat visited the east coast of America to gain first-hand experience of outpatient abortion centres. In its Report, the Committee concluded that

> 'The provision of adequate facilities for early day-care abortions
> could provide a useful step towards the solution of many other
> problems in the working of the Abortion Act and would
> remove some of the pressure from gynaecological wards while
> at the same time keeping abortion within the mainstream of
> gynaecology.
> The speed of the procedure should enable waiting lists to be
> reduced and thus make it possible to operate earlier in the
> pregnancy when the risks of mortality and morbidity are lower.
> This is one of the forms of minor surgery in which suitably

trained general practitioners might usefully participate. The provision of nursing care might be attractive to nurses and midwives who do not wish to work at night or at the weekend.

Early experience of the working of the Kingston gynaecological daycare unit has shown that both suggestions work well in practice. The pay of general practitioners working as clinical assistants is so low that it could not be held to constitute a financial incentive towards abortion-operating. Yet it has proved possible to recruit experienced and deeply committed doctors. There is even a waiting list of nurses wishing to work in the unit, although it is situated in an area where all the NHS hospitals suffer from severe nursing shortages. The financial advantages to the NHS of daycare are obvious. Fewer nurses are required since the woman is only in hospital for a few hours and there is no need for a 24-hour nursing staff. The consultants are involved only in a supervisory capacity and a clinical assistant is a far less expensive doctor to employ. Many, if not most, cases can be performed in a procedure room rather than in a specialised and specially staffed operating theatre and local rather than general anaesthesia will often be preferred – both are factors that lead to considerable financial savings.

The Lane Committee pointed out that 'The great majority, 87 per cent, of the women having abortion saw a doctor before nine weeks had elapsed since their last period. This means that, if patients were referred straightaway by the first doctor they contacted, the techniques that have to be applied in early pregnancy could be used for most patients currently having abortions.'

Counselling

The woman with an unwanted pregnancy turns to her advisors for help, not only as to the possibility of abortion but also about how she may avoid a similar situation in the future, and at such a time she is peculiarly receptive to contraceptive advice. The Lane Report recommends that adequate counselling should be available to all women undergoing abortion. The need for such services was appreciated early in the USA when liberal abortion became available, and a whole spectrum of abortion counselling developed in which the woman came into close personal contact with her counsellor, who not only explained and discussed all the facilities available but remained physically with the woman throughout her stay in the abortion clinic and, in co-operation with the operating doctor, advised on future contraception.

In the UK the woman's own practitioner could be potentially the foundation of a superior system of counselling and support. He knows the woman's family, her social situation and medical history. When he recommends abortion he should discuss contraception or even sterilisation at the same interview. After operation the woman returns to his continuing care and supervision so that really adequate follow-up is feasible without cost to the woman.

Unfortunately, not all general practitioners have yet been able to accept this role. Often the woman reaches hospital or clinic without having fully discussed all the possibilities open to her in a relaxed atmosphere. Up to the present time, there has been no provision for abortion counsellors within the NHS. There have been model schemes using fully trained social workers and the PASs have used selected and trained lay counsellors for some years.

The need to provide an adequate counselling service is now widely appreciated but argument continues about which is the best way to do this. There is clearly a great deal of difference in the counselling needs of an older married woman whose unwanted pregnancy has resulted from contraceptive failure compared with those of the young unmarried girl. In the first case, abortion possibly accompanied by sterilisation or by improved contraception is often all that is required. In the second, the young girl may need considerable help in accepting the problems of her own sexuality and, unless enabled to achieve this, may even refuse to acknowledge that she will have a need for contraception in the future.

The present position of counselling is unsettled and controversial. The high-pressure system appropriate to an American clinic, where the woman is seen for the first and probably the only time on the day of her abortion, is unlikely to be necessary within the British NHS. The charitable pregnancy advisory services may be able to provide some degree of follow-up as well as pre-abortion counselling, since in Britain it is rare for residents to be aborted on the day they are first seen. Because of the wide variations between the NHS, PAS and the private sector, it is probably wise to avoid counselling services becoming too stereotyped or formalised now.

Madeleine Simms in her *Report on Non-Medical Abortion Counselling* has summarised the position succinctly when she says, 'the object of counselling generally is to help the client to a greater awareness of the nature of her difficulties so that she is able to find an acceptable way to resolve them. Provided, that is, she really has difficulties. Many abortion clients are simply careless or even unlucky. They may need some support through a stressful complication in their lives. They may not need much more.'[29]

Evaluation

In the eight years since the 1967 Act passed through parliament several important lessons have been learned. The abortion rate for British women appears to have levelled off at approximately two per 1000 of the population per year. In 1973 the number of

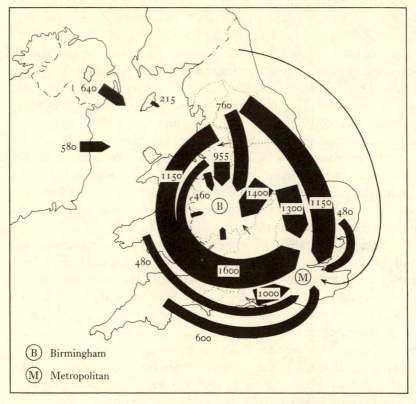

Fig. 41. Migration of women seeking legal abortions (mostly in the private and charitable sectors) between regions. (England and Wales 1971, residents of the British Isles only.) (See also Figs. 39 and 40.)

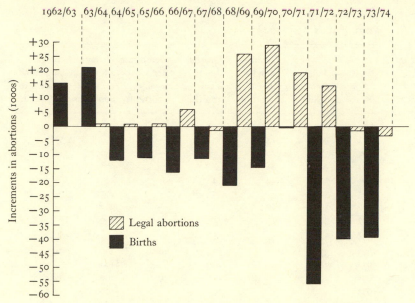

Fig. 42. Annual increments in legal abortions (England and Wales residents only) compared with changes in total number of births.

abortions in England and Wales plateaued and fell by 2.4 per cent in 1975[30] and a further 6 per cent in 1976 (Figs. 38 and 42).

The cumulative total number of legal abortions has now reached over one million, with more than 700000 performed on British residents. The birth rate fell slowly in the late 1960s and rapidly in the 1970s. When the year-by-year increments in legal abortions are plotted beside the annual fall in total number of births (Fig. 42), it is apparent that, in the second half of the 1960s, the birth rate was declining more rapidly than the abortion rate was climbing. For three years after the change in the law, the annual jump in abortions more than accounts for any fall in the birth rate, but after 1971–72, the fall in births exceeds the annual increment in legal abortions. The analysis is a crude one; more than one abortion is required to avert a full-term birth and delivery usually occurs six months later than would an abortion, yet it is strongly suggested that contraceptive practice is improving. Among married women under 20 years of age, who represent the least experienced group in terms of contraception, total deliveries fell by 14000 in the decade 1965–74, but legal abortions only rose by 800. The alternative explanations

Table 25. *Deaths due to legal and illegal abortions (England and Wales 1960–74)* [a]

Year	Total abortion deaths	Deaths due to illegal abortions	Deaths due to legal abortions	Death rate per 100000 legal abortions	Hospital admissions for septic abortions	Illegal abortions known to the police
1960	62	30	—	—	—	—
1961	54	23	3	—	—	—
1962	57	29	4	—	2500	—
1963	49	21	4	—	2700	—
1964	50	24	4	—	2950	—
1965	52	21	5	—	2950	—
1966	53	30	4	—	2600	—
1967	34	17	1	—	2600	—
1968	50	22	5	21.2	2290	—
1969	35	15	10	18.2	2000	257
1970	32	11	10	11.5	1900	212
1971	27	6	12	9.4	1200	80
1972	26	—	10	6.25	1000	62
1973	—	—	6 [b]	3.6	—	36
1974	—	—	6	3.6	—	—

[a] The Act was implemented from 27 April 1968.
[b] From 1973, deaths within one month of operation are included, some of which were from concurrent disease such as carcinoma.

that could account for a fall in birth rate, namely a rise in illegal abortions or a change in sexual habits, are not supported by any observational data.

Deaths due to septic abortion and hospital admissions due to the same cause have both fallen since the 1967 Act was implemented. The decline has not been so unequivocal as in the USA (p. 89) and the numbers are so small that minor ambiguities in the statistics become important. However, the trend is consistent (Table 25, p. 320 and more marked than in the case of maternal mortality rates. Godber (1972) stated that it is 'beyond dispute that deaths attributed to abortion are now at a sustained low level compared with the years 1961–6'.[31] Regression analysis of abortion and delivery deaths invalidates the hypothesis that the fall in abortion deaths is merely a reflection of improved clinical care.[32] The confidential enquiries into maternal deaths (which cover 89 per cent of maternal deaths in England and Wales) show that deaths from illegal abortion fell dramatically in the years 1968 to 1972.[33]

Age-specific analysis of live births highlights differences in the use of legal abortion by different age and marital groups. Between 1969 and 1973, annual births to married women aged 35 years and over fell by 23029 while legal abortions only rose by 8716. By contrast, the annual rate of illegitimate births to women under 25 fell by 5875 while registered abortions to unmarried girls in the same age group rose by 30780. Within marriage, legal abortion has been largely used by women with several children. Among married women under 20 in the 1970s, the ratio of live births to legal abortions was 147:1 for women pregnant for the first time but 1:1 for those having a third pregnancy. For married women in the 25–39 age group the ratios were 15:1 and 2:1, respectively. Outside marriage there has been a rise in both the number of deliveries and legal abortions in the decade 1965–74, although since 1971 the total number of illegitimate births has fallen and the trend in registered abortions among cohorts of girls born in 1945 and 1950 and aged 22–24 at the time of the termination has begun to fall, although not yet in younger groups.[34]

The need to review abortions of married and unmarried women separately has been commented upon several times in this book. In contemporary Britain, contraceptive practice among married women appears to be improving in the presence of liberal abortion legislation: the law happens to have been altered at the time of changing sexual practice among the unmarried. When reviewing illegitimacy statistics it should also be noted that the Family Law Reform Act (1969) lowered the age of majority and some early marriages, which previously parents might have forbidden, may have taken place, altering the ratio of legitimate to illegitimate births or removing the pressure for abortion.

It has been said that, since abortion became readily available, infertile couples have found it harder to adopt a baby. In fact, the total number of adoption orders has remained constant in recent years and only healthy babies of Anglo-Saxon parentage are hard to find. By the 1970s the Church of England Children's Society was closing 17 of its 95 mother-and-baby homes.[35] 'It is a shame,' said one Matron, 'we will have to close because there is not the supply of babies.' The fall in the total number of babies for adoption assisted the settlement of difficult-to-place children. 'The supply of Roman Catholic, coloured or handicapped children continues to exceed demand.'[36] The total number of adoption orders made rose slightly between 1972 (21603) and 1974 (22502).[37]

Overall, the Lane Committee concluded that 'by facilitating a greatly increased number of abortions, the Act has relieved a vast amount of individual suffering'. The Committee was also 'unanimous in supporting the Act and its provisions', and whilst recognising that it had disadvantages and had been criticised, it suggested that professional and administrative solutions should be sought, not a restrictive amendment of the Act, because 'to do so when the number of unwanted pregnancies is increasing and before comprehensive services are available to all who need them would be to increase the sum of human suffering and ill-health, and probably to drive more women to seek the squalid and dangerous help of the back-street abortionist.'

In comparison with other countries, such as Japan, Britain still has an unsatisfactory proportion of second-trimester abortions. It is for this reason that British mortality and morbidity rates are higher than they should be. The earlier the abortion the safer it is. International experience shows that there are two important factors which promote early abortion. The first is the provision of adequate and acceptable services, free from undue administrative delays,[38] and this is why the Lane Report recommended expanding daycare abortion services. The second is that the couple should know that if they seek abortion they are likely to obtain it. Delays occur when emotional and psychological hurdles have to be surmounted and the paternalistic, judgemental attitudes of doctors can be strongly inhibitory to early consultation.

Absorbing the load

The total load of legal abortions has been accommodated in the NHS and the private sector without any nationwide increase in gynaecological waiting lists, but the number of abortions by the NHS has remained almost stationary for five years. Future options include a further expansion of the charitable services, possibly by their becoming agents of the NHS, as occurred in the evolution of contraceptive services, or by a quantum jump in NHS numbers, as could easily occur with the introduction of general-practitioner staffed daycare units in, or attached to, area hospitals.

When the need is so obvious and the most economical and rational solution so clear, it may be asked why more NHS hospitals do not set up daycare abortion units. The answer lies in the open-ended nature of the contract between the NHS and the community.

It is easy to show that daycare abortion units provide more efficient (because many delays are eliminated) and cheaper services than does the normal gynaecological referral system with its outpatient appointments, waiting lists, hospital admission and inpatient care: but it would be false to suggest to the Hospital treasurer that by setting up such a unit he can save money. He well knows that the outpatient clinic appointments and the ward beds left vacant when the new unit functions will at once be filled by new patients seeking other gynaecological help.

The savings and convenience of daycare operations also apply to the charitable and private sectors. The PASs are ready to make the necessary investment of skill and money and the Minister of Health, Dr David Owen, announced in 1975 that he would consider permitting the charities to perform daycare abortions within the safeguards set out in the Lane Report.

Getting cases early

Most people do not see themselves in the position of requiring an abortion until the unexpected happens. They do not store details about abortion services in the way they record the telephone numbers of plumbers and electricians.

Modern advertising is a powerful weapon, and there are those who would like to see its powers of persuasion harnessed to public health needs and slogans such as 'If you are late, come early' or 'What's worse than the curse?' put about. In England this is not possible, and a journey on the London underground is much less informative in relation to abortion services than one in the New York subway. Advertising practice is regulated more by commercial codes and the political problems of obtaining space, than by statute. London Transport, for example, has bracketed family planning advertising with politically and racially disruptive messages. It is paradoxical that in a decade of increasingly free use of sexual imagery in relation to selling everything from films to toothpaste, only euphemisms are permitted in relation to abortion services. The Lane Committee noted that one of the most worrying abuses of the 1967 Act could be that foreign women who came to England did not know where to go and ended in the hands of unscrupulous operators. The logical solution of this problem is to permit responsible services to advertise adequately.

Abortion (Amendment) Bill 1975

In February 1975 a Bill to amend the 1967 Abortion Act passed its second reading by a two to one majority. The Bill attempted to neutralise the original Act by the fine print of clauses and regulations, rather than by direct assault on the fundamental principles of the 1967 Act, such as the doctor's right to take into account the total environment of the woman seeking an abortion.

The draft Bill added the words 'grave' and 'serious' in the clauses dealing with the woman's mental and physical health, and attempted to restrict decision-making to two doctors who were not in practice together and where one had been registered for at least five years. It was suggested that surgeons performing abortion should be under the control of a consultant gynaecologist, or someone with consultant status. A number of elliptically phrased clauses proposed that advice on termination could only be given by a registered medical practitioner in specified referral agencies. It was proposed that girls under 16 could only be counselled in the presence of a parent or guardian.

One of the constructive items in the Bill was a proposed system of registering abortion referral agencies, but a suggested resident qualification of 20 weeks presented unusually difficult administrative problems in the UK, with its numerous overseas connections and its recent entry to the European Economic Community. The most astonishing clause of the Bill was one that, contrary to hundreds of years of British justice, assumed the practitioner to be guilty until he had proved his innocence.

The draft Bill would have cut down the constituency of doctors legally able and professionally willing to advise or perform abortions, thus creating delays in operating. The administrative regulations would have created further hold-ups. The proposals about counselling girls under 16 would have inhibited some girls from seeking help *and* have allowed parents to pressurise a teenager into having an abortion she did not herself want. James White (Labour, Glasgow Pollok) who introduced the Bill commented: 'I never thought about abortion until the 1970 election. But on polling day a Glasgow paper showed a picture of my Tory opponent with a group of nuns calling the Labour Government immoral for working the Abortion Act. How would you like it if you were fighting a marginal seat with a strong Catholic vote?'[39]

The Bill was largely drafted by Leo Abse (Labour, Pontypool), a lawyer from Wales, with great experience of parliamentary affairs and an emotional opponent of abortion, and George Crozier, Chairman of the Glasgow Lay Council of the Roman Catholic church.

The debate on the second reading of the Bill (7 February 1975) was confused.[40,41] Abse pre-empted normal parliamentary procedure in a television talk-show the night before the debate by announcing the government's intention to set up a Select Committee to review the Bill. David Owen, Minister of Health, perhaps in an effort to shunt the Bill into a siding, agreed to the Select Committee, but eventually the House voted both for the Select Committee (218 to 45) and the Bill (203 to 88). This surprisingly high majority was partly because a fevered campaign built up around an improbable book entitled *Babies for Burning*.[42] It was a paperback produced by two journalists who attended a number of pregnancy referral agencies, claiming that they were not married (which indeed was true), had been sleeping together and that the girl was pregnant and sought an abortion. They carried a taperecorder. Instead of transcribing evidence, which in some cases may well have demonstrated a somewhat cavalier treatment of women, they loaded their descriptions with vulgar journalistic phrases and comments on the Fascist nature and supposed interests of some of the people they interviewed. One doctor, who unlike most of the others goes unnamed, was claimed to have disposed of fetuses to a soap factory. The same doctor is also supposed to have confessed to killing viable fetuses: 'One morning I had four of them lined up and crying their heads off. I hadn't time to kill them there and then.' It was the second book published by the Serpentine Press. A receiver was appointed for the Press in June 1975 – a factor which may have discouraged libel actions.

Setting aside the biological fact that even a second-trimester fetus has no subcutaneous fat to act as a raw material for soap, the accounts were unusual. The authors were not available to help Scotland Yard investigate the allegations of murder. Curiously a tape of this key conversation did not exist. Gillie, Wallace & Ashdown-Sharp & Zimmerman of *The Sunday Times* tracked down the doctor, who recalled being interviewed by a man seeking fetal material for research.[43] The doctor concerned had been imprisoned in Dachau and Buchenwald and his wife and son died in Auschwitz.

The General Medical Council cleared two doctors named in *Babies for Burning* and the Director of Public Prosecutions 'decided that the evidence is not sufficient to justify proceedings against any person'. It was a repetition of the story of live fetuses used for research (p. 312).

The public and parliamentary debate of the 1975 Abortion (Amendment) Act saw a reversal of some of the political alignments surrounding the 1967 Act itself. Partly as a result of *Babies for Burning*, whose authors were described by Leo Abse[41] as 'virginal and pristine', and similar publicity of abortion abuses and supposed abuses, members of parliament were more receptive to the idea of restriction of the 1967 Act. But professional opinion had swung much more solidly in favour of liberal legislation. The Royal College of Psychiatrists called the White Bill 'loosely drafted, in some respects impractical, restrictive and in danger of putting the clock back'. The Royal College of Pathologists used the unacademic description 'quite ludicrous' and the Association of Anaesthetists pointed out that it would hamstring ethical doctors 'while providing plenty of loopholes for continued abuse by an unscrupulous minority'. Even the British Medical Association said the Bill presented 'very practical difficulties' and opposed it 360 to 4 at a conference of local representatives. In May 1975 a small group of doctors had been sufficiently frustrated with the BMA's previous attitude that they physically took over part of BMA House.

After a slow start, public opinion in favour of abortion began to return. A joint report by the Church of England and the Methodist Church looked sympathetically at the abortion problem but it was diagnostic of the confused opinions of the mid-1970s that the Board of Social Responsibility 'did not approve its publication'. A public demonstration by the National Abortion Campaign in June 1975 attracted an estimated 15 000–20 000 people, while a rival meeting of the Order of Christian Unity and Festival of Light, on the same day, was attended by fewer than 300 people. However, an anti-abortion demonstration in October gathered upwards of 50 000 people.

The 1975 Hastings Congress of Women Trade Unionists voted overwhelmingly for *further* liberalisation of the abortion law. The potent parliamentary lobby group that ALRA had once represented came out of hibernation. Reason, A Woman's Right to Choose and The National Abortion Campaign began to counter SPUC.

A poll of 1221 general practitioners in 1973 showed 52 per cent supported the 1967 Act and equal numbers of the rest wanted some restraint or further liberalisation. Only 6 per cent of all respondents would never refer a woman for abortion, while a third would act on request. By 1975 only 14 per cent of 600 general practitioners thought the 1967 Act was a 'tragic mistake', while 60 per cent believed it a 'reasonable compromise' and 22 per cent 'a major advance'.

The constitution of the Select Committee set up to review the White Bill followed normal parliamentary practice and reflected the vote in the Chamber of the House, but the under-representation of women members (3 out of 15) was so great that a group of Labour members threatened the unusual parliamentary procedure of a strike, if the selection was not reviewed. The Committee nevertheless struggled on totally and unequally split.[40,41] Finally, it issued a Special Report at the end of the 1974/75 session, summarising the few points of agreement that had emerged: counselling should be encouraged, private-sector fees should be controlled, doctors signing certificates should examine the woman and referral agencies should be approved in the same way as nursing homes. These recommendations are now being implemented. Among the changes involved is an important one of principle: should information required for statistical analysis be disclosed when a doctor falls under suspicion of possible misconduct?

The White Bill fell for lack of parliamentary time at the end of the session. The Select Committee, like the grin on the Cheshire cat, was reconvened in February 1976 by a vote of 313 to 172.

Conclusions

We believe the 1967 Abortion Act has worked well.[44-50] Approximately one in ten women of fertile age in Britain have now taken advantage of the freedom granted by the Act. Nevertheless, many criticisms of the new law and its implementation persist. Undoubtedly, the Act could be made to work even better. It is ill-informed reaction to the liberal legislation that has prevented its better implementation. Fear of criticism has made the DHSS reluctant to permit innovating services and has stifled the dissemination of responsible information.

In 1974 the Lane Committee explicitly recommended the extension of daycare facilities, but such facilities had remained legal only within the NHS, and the DHSS refused to allow non-NHS clinics to perform routine daycare abortions even though the limited NHS experience had been highly satisfactory. Only in February 1976 did the Department first give permission, and even then only on a trial basis, exclusively to the charitable PASs. In fact the provision of daycare facilities in the NHS, the charitable sector and the private sector would undoubtedly encourage earlier abortions and improved safety. It is the regrettably slow reduction in the burden of second-trimester abortions which has left Britain with a higher mortality for legal abortion than countries such as America. In a very real way the backlash against the 1967 Act has harmed the very people it was intended to help because it has been responsible for the late abortions to which it gives so much publicity.

At the root of many of the remaining problems concerning legal abortion in Britain is a basic one of philosophy. Everyone is agreed that the decision to have an abortion is a weighty one. Many general practitioners, gynaecologists and others with experience in abortion counselling have come to believe that the woman herself, when adequately informed of the possible options, nearly always understands the problems confronting her more clearly than is possible for any second party.

Unfortunately the woman seeking abortion is all too often put in the position of having to make out a case and to plead with a doctor whom she feels is reluctant to grant her request. Doctors find themselves in an unsought position of power in deciding issues that are not medical and for which they have had no special training. They are open to being accused either of unreasonably withholding abortion or of practising abortion on demand.

British law permits abortion when it is safer than allowing the pregnancy to continue. Normally this situation exists until at least the twelfth week of pregnancy. We therefore believe that if the woman has made a sober and reasoned decision to seek abortion in early pregnancy, fully understanding the alternatives open to her and having been informed about the nature of the operation, then it is reasonable that she should expect to have her pregnancy terminated. Such a philosophy allows women to obtain abortion in early pregnancy with dignity and compassion and removes the basis for much of the emotional reaction against the 1967 Act.

References

Detailed clinical and sociological studies of legally induced abortion in Britain have been conducted in Aberdeen and are reviewed in *Experience with Abortion: A case Study of North-East Scotland* (1973), ed. G. Horobin. Cambridge University Press, London.

1 *Report of the Committee on the Working of the Abortion Act* (1974), Chairman The Hon. Mrs Justice Lane: vol. I *Report*; vol. II *Statistical Volume*. HMSO, London.

2 Brooks, E. (1973). *This Crowded Kingdom*. Charles Knight & Co., London.

3 Buckle, A. E. R. & Anderson, M. M. (1972). Implementation of the Abortion Act: report on a year's working of abortion clinics and operating sessions. *British Medical Journal*, **3**, 381.

4 Hull, M. G. R., Gordon, C. & Beard, R. W. (1974). The organisation and results of a pregnancy termination service in a National Health Service Hospital. *Journal of Obstetrics and Gynaecology of the British Commonwealth*, **81**, 577.

5 Lewis, S. C., Lal, S., Branch, B. M. & Beard, R. W. (1971). Outpatient termination of pregnancy. *British Medical Journal*, **4**, 606.

6 Maresh, M., Barber, N., Adshead, D. & Rowlands, S. (1974). Why admit abortion patients? *Lancet*, **ii**, 888.

7 Farmer, C. (1971). Mechanism of selection and decision-making in therapeutic abortion. *Journal of Biosocial Science*, **3**, 121.

8 McCance, C. & McCance, P. F. (1971). Abortion or no abortion – what decides? *Journal of Biosocial Science*, **3**, 116.

9 Olley, P. C. (1971). Personality factors and referral for therapeutic abortion. *Journal of Biosocial Science*, **3**, 106.

10 Parry Jones, A. & Grimoldby, M. R. (1973). Abortion Act in Somerset. *British Medical Journal*, **3**, 90.

11 Eames, J. R., Jamieson, J. A. & Hall, J. (1971). A general-practitioner survey of the Abortion Act 1967. *Practitioner*, **206**, 227.

12 Williamson, J. (1972). The problem of abotion. *Journal of the Royal Society of Health*, **2**, 85.

13 Todd, N. A. (1971). Psychiatric experience of the Abortion Act (1967). *British Journal of Psychiatry*, **119**, 489.

14 Ingram, I. M. (1971). Abortion games: an inquiry into the working of the Act. *Lancet*, **ii**, 1197.

15 Compton, P. A., Goldstrom, L. & Goldstrom, J. M. (1974). Religion and abortion in Northern Ireland. *Journal of Biosocial Science*, **6**, 493.

16 Cartwright, A. & Waite, M. (1972). General practitioners and abortion. *Journal of the Royal College of General Practitioners*, **22**, *Suppl.* no. 1.

17 Jeffcoate, T. N. A. & Gibson, H. (1970). *The Times*, 12 February.

18 Lewis, T. L. T. (1969). The Abortion Act. *British Medical Journal*, **1**, 341.

19 *Lancet*, **i**, 26 April 1969.
20 Jeffcoate, T. N. A. & Foot, P. (1970). In *Morals and Medicine*, p. 29. BBC, London.
21 ALRA (1972). Written evidence submitted to the Lane Committee.
22 Kestleman, P. (1970). Personal communication.
23 Diggory, P. C. L. (1969). Some experiences of therapeutic abortion, *Lancet*, **i**, 873.
24 Ingham, C. & Simms, M. (1972). Study of applicants for abortion at the Royal Northern Hospital, London. *Journal of Biosocial Science*, **4**, 351.
25 Goodhart, C. B. (1970). Abortion problems. *Proceedings of the Royal Institution of Great Britain*, **43**, 378.
26 *Catholic Herald*, 22 May 1970.
27 Simms, M. (1970). The great foetus mystery. *New Scientist*, **48**, 592.
28 *Report of the Committee on the Working of the Abortion Act* (1974), Chairman The Hon. Mrs Justice Lane: vol. III. *Survey of Abortion Patients for the Committee on the Working of the Abortion Act* by Ann Cartwright and Susan Lucas. HMSO, London.
29 Simms, M. (1973). *Report on Non-Medical Abortion Counselling*. Birth Control Trust, London.
30 *OPCS Monitor*, November 1975. Office of Population Census and Surveys, London.
31 Godber, G. E. (1972). Abortion deaths. *British Medical Journal*, **3**, 424.
32 Soskice, D. W. & Trussel, T. J. (1973). Effects of the Abortion Act. *British Journal of Hospital Medicine*, **9**, 299.
33 Lewis, E. M. (1975). The report on confidential enquiries into maternal deaths, England and Wales, 1970–72. *Health Trends*, **9**, 51.
34 Thompson, B. (1975). Statistics of abortions in the U.K. (In preparation.)
35 *Windsor Weekly Express*, 16 November 1970.
36 *The Times*, 21 September 1970.
37 *Hansard* (1975). **886**(73), cols. II 505–6.
38 Chalmers, I. & Anderson, A. (1972). Factors affecting gestational age at therapeutic abortion. *Lancet*, **1**, 1324.
39 Ashdown-Sharp, P. (1975). Abortion: how we won the battle and nearl, lost the war. *Nova*, October, 62.
40 Munday, D. (1975). The abortion debate. *Family Planning*, **24**, 17.
41 Simms, M. (1975). The progress of the Abortion (Amendment) Bill. *Family Planning*, **24**, 32.
42 Litchfield, M. & Kentish, S. (1973). *Babies for Burning*. Serpentine Press, London.
43 Gillie, O., Wallace, M., Ashdown-Sharp, P. & Zimmerman, L. (1975). Abortion horror tales revealed as fantasies. *Sunday Times*, 30 March.
44 Diggory, P. L. C., Peel, J. & Potts, D. M. (1970). Preliminary assessment of the 1967 Abortion Act in practice. *Lancet*, **i**, 287.

45 Baird, D. (1970). *The Abortion Act: The Advantages and Disadvantages*. Royal Society of Health, London.

46 Diggory, P. L. C. & Simms, M. (1970). Two years after the Abortion Act. *New Scientist*, **48**, 261.

47 Potts, D. M. (1971). Impact of English abortion laws on the practice of medicine. *Advances in Planned Parenthood*, **6**, 145.

48 Lafitte, F. (1972). *Abortion in Britain Today*. British Pregnancy Advisory Service, Birmingham.

49 Simms, M. (1973). How do we judge the Abortion Act? Reflections on the Lane Committee and the 1967 Abortion Act. *Public Health, London*, **87**, 155.

50 Simms, M. (1974). Abortion law and medical freedom. *British Journal of Criminology*, **14**, 118.

10
The American revolution

The changes which took place in Britain and the Commonwealth during the 1960s and early 70s, while rapid compared with previous experience, were tortoise-like beside events soon to follow in the USA. The movement for liberal abortion started more slowly there, but in the space of six years went from modest reform, in some states, to total repeal in others and ended with a revolutionary judgement by the Federal Supreme Court. The Supreme Court strongly asserted the rights of the pregnant woman and carefully limited the role of the State with respect to the woman and her fetus, producing a profoundly new abortion situation in the USA – and the world.

A key factor in the choice of the Supreme Court Justices, when they were presented with strongly held and apparently irreconcilable views, lay in the eighteenth- and nineteenth-century history of abortion law and practice.

The Constitution (1789) and the Bill of Rights (the first ten Amendments) speak of 'persons' who have 'constitutional rights', and it is reasonable to ask if a fetus is such a 'person'. This does not appear to have been the intention of the first Congress. The American colonies had taken over the public and legal practice of England and for several decades after the ratification of the Constitution there was no prohibition against abortion prior to quickening. Moreover, the first census in 1790 required the 'whole number of persons' in each state to be counted and to be enumerated according to sex: clearly fetuses were not counted. An effort to insert the phrase 'from the moment of conception' after the word 'person' was defeated on a voice vote in the Constitutional Convention of 1967. After quickening, some legal rights are implied and New York State laws still carry a statute requiring that a woman whose fetus has quickened is not to be executed until she has delivered. If a fetus is injured, a wrongful death action is possible, but it brings benefits to the parents not the fetus. A legal fiction is used with respect to property rights, which are partly recognised by American law, but can only be enjoyed when the fetus is born alive.[1,2]

Abortion appears to have remained a legal, but rarely used, possibility in a number of states early in the nineteenth century. Christopher Tietze, the medical epidemiologist and member of the Population Council, and Cyril Means, professor at New York Law School, were largely responsible for unravelling the early nineteenth-century history of abortion attitudes and Mr Justice Blackmun, who drafted the Supreme Court judgement, has commented upon the significance of this evidence in the Justices' conclusions. When most criminal abortion laws were first enacted, the procedure was a hazardous one for the woman. In New York State between 1803 and 1828 eight therapeutic terminations were performed. In three cases the women died, representing a mortality rate ten times greater than that found in hospitals dealing with obstetric complications due to childbirth. It is not surprising that it was for reasons of safety, rather than for moral reasons, that the state abortion legislation was made more restrictive in 1828.[3] In fact, the legislative report that led to the Act recommended banning most types of surgery. As late as 1858 a New Jersey judge stated that the role of abortion legislation was 'not to prevent the procuring of abortions so much as to guard the health and life of the mother against the consequences of such attempts'. Sauer,[4] quoting Storer's book of 1860 *On Criminal Abortion in America*, writes, 'the common law and many State laws almost wholly ignored early fetal life and viewed abortion as an offence against the mother'.

The US Supreme Court in reviewing the evolution of abortion laws in various states concluded:

> it is thus apparent that at common law, at the time of the
> adoption of our Constitution, throughout the major portion of
> the nineteenth century, abortion was viewed with less disfavour
> than under most American statutes currently in effect. Phrasing
> it another way, a woman enjoyed a substantially broader right
> to terminate a pregnancy than she does in most states today. At
> least with respect to the early stage of pregnancy, and very
> possibly without such a limitation, the opportunity to make
> this choice was present in this country well into the nineteenth
> century.[5]

The Supreme Court argued that restrictive abortion laws discriminate against women, violating the Fourteenth Amendment to the Constitution, which grants equal rights to all citizens. However, Rehnquist, one of the dissenting judges in the Supreme Court ruling, pointed out that the Fourteenth Amendment was passed in 1868, while the first restrictive abortion legislation took place in Connecticut in 1821. Thirty-six states had anti-abortion laws by the time of the Fourteenth Amendment, and apparently there 'was no question concerned in the validity of this provision or of any of the other State Statutes when the Fourteenth Amendment was adopted.'

The American Medical Association (AMA) was more active than its British counterpart in reviewing the problem of illegal abortion in the ninteenth century. A Committee on Criminal Abortion reported to the annual meeting of the Association in 1859 after two years' analysis. It found it to be a problem of 'frightful extent'. The Committee continued to make submissions and in 1871 recommended that it should 'be unlawful and unprofessional for any physician to induce abortion or premature labor, without the concurrent opinion of at least one respectable consulting physician, and then always with a view to the safety of the child – if that be possible.'[6] The report, like the earlier one, was one in which concern for morality overcame concern for epidemiology. The medical profession was exhorted to join hands with clergymen in denouncing 'the perverted views of morality entertained by a large class of females – aye, and men also – on this important question'. It concluded with the words, 'We had to deal with human life. In a matter of less importance we could entertain no compromise. An honest judge on the bench would call things by their proper names. We could do no less.'

American professional attitudes a century ago were summed up by Hodge: 'If. . . the profession in former times, from the imperfect state of their knowledge had, in any degree, undervalued the importance of fetal life, they have fully redeemed their error and now they call upon the legislatures of our land. . . to stay the progress of this destructive evil of criminal abortion.'[7]

Eventually restrictive laws were enacted in every state, beginning with Missouri, 1835; Ohio, 1841; Iowa, 1834; and West Virginia, 1848. The details differed: in Kansas the guilty abortionist was imprisoned for one year, in Mississippi for 20 years. In 15 states the pregnant woman herself could be found guilty. In some states, health considerations continued to figure in statutes and, for example in the District of Columbia, abortion was allowed to preserve the woman's 'health' as well as her 'life'. The movement reached its apogee in the late nineteenth century under Anthony Comstock, who tried to impose his own brand of morality and in particular his hatred of any aspect of birth control – contraception as well as abortion – on his fellow citizens by legislation.

As in Europe, the anti-abortion legislation was weakly enforced; the rich bought the services of doctors, but the poor suffered heavily. It was this suffering which inspired Margaret Sanger in her crusade for contraception (p. 11). She, and other far-sighted Americans, slowly made family planning acceptable to the lay public and medical profession. She went on to become the first president of the International Planned Parenthood Federation. However, the movement for abortion law reform ran more than a generation behind that for contraceptive availability. In the 1960s one hospital in California performed less than one abortion per 1000 deliveries. It was felt the abortion review committee at the hospital reduced 'the number of requests for therapeutic abortion and provides impersonal judgement on applications'.[8] In 1966 the Downstate Hospital in New York, which serves a populous but poor area, performed five therapeutic abortions: in the same year there were 5848 births and 2436 abortion admissions in the hospital, many of which were known to be the result of illegal operations.

Movement for reform

The first American known to have justified therapeutic abortion on social grounds in the twentieth century was W. J. Robinson.[9] In 1911 he spoke of the need to abort some premarital pregnancies, and in 1933 he went so far as to suggest repeal of all restrictions on abortion, except those relating to health – the stance to be adopted by the Supreme Court exactly 40 years later.

State responsibility for abortion legislation made attempts at reform appear a formidable undertaking but groups of interested people began to lobby for reform in the 1950s. In the 1960s the Association for the Study of Abortion assumed national leadership, bringing a high standard of academic analysis to bear on the problem.

A great deal of interest and public sympathy was aroused in 1962 by the case of Sherri Finkbine, a television personality from Phoenix, Arizona, who sought an abortion because she had taken thalidomide. Refused in the USA, she was eventually terminated in Sweden.[10] Over the next two years many thousands of congenitally abnormal babies were born during a rubella (German measles) epidemic, further focusing attention on the abortion issue. This time (1962) the American Law Institute (ALI) suggested a model penal code to legalise abortion: 'that continuation of pregnancy would greatly impair the physical or mental health of the mother, or that the child would be born with grave physical or mental defect, or that the pregnancy resulted from rape, incest or other felonious intercourse.'[11] The model code became accepted as a goal by many reform groups.

The year 1967 became the turning point in the USA as it was in the UK. Colorado passed a reform Bill based on the ALI recommendations. The foundations of public support for reform were widened, and a resolution passed by the Central Conference of American Rabbis in June of that year is typical: the Conference considered it 'religiously valid and humane' to seek legislative changes and called upon 'our members to work towards this end'. 'The preservation of a mother's emotional health' was considered to be 'as important as her physical well-being'. But while the ALI model code was receiving support, a new and more radical series of arguments began to be heard. In the middle of 1967, the American Civil Liberties Union discussed abortion law reform. Their model statute was a radical departure from the traditions embodied in the ALI model statute, stating, 'It is a civil right of a woman to seek to terminate a pregnancy, and of a physician to perform or refuse to perform an abortion, without threat of criminal sanctions. Abortions should be performed only by doctors, governed by the same considerations as other medical practices.'

In 1973 this argument became the main plank in the Supreme Court ruling which struck down all restrictive abortion laws in the USA.

As thinking on abortion developed, practical innovations also began to evolve. Early in 1967 Rev. Howard Moody began the first Clergy Counseling Service in New York involving Protestant and Jewish clergy in giving practical assistance (including referral, if necessary) to doctors operating outside the law. It was an event that aroused public sympathy, assisted in the education of professional groups and greatly aided the implementation of changes in the law, when these occurred. Later the same year, Rev. Hugh Anwyl, a Welsh-born Congregational minister who had moved to Hollywood, opened a Clergy Counseling Service for Problem Pregnancies in Los Angeles. On the day it opened, 293 telephone calls were received and in the first 10 days 175 women had been counselled.[12] Experience in these services exposed many clergymen to a problem that previously had been partly invisible and the volume of work itself created a pressure for reform. Roman Catholic priests were amongst those who referred women to the Counseling Services. However, the involvement of the clergy was not always without its tensions and did not always validate the enterprise.

Reform and repeal

For four years, State laws on abortion changed more rapidly than the figures on a cricket score board. Between 1967 and 1971, 17 states either reformed or repealed their laws. Some variation in the duration of pregnancy that could legally be terminated, in the need for consent by third parties and in residency requirements arose. But, during the first three years of change, a major element in the new legislation was always some, or all, of the ALI recommendations. The influence of British legislation was also apparent, both in the timing of reforms and in the wording of the new laws. In Oregon, for example, the law used the British phrase, 'account may be taken of the mother's total environment, actual or reasonably foreseeable'.

California was the most important amongst the first generation of reformed state laws. It was also the state where some of the weaknesses of the reformed laws came to be much publicised. On the whole, the medical profession interpreted the new laws cautiously and some legislators, and many women, were disappointed at the small number of legal abortions performed, especially as these did not appear to relieve the burden of criminal abortions. For example, in Colorado the number of legal terminations rose from 50 to 1000 per annum, but the criminal abortion rate remained at an estimated 10000 per annum. In Georgia fewer legal abortions were performed after the reform of the law than before. Some hospitals set up abortion committees to deliberate on individual cases, thereby causing unreasonable delays. Generally therapeutic abortion continued to be more common among the socially privileged than among the medically indigent.[13]

However, almost before the new laws had come into being, a second generation of legislation was being canvassed. Instead of defining the grounds under which abortions could be performed, a movement towards the total repeal of abortion legislation got under way. Abortion was now to be a matter for decision between a woman and her physician alone. A burst of repeal legislation was introduced in Georgia, Massachusetts, Michigan, Pennsylvania, Oklahoma, Maryland, Hawaii, Alaska, New York and Washington States. Hawaii was the first state to repeal its law, doing so on 24 February 1970. Abortion was limited to women who had resided in the state for three months or longer. In Alaska and Maryland, repeal bills also passed the state legislatures. On 18 April 1970 Governor Miller of Alaska vetoed the new legislation, but his veto was later over-ruled. Colorado, which had pioneered reform, saw a repeal law defeated by only one vote. In Maryland, which also had reformed its law in 1968, a repeal notion was passed by 23 votes to 18 in the Senate and by 78 votes to 43 in the House of Delegates, only to be set aside by the Governor Mandel on a technicality.

New York State

The most spectacular events of all took place in New York and Washington States. The state legislatures in the USA have some of the characteristics of the eighteenth-century British parliament. Some meet for only limited periods of the year, members often combine their office with more or less full-time employment and statesmanship is not always of the highest quality. In New York in 1959 a reform Bill based on the ALI recommendations failed to progress, partly as a result of a very emotional speech by a Republican member who was confined to a wheel chair because of poliomyelitis (and not, as some newspapers suggested, because of congenital deformity).

Probably the strongest single political voice for reform was that of Governor Rockefeller, later to become Vice-President of the USA. He pressed for change behind the scenes. Rockefeller's concern with abortion went back several years. In 1968 he appointed a Commission to examine and recommend changes in the state abortion law. Dr Alan F. Guttmacher, president of Planned Parenthood/World Population, was a persuasive and important member of that Commission and he recalled how Rockefeller convened the first meeting with the words, 'I am not asking *whether* New York's abortion law should be changed, I am asking *how* it should be changed.'[14] Rockefeller persuaded the leader of the Senate, Bridges, to draft a repeal Bill (Bridges himself was a Catholic and was to vote against the measure).

Both opponents and supporters were surprised in the middle of March 1970 when the repeal Bill passed by 31 votes to 26 in the State Senate and was only defeated by 73 votes to 71 in the State Assembly. Two members who supported the Bill then had their votes declared void by the Speaker, Mr Duryea, because they were not in the chamber, despite the well-established tradition of the New York State Assembly that waives the need for members to be in their seats when a vote is taken. Paradoxically, Duryea himself had promised to vote for the Bill in the event of a tie. The opponents tried to prevent a second vote and once again the action of the Speaker was crucial. This time he made the unique demand that every Assemblyman should be present and requested 12 absent members to be rounded up 'by whatever force necessary'. The assembly dissolved in confusion. When the full house did assemble and voted for a second time the repeal Bill passed by one vote, George M. Michaels, his hands trembling, declared: 'I realise, Mr Speaker, that I am terminating my political career, but I cannot in good conscience sit there and allow my vote to be the one that defeats this Bill – I ask my vote to be changed from "no" to "yes".' He continued sobbing: 'my son called me a whore for voting against the Bill and my other son begged me not to let my vote be the one that defeated the Bill'.

Earlier in the debate a woman had had to be removed for shouting from the public gallery: 'Murderers. You are murderers, that's what you are. God will punish you.' When the Bill passed, however, the onlookers applauded. Voting cut across political parties but, as in Britain, the vote of the left (18 out of 24 Democrats voted 'yea') was larger than that of the right (13 out of 33 Republicans voted 'yea').

The repeal movement in the State Assembly had been led by Mrs Constance Cook, a Republican member and a calm, patient woman of 50, married with two children. She was assisted by a Democrat, Al Blumenthal. Opposition came from the Catholic Church, and

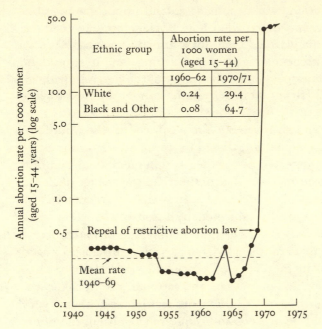

Fig. 43. Legal abortions in New York City (1940–74). (Note that the annual abortion rate is plotted on a log scale.)

State Medical Society and others. As had been the case in Britain, opposition groups to abortion reform attempted to mobilise public opinion too late. A pastoral letter read in 1700 churches between the two votes strongly condemned those who had voted for the Bill, which incidentally included some Catholics.

Following the Bill, George Michaels lost his seat – as he had predicted. So did Senator Dominick, the chief sponsor of the Bill in the upper House. A Bill repealing the Blaine Amendment (which forbade public money to be paid towards the support of religious schools) was passed and it was rumoured that political 'horsetrading' involving this and the abortion legislation occurred.

Washington State

The change of the abortion law in Washington State, later in 1970, was less dramatic than it had been in New York, but more revealing of public attitudes. The constitution of this north-western state of America allows the voter a great deal of participation in decision-making. Citizens can initiate public ballots, or the state legislature can pass on an issue for public decision. Anxious to avoid deciding on a controversial issue, the legislature handed over to referendum a Bill to reform the then current 1909 abortion law. The Bill permitted abortion up to 16 weeks of pregnancy for any state resident, providing the operation was performed in an accredited hospital or approved place, and if the husband (or guardian in the case of an unmarried girl under 18) gave permission. Aware that a unique test of contemporary public opinion on abortion was to be carried out, supporters and opposition mounted a vigorous campaign the Non-Sectarian Committee for Life, the Voice for the Unborn, the Washington Citizens for Abortion Reform, the Planned Parenthood/World Population and Population Dynamics all entered the arena. The last used newspaper advertisement with the simple slogans such as 'Isn't it Crazy – It's *Your* Vote but *Her* Pregnancy?' The Non-Sectarian Committee for Life was more poetic in its copy: 'Women do not create human life – together with man they merely pass on, from century to century, from conception to death, The Walk of Mankind through Time.' The Voice for the Unborn took large billboards for its posters, which displayed a four-month human fetus held in an adult hand with the words 'Kill Referendum 20 Not Me!'

The need to reform the abortion law was argued in the Official Voters' Pamphlet as a basic human right, as an end to hypocrisy, as 'prevention of cruelty to mothers' and to children, and as a socially humane measure which had the support of doctors, lawyers and clergy. It was opposed as 'a giant step backward for mankind'. The experience of abortion law in Britain was quoted in campaign literature, and speeches by Sir John Peel, President of the Royal College of Obstetricians and Gynaecologists, London, were reproduced by the Voice for the Unborn.

On 3 November 1970 the 1 260 000 voters of Washington State, in a democratic orgy, chose 47 State Representatives, 4 State Senators, a Federal Representative and decided on such issues as to whether 'non-refundable beverage receptacles' should be prohibited or the voting age lowered to 19. Nine hundred thousand people voted on abortion and the law passed by a majority of 56 per cent. Details of the ballot are, of course, secret, but inspection of the trial polls showed that people were expressing genuine conviction, largely uninfluenced by religion. However, abortion is a complex topic, even at the time of a secret ballot. In Spokane County, unlike most

others in the State of Washington, a majority (58 per cent) voted
against liberal abortion. But since repeal, the inhabitants of Spokane
have had an above average recourse to the law they opposed (222
legal abortions to 1000 live births versus a state average of 193).[15]

The end of state reform

As the number of states permitting liberal abortion increased
and the number of legal abortions performed climbed, so the pressure for abortion law reform in the remaining states slackened. In
addition, a politically effective counter movement arose. In 1972,
only one state, Florida, enacted liberal legislation. The bitterness
of the battles that took place increased, including harsh personal
allegations. For example, Pennsylvania State is 35 per cent Catholic,
and in 1972 two Bills were presented to the legislature: a liberal
reform Bill and a conservative Bill restricting abortion to cases where
three physicians certified the operation necessary to preserve the
woman's life. Cardinal Krol supported the Bill permitting abortion
to save the mother's life as a political manoeuvre to defeat the more
liberal legislation. The ploy succeeded, but the liberal Democratic
Governor Milton Shapp, vetoed the legislation in December 1972
as 'unsound, unenforceable and totally unfair'. During the public
debate on the issue, a local female politician, Patricia Arney, revealed
that she had had an affair with Catholic State Senator Henry
Cianfrani, a notable opponent of the liberal Bill and that he had paid
for her to have an abortion in 1970. Cianfrani denied the allegation,
but admitted giving Arney money.[16]

In February 1972 the American Bar Association drafted a Uniform
Abortion Act, which was approved by the Conference of Commissioners on Uniform State Laws, but it did not lead to anything.
One attempt was made to change abortion laws by Congressional
action. Republican Senator Robert Packwood from Oregon, proposed a Federal abortion law using the Ninth Amendment to the
Constitution (which assures the citizen's fundamental right to
privacy) to over-rule state laws, but the approach failed and nationwide uniformity, when it arrived, came from another quarter.

The courts

The Federal Supreme Court has the capacity to over-ride decisions made by state courts and, if appropriate, to declare statute laws unconstitutional. In the case of the anti-contraceptive legislation, important precedents were set when higher courts declared certain state laws to be unconstitutional (*Griswold* v. *Connecticut* and *Baird* v. *Massachusetts*). Proponents of abortion law reform were eager to use court decisions to help change attitudes and practice and, in particular, to use the Supreme Court to alter practice throughout the nation at a stroke.

The first important decision at state level was made in the case of *Belous* v. *California*. Dr Leon Belous had been convicted of referring a patient to a doctor performing illegal abortions, but in September 1969 the State Supreme Court reversed the sentence of the lower court on the grounds that the Californian law was unconstitutional. However, such was the pace of change that the law under which Belous had been convicted had been reformed before the case was heard. The Federal Supreme Court refused to review the case and therefore the precedent was of only tangential significance. The California judiciary also over-ruled an action taken by the State Board of Medical Examiners in disciplining nine gynaecologists for terminating pregnancies in women who had rubella. It was held that the Board of Examiners had violated the Fourteenth Amendment.

During 1970 and 1971, an avalanche of cases came before all levels of courts, some attempting to create a more liberal situation and others attempting to halt or reverse changes taking place. In Michigan, South Dakota, Georgia, Wisconsin and Texas, laws were challenged as unconstitutional and stuck down by at least one level of jurisdiction. In Wisconsin the law was also found to infringe the right to privacy granted under the Ninth Amendment.

Late in 1969, Judge Gesell in the District of Columbia (the administrative area containing the capital, Washington) declared that the existing abortion law was 'unconstitutionally vague' in the case of *US* v. *Vuitch*. The case allowed Preterm Inc., one of the most efficient and humane abortion clinics in the USA, to open within a few blocks of the White House.

In October 1972 the US Court of Appeals over-rode an attempt to restrict abortion procedures to facilities that could ensure a 24-hour stay for the woman, as it might 'result in irreparable injury to the parties at whom the Regulation is directed'.

Jane Roe and Mary Doe

By 1971, 17 cases relating to abortion had been referred to the Supreme Court. The Supreme Court chose to consider the constitutional challenge presented by the Texan law an abortion, which had been in effect for approximately a century and typified nineteenth-century attitudes towards termination of pregnancy, and the Georgian statute, which had been passed in 1968 in the first wave of reform and was similar to the 1967 British Act. Despite the liberal precedents that had been established in the previous three years, most observers were unprepared for the ruling given on 22 January 1973.[5] One of the Justices forming the majority opinion, William Brennan, was a Roman Catholic.

An anonymous unmarried woman (known in the Supreme Court under the pseudonym of Jane Roe) in good health from Dallas, Texas, claimed that the Texas statutes were 'unconstitutionally vague' and that they took away her right to personal privacy as protected in the First, Fourth, Fifth, Ninth and Fourteenth Amendments of the Constitution. The case was supported by a married couple, in which the wife was suffering from 'a neuro-chemical' disorder, where pregnancy would not threaten her life but should be postponed. Of course the pregnancies concerned had finished by the time the cases had completed their legal gestation and the Supreme Court pointed out that if the end of pregnancy made 'a case moot, pregnancy litigation seldom will survive much beyond the trial stage, and appellate review will be effectively denied. Our law should not be that rigid.'

The Supreme Court reviewed the laws with respect to the Fourteenth and Ninth Amendments. They concluded 'that the right of personal privacy includes the abortion decision, but that this right is not unqualified and must be considered against important state interest in regulation'.

The Supreme Court had to consider the appellant's contention that the fetus is a person 'within the language and meaning of the Fourteenth Amendment'. The Court pointed out that the Constitution only uses the word 'person' in situations where it is unequivocally referring to an individual already born and concludes, considering the historical background of the situation already referred to above, that 'the word "person", as used in the Fourteenth Amendment, does not include the unborn'. They tempered this conclusion with the observation that 'It is reasonable and appropriate for a state to decide that at some point in time another interest, that of the health of the mother or her potential human life, becomes significantly involved. The woman's privacy is no longer sole and any right of privacy she protests must be measured accordingly.' With wisdom the Court decided, 'we need not resolve the difficult question of when life begins. When those trained in the respective disciplines of medicine, philosophy and theology are unable to arrive at any consensus, the judiciary, at this point in the development of man's knowledge, is not in a position to speculate as to the answer'.

In a separate statement Mr Justice Clark wrote:

> to say that life is present at conception is to given recognition to the potential, rather than the actual...but the law deals in reality not obscurity – the known rather than the unknown. When sperm meets egg, life may eventually form, but quite often it does not. The law does not deal in speculation. The phenomenon of life takes time to develop, and until it is actually present, it cannot be destroyed. Its interruption prior to formation would hardly be homicide, and as we have seen, society does not regard it as such. The rites of baptism are not performed and death certificates are not required when a miscarriage occurs. No prosecutor has ever returned a murder indictment charging the taking of the life of a fetus.

The Court drew upon the field of tort to show that, prior to viability, courts had been reluctant to recognise legal rights for the fetus. It summarised much of its thinking in the following paragraph:

> We do not agree that, by adopting one theory of life, Texas may override the rights of the pregnant woman that are at stake. We repeat, however, that the state does have an important and legitimate interest in preserving and protecting the health of the pregnant woman, whether she be a resident of the state or a non-resident, who seeks medical consultation and treatment there, and that there is still *another* important and legitimate interest in protecting the potentiality of human life. These interests are separate and distinct. Each grows in substantiality as the woman approaches term and, at a point in pregnancy, each becomes 'compelling'.

The Court considered that these interests become 'compelling' at the end of the first trimester. At this point the state may set up regulations concerning the qualifications of the person to perform abortion and facilities where it is performed. Prior to that time the attending physician, 'in consultation with his patient, is free to determine, without regulation by the State, that in his medical judgment the patient's pregnancy should be terminated. If that decision is reached, the judgment may be effectuated by an abortion free of interference by the state'. The Court further ruled that, 'if the state is interested in protecting fetal life after viability, it may go as far as to proscribe abortion during that period except when it is necessary to preserve the life or health of the mother'.

The Court took into account its ruling on Jane Roe when considering Mary Doe and the Georgia statutes. Mrs Doe had three children and was pregnant again by the age of 22, she lived in poverty and her older children were in care. An abortion was sought on the grounds that she could not support a new child, but rejected by the Abortion Committee of the Grade Memorial Hospital, Atlanta. Problems concerning the Joint Commission on Accreditation of Hospitals, of abortion committees and of two doctors being concurrent in a procedure were all raised, and each one was ruled unconstitutional. The court quoted a study that showed that the mean time for preparing documentation on a woman seeking an abortion was 15 days. The Georgia law involved a residency requirement which was also declared unconstitutional. The Court rejected the argument that the nineteenth-century laws were designed to discourage illicit sexual conduct, pointing out that they failed to distinguish between the married and unmarried mother.

Mr Justice Blackmun, a Republican appointed to the Supreme Court by President Nixon in 1970, drafted and delivered the decisions in the Georgian and Texan cases. As noted earlier, he had been influenced by the historical arguments presented by the appellants. He researched much of the literature himself, working in the library of the Mayo Clinic, Minnesota, and in the Royal Society of Medicine, London. There is an apocryphal story that when he circulated the draft he suggested that his colleagues avoided modifications because he had worked every detail so thoroughly. It is said that the Justices, on reviewing the evidence, felt they 'had no choice' but to arrive at the judgement they did.

Mr Justice Douglas, 75, the oldest member of the Court and a

Democrat, concurred in the Texas and Georgia opinions and added comments from the celebrated Griswold case on contraception and the Vuitch and Belous cases on abortion. Douglas placed the freedom to have an abortion beside the freedom to choose one's own marriage partner, the right to procreation, the liberty to direct the education of one's children and the privacy of marital relations. He wrote:

> elaborate argument is hardly necessary to demonstrate that childbirth may deprive a woman of her preferred life style and force upon her a radically different and undesired future. For example, rejected applicants under the Georgia Statute are required to endure the discomforts of pregnancy; to incur the pain, higher mortality rate and after effects of childbirth; to abandon educational plans; to sustain loss of income; to forgo the satisfaction of careers; to tax further mental and physical health in providing child care; and in some cases, to bear the lifelong stigma of unwed motherhood, a badge that may haunt, if not deter, later legitimate family relationships.

Two Justices, Mr White and Mr Rehnquist, the former a Kennedy and the latter a Nixon nominee, dissented. They called the judgement 'an improvident and extravagant exercise of the power of judicial review which the Constitution extends to this Court'. Rehnquist claimed that that Court departed from the long-standing admonition that it should never 'formulate a rule of Constitutional law broader than is required by the precise facts to which it is to be applied'. The two dissenting Judges found:

> nothing in the language or history of the Constitution to support the Court's judgment. The Court simply fashions and announces a new Constitutional right for pregnant mothers and, with scarcely any reason or authority for its action, invests that right with sufficient substance to override most existing State abortion statutes. The upshot is that the people and legislators of the 50 States are Constitutionally disentitled to weigh the relative importance of the continued existence and development of the fetus on the one hand against the spectrum of possible impact on the mother on the other hand.

Cardinals Cooke and Krol reacted to the Supreme Court decision in public statements. Krol said 'it is hard to think of any decision in the 200 years of our history which has had more disastrous implications for the stability of a civilized society'. He called the ruling 'bad logic and bad law'. Cooke asked the question 'how many millions of children prior to their birth will never see the light of day because of the shocking action of the majority of the United States Supreme Court today?'

Tort and contract

A potent legal force for limiting practice in the USA is less obvious, but most important. Increasingly, medical practice in America is influenced by the possibility of the patient suing the doctor on grounds which, in most countries, would not be considered evidence of negligence. Unnecessary medical tests are commonly carried out because past legal suits, rather than strictly medical indications, have established certain procedural patterns. Attorneys specialise in advising patients in litigation against doctors, and the successful obstetrician may pay over $20000 annually in insurance against malpractice suits. If any significant tradition of suing following the unpredictable hazards of termination arises, the paradox may yet come about where physicians look back wistfully to the old restrictive, but poorly enforced, legislation. It is, after all, very difficult for a patient to bring a malpractice suit against an illegal abortionist.

Implementation

The practical way in which the new American legislation was implemented was even more remarkable than the rate and degree of change in law and attitudes (Fig. 44). By mid-1971 in New York State alone, one year after the repeal, more legal abortions had been performed than had been carried out in the whole of Britain during the three years after the 1967 Act.

In nearly all states where records are available the legal abortion rate doubled in 1970 (Fig. 18, p. 76). This was true where the ratio of abortions to deliveries had been high for some time, as in Oregon, or where it had always been low, as in Georgia. Hawaii proved to be an exception in the legal abortion rate and the number of operations rose to a plateau almost as soon as the law was repealed.[17] However, even here medical attitudes continued to relax, and four months after repeal, 10 hospitals were performing abortions, while after 9 months there were 13.

The availability of abortion on request in New York State was

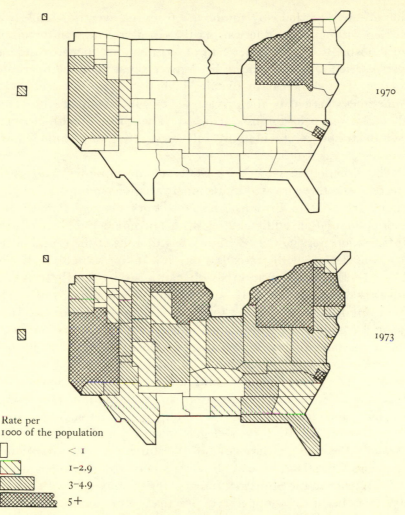

Fig. 44. Rate of legal abortions per 1000 women (aged 15–49) in the USA (1970 and 1973), by state of residence. The area of each state is proportional to the population. Total legal abortions in 1970 = 900 000.

influential throughout the country. Women from every other state of the Union, as well as from a number of foreign countries, came to New York. In 19 of the eastern states the ratio of legal abortions to deliveries was over 1 : 10, largely as a result of terminations obtained by residents of those states who travelled to New York. In another eight states the ratio exceeded 1 : 20.

The very heavy load of termination cases in New York, which

literally arrived daily by jumbo jet from all over the USA, was carried without an undue waiting list. In March 1971 in the municipal hospitals, where 99 per cent of terminations on state residents were carried out, the waiting list between first visit and operation was 12 to 14 days. As in Britain, high fees ($250 upwards) were sometimes charged in the private sector, but about one in five of all cases was paid for by Medicaid. The City's Health Services Administrator commented in July 1971, 'the catastrophe many foresaw a year ago failed to materialize.'

The situation in New York State set up nationwide pressures analogous to those created by regional variations in implementation of the 1967 Act in Britain. The New York Planned Parenthood/World Population affiliation set up a telephone Family Planning Information Service that, within a few months of the repeal of the law, was dealing with 300 calls a day at a 16-line switchboard. The City Health Administration also began a service and both bodies advertised on the New York subways in English and Spanish. The most original service was set up by Zero Population Growth Inc., using a computer to store data about operating doctors and, with the American panache for acronyms, called AID Bank (Abortion Information Data).

As already noted, Clergy Counseling Services were important in changing attitudes towards abortion, and they continued to provide a responsible channel of referral under the new laws. By mid-1971 it was estimated that 75000 legal abortions had been obtained through the Clergy Services. In Washington State the Young Women's Christian Association was a site of abortion referrals.

Even prior to the Supreme Court ruling, some states with restrictive laws began to adopt liberal practices. For example, in Pittsburgh, Pennsylvania, one big hospital had a 23-fold increase in terminations in a three-year period, solely because of changes in medical attitudes. Interestingly, the operations performed were done by only 4 out of 63 staff obstetricians and 5 out of 158 consultants.[18]

Administration

Hospital services in the USA can be divided into two main categories. First, there are government hospitals run by the community, state or Federal agencies, non-sectarian voluntary hospitals run by a board of directors, and hospitals run by religious groups.

None of this group of hospitals is run for profit, and patients pay either full or reduced fees, which may be wholly or partially covered by insurance. Within this group it is up to the individual hospital to determine its attitude towards abortion and a great deal of variation is found. Secondly, there are proprietary hospitals where patients pay standard fees and the hospital is run at a profit to those who invested in setting up the services. In general, these hospitals tend to adopt more liberal attitudes to abortion than the municipal hospitals.

The cost of termination has often been high and no doubt has been a cause of hardship for many, forcing some women to seek an alternative solution to their problems. However, this problem is a recurrent one in American health care and has been no worse, and perhaps in some cases slightly better, in the field of abortion than for many other operations. Some private charitable organisations have run clinics charging $100–$250. In Hawaii the normal cost for the paying patient is $300.

In April 1971, the New York State Social Services Commissioner, G. K. Wyman disallowed Medicaid payments to hospitals for abortion cases on situations other than to save a woman's life. However, in August 1972, after legal arguments conducted at a number of levels, a three-judge Constitutional Court ruled that to stop Medicaid 'would deny indigent women the equal protection of the laws to which they are constitutionally entitled . . . no interest of the state is served by the arbitrary discriminations'. The Court also upheld an earlier precedent that the fetus *cannot* receive legal protection under the American Constitution. Some personal health insurance plans provided for abortion, although unexplained geographical anomalies arose (for example, Blue Shield insurance in Dallas covers abortion, but in many other areas does not). All Federal employees' health benefit programmes, which cover about eight million people, allow for expenses in connection with legal abortions.[19]

The incentive to watch costs is far greater and more direct in the USA than in Britain and may be the reason why technical innovations that save time and money have been more readily accepted in the USA. Within the British National Health Service the choice of technique and bed usage is wholly under the jurisdiction of the hospital consultant and he is not responsible for costing the services provided. Indeed, in a London teaching hospital in 1971, the management committee refused a senior surgeon's request to experiment with outpatient abortions, while in New York hospital managements have actively encouraged doctors to use the simplest techniques. Constant attention to costs may not always lead to good medicine, but in the case of abortion it happens to have had a constructive influence.

The American Public Health Association recommended standards for abortion services in October 1970. Among other things it emphasised that 'psychiatric consultation should not be mandatory' but noted that 'counseling is an integral part of abortion services'.

Free-standing clinics

Clinics specialising in early terminations, but not physically linked with a hospital, evolved with remarkable speed as legislative changes paved the way for clinical innovation. By the end of 1971 there were 18 free-standing clinics in New York City. Their most important achievement was to contribute to the rising number of operations performed before twelve weeks of pregnancy. The best outpatient clinics, such as the Women's Medical Center in New York and Preterm Inc. in Washington D.C. had personnel and premises which met high standards, charged moderate fees (remitting costs for poor women), performed 25 to 150 procedures a day and provided counselling for every woman prior to the operation.

Before the Supreme Court ruling, outpatient or daycare clinics were able to deal with women who had telephoned for appointments from 3000 miles away. In order to work well, the free-standing clinics had to exclude all women more than 12 weeks from their last period, and those with any complicating medical or gynaecological condition.

Preterm Inc. was one of the first and best of such clinics. It handled 10 women an hour, or 300 weekly. It is organised as a non-profit, tax-exempt corporation and was initially supported by individual donations. A full-scale counselling service is afforded to each woman and begins with discussion of the alternatives to abortion, collects information designed to help the doctor, and concludes by a detailed explanation of all the medical procedures. Counselling provides psychological support and each applicant is encouraged to discuss her attitude towards her own sexuality. A complete contraceptive service, including the opportunity of vasectomy for the male partner, is available. After the operation there is an opportunity to rest, to take light refreshment and to talk with fellow 'patients' or counsellors. The average time spent at the centre is two and a half to three hours. Post-treatment instructions and a referral letter to the follow-up physician or clinic are provided. The woman can be in telephone contact with Preterm at any time of the day or night. During operating schedules, at least two physicians are present. Emergency drugs and equipment, including an electrocardiogram, aspirator, intravenous drip fluids, a stretcher and vehicle to take a woman to a nearby hospital, are available on a standby basis at all times. Each physician has three treatment rooms available for use, and performs three to four procedures per hour. Although the full-time staff carry out selected termination procedures, most are done by one of a roster of physicians attending on a sessional basis.[20]

In New York, a parallel facility, the Women's Medical Service, performed over 100 terminations a day in mid-1971 and completed over 20000 operations, without a known maternal death in the first year of activity (see p. 143). Many hospitals have also run outpatient abortion clinics. The estimated cost at municipal hospitals, where services are free to the woman, are as low as $100 per case.

The National Women's Health Coalition created innovative services involving a good deal of self-help and assistance from feminist groups. Very early, atraumatic techniques of terminating pregnancy (menstrual regulation) were made available. The service also reached out beyond the need for safe cheap abortions and, under the leadership of Ms Meryl Goldberg, set up a total female health care system, including access to abortion, ante-natal care, venereal disease advice and routine pelvic and breast examination for an annual fee of $90.

Planned Parenthood/World Population, the American sister of the British Family Planning Association, opened a clinic in Syracuse in 1970 and two more in New York in 1971. The Syracuse clinic performs six outpatient abortions in one three-hour session with one doctor and two nurses in attendance.[21] A Planned Parenthood/World Population outpatient clinic, affiliated to a New York hospital, can handle 10000 patients a year at a cost of around $100 per patient.

Outpatient clinics on the eastern seaboard of the USA were visited by representatives of the Lane Committee from Britain and influenced the conclusions of its report.

The advantages of daycare abortion are not only a reduction in surgical risks, but the creation of administrative flexibility. Inpatient care is tied to bed availability and therefore waiting lists are created once the decision to operate has been made and before a bed is available. Delay raises the maternal mortality and morbidity, besides putting a considerable strain on the woman. A survey in Yugoslavia has shown that women worry over the interval following the decision to have an abortion and preceding the operation more than about the procedure itself.

Results

The widespread availability of abortion on request led to a reduction in illegal abortion and in maternal and infant deaths and to a fall in the number of unwanted children. There was a very low mortality rate for the operation itself.

Statistics from New York and California concerning the decline in illegal abortions have been noted elsewhere (p. 140). Tietze estimated in New York that four out of five legal abortions replaced illegal operations, while one in five terminated an unwanted conception that would previously have gone to term.[22] Maternal mortality in New York dropped from 5.3 per 10000 live births in 1969 to 2.9 in the first 12 months of the new law. A part of this decline could have been expected, because of improving obstetric care, but much of it is likely to have been the result of a reduction in high-risk pregnancies: 7 per cent of legal abortions in New York in the first year were on girls under 17, and 10 per cent on women over 35, and both groups are examples of women with above-average risks during delivery. Infant mortality also declined. Deaths between 1 month and 12 months of age dropped from 24.4 per 1000 live births in 1969 to 20.7 in 1971. Again the availability of abortion, by cutting down the number of high-risk deliveries (such as those to unmarried mothers and highly parous women) seems to have contributed to this welcome fall. Illegitimate births fell by 9 per cent in the first year of the new law. As the rate had been rising by 5 per cent per annum in previous years the real decline is likely to have been higher. A number of homes for unmarried mothers closed and homes that once had a waiting list turned to placing advertisements on radio stations. Yet others, in the phrase of the *Wall Street Journal*, undertook some degree of 'diversification' – for example, taking-in emotionally disturbed teenagers. Guttmacher told of a medically qualified abortionist with 25 years' experience of illegal practice who complained after the passage of repeal legislation that he had not 'seen a single patient for the past two weeks.'

Table 26. *Mortality associated with legal abortion in New York City (July 1970–June 1972)*

	Number of abortions	Deaths New York City	Deaths Elsewhere USA	Mortality rates per 100 000 legal abortions
Residents	142 500	11	0	7.7
Non-residents	259 500	5	4	3.5
Total	402 000	16	4	5.0
12 weeks or less	321 500	4	2	1.9
13 weeks or more	80 500	12	2	17.4
Vacuum aspiration	261 700	3	2	1.9
Hysterotomy	2 400	5	0	208.3

The maternal death rate due to legal abortions in New York City was lower than in Scandinavia or the UK and only slightly higher than in eastern and central Europe or Japan. This is surprising because the law permitted termination up to 24 weeks of gestation, and for the first three and a half months of the new law an unknown number of operations were performed in doctors' surgeries (often with poor and occasionally with inadequate facilities). Many saline inductions were carried out, sometimes as outpatient procedures.

The passage of so many women from all over the USA to New York City in order to obtain legal abortions created difficulties in monitoring the complication rate. A nationwide search by Tietze and his colleagues[23] traced deaths that had occurred in New York and deaths that had occurred in other states, but were related to procedures that had been carried out in New York City (Table 26).

Repeal brought equality as between different ethnic groups. In one series of 200 women receiving therapeutic abortions in 1968–70, 92 per cent were white.[24] After repeal, the highest legal abortion rates were among black women. Kramer summarises the statistics (over 1970–71) and their implications:

> Prior to liberalization of New York's abortion law, the total fertility rate of blacks was 2.85, as compared to 2.15 for whites. . . In the course of just 18 months, the. . .rate of blacks fell to 2.11, the replacement level, while white fertility declined much more modestly to 1.84. . .The evidence is compelling that. . .by enabling blacks to avert what must have been a

substantial number of unwanted births, and thereby to reproduce at a rate more compatible with the well-being of the family unit, abortion legalization may rank as one of the great social equalizers of our time.[25]

The law, and the rapid evolution of services, enabled an increasing number of operations to be performed before 12 weeks. In New York, two months after repeal, 68.7 per cent of women received their abortions within 12 weeks of the last menstrual period; six months later the proportion had risen to 77.3 per cent, one year later to over 80 per cent, and there seems no reason why it should not exceed 95 per cent in the long term. The American characteristic for business-like efficiency in the face of challenge enabled the bulk of legal abortions to be performed at an earlier stage in pregnancy than was the case in Britain or Scandinavia.

In 1973 at least 745 400 legal abortions were performed in the USA. The Supreme Court ruling was associated both with a rise in the total number of legal abortions and with a redistribution of services. States that had previously had a restrictive attitude witnessed a two- to three-fold jump in legal abortion numbers. States that had a middle-of-the-road attitude, and often limited abortion to local residents, experienced a 70 per cent increase. While states such as New York and Washington, which had previously served many out-of-state women, did approximately a quarter fewer abortions.

The climb in abortion numbers mainly occurred in free-standing clinics and such clinics now carry out the majority of the abortions in the USA. A small number of large-scale clinics accounted for more than half the total abortions performed in the first quarter of 1974. A mere 118 hospitals and clinics, which performed 500 or more abortions in the three-month interval, accounted for 57 per cent of the nation's total operations, although they only comprised 7 per cent of all facilities offering abortion.

In 1973 the legal abortion rate per 1000 of the population was 3.5 and the ratio of abortions to live births was 19.1 : 100.[26]

Public opinion and medical attitudes

The size and diversity of the USA produced a wider range of attitudes within religious and professional groups than occurred in Britain. The deciding issues in the abortion debate changed with time: a pragmatic discussion of the public health aspects of legislation came into greater prominence and discussion of the sanctity of life became relatively less important, although remaining the single issue discussed most often in public and private.[27] In the Belous case, the phrase 'the fundamental right of the woman to choose whether to bear children' was used. It was an issue which was to become increasingly important.

Feminist groups

Feminist organisations adopted the cause of abortion law reform or repeal as a rallying point. In the social history of the movement, abortion may have been as significant as a unifying goal to the movement as the movement was to changing abortion attitudes.

Some legislators claimed to have been embarrassed by this intervention and politically it may have been a double-dged weapon. Individual feminists, however, became invaluable lobbyers, organisers or, like Dr Emily Moore, sustained a useful and informed academic commentary on many aspects of abortion. Women's Groups continued to be creative in New York and other places after the repeal of the law. They helped by their control of medical facilities to lower prices – perhaps an experiment in the role of consumer-advocate that will be extended to other areas of medicine.

Roman Catholic attitudes

Many Catholics attempted to distinguish their own deep convictions from the right of the community to freedom of action. The Bill repealing the abortion law in Hawaii was sponsored by Senator Vincent Yano, a Roman Catholic with ten children, and allowed to pass by a Roman Catholic Governor. In October 1970 the *Catholic Medical Quarterly* discussed the possibility that refusal to abort a woman might be interpreted as denial of that woman's rights under the law. In Pennsylvania a local group was formed called Roman Catholics for the Right to Choose. It claimed 500 members in 1971, and a spokesman said, 'our Church should not attempt to use civil law to impose its moral philosophy upon our non-Catholic neighbors'. In June 1972, a Gallup poll found 56 per cent of Catholics believed that 'the decision to have an abortion should be made solely by the woman and her physician'. Dr Mary Daly, Professor of Theology in Boston College, was willing to testify on behalf of abortion law repeal before the Social Welfare

Committee of the Massachusetts legislature in 1971. Several Catholic legislators in New York State voted for the repeal Bill, and that extraordinary piece of legislation would not have passed without their support. A colourful individual incident was well publicised in 1974 when a Massachusetts priest refused to baptise a baby of Catholic parents who supported the right of American women to abortion. A New York Jesuit and director of Catholics for a Free Choice later performed the baptism on the steps of the Church of the Immaculate Conception. He was dismissed from the Order, although other Jesuits continued to campaign.

Among individual thinkers, Daniel Callahan, formerly editor of *Commonweal*, greatly advanced the thinking of Roman Catholics (and of many others) with his book, *Abortion: Law, Choice and Morality*.[28] Published in 1970, it won the Thomas More Association Medal for the year's most distinguished contribution to Catholic literature. The citation stated that it provided 'a desperately needed perspective for legislators, moralists, civic leaders, doctors, nurses and parents'. Callahan argued for the repeal of abortion laws.

Medical opinion

The evolution of medical attitudes, like the pace of legal change, was faster in the USA than in Britain. A national conference on abortion in the 1950s mainly concentrated on epidemiology.[29] Early in the 1960s the USA was more conservative than Britain in medical opinion regarding abortion and had a lower rate of therapeutic abortions. In a mere five years it caught up with, overtook and arrived at a point not even considered possible in Britain at the time of the 1967 Act. At the point when the changes became most rapid, a number of surveys of doctors' opinions were conducted; indeed the sudden multiplication of surveys in 1967 was about as sensitive a marker of change as the content of the surveys themselves.

In the late 1960s Tietze had estimated a rate of 1.9 therapeutic abortions per 1000 deliveries.[30] Eliot and his colleagues in a survey sponsored by the American College of Obstetricians and Gynecologists and the American Public Health Association and carried out in 1967, found that 90 per cent of non-Catholic hospitals did some terminations, but also confirmed Tietze's study that rates were very low (2.4 per 1000 deliveries – usually less than five terminations per hospital per year).[31] The indications for operation were usually strictly medical and private patients were three times as likely to receive an abortion as others. There was a strong positive correlation between the degree of development of contraceptive services and the likelihood of the hospital granting an abortion.

Guttmacher said it took him 45 years to accept the idea of abortion at the request of the pregnant woman, and he was the most far-sighted American physician in this field. When change did take place, it came late and was rapid. This is well illustrated by the paper by Eliot *et al.* cited above. When they collected data for the paper in 1967, only one in ten chiefs of obstetrics believed that the existing laws should be abolished; when the paper was actually presented at the Hot Springs Conference on Abortion in 1968, reform had only made a timid beginning and no repeal legislation had been moved, but, by the time it left the printers in 1970, Hawaii, Alaska and New York State allowed abortion on request.

Sometimes, physicians questioned individually gave different answers to those given when they were observed playing a defined role as part of a medical group. A hint of future change came in a poll by *Modern Medicine*, also in 1967,[32] which found that 80 per cent of physicians favoured some degree of abortion law reform, including half the respondents who identified themselves as Catholic. Indeed, a Harris poll of Catholic doctors showed that many were overtly opposed to traditional Church teaching. However, opinions were ahead of practice.

Further liberalisation of medical attitudes took place in the wake of law reform in the late 1960s. By 1970 the American College of Obstetricians and Gynecologists relaxed their rules for consultation prior to sterilisation or abortion and stopped listing medical indications for termination – which previously had been along ALI lines. The American Public Health Association adopted a liberal policy in 1969 and widened it in 1971. The American Psychiatric Association, like its British counterpart, favoured legal changes as did many state medical associations.

Surveys of a sample of New York State physicians were carried out in July 1970 (the time of repeal) and January 1971. In the initial survey 58 per cent of obstetricians and gynaecologists unreservedly approved of the new situation and a further 14 per cent approved but expressed some technical reservations concerning, for example, the duration of the pregnancy on which the operation might be performed. The impact of the law on Roman Catholic doctors is interesting and those favouring the change increased from 23 per cent to 31 per cent in the first half-year of its operation. Ninety eight per cent of Jewish physicians and 86 per cent of Protestants approved of the law. One-quarter of the total sample disapproved of the repeal and 8 per cent said they would neither perform an abortion or refer a woman elsewhere for advice. On average, the doctors were receiving 4.2 abortion requests a week and most did not feel this level overburdensome. Most were familiar with the newer techniques, such as vacuum aspiration, and 45 per cent agreed that outpatient clinic terminations were responsible if limited to pregnancies of less than 12 weeks' gestation. Oral contraceptives were the preferred method recommended after abortion, and 96 per cent of physicians claimed to recommend some form of contraception post-abortion.[33,34]

The changes which have occurred in the opinion of doctors generally, and of gynaecological specialists in particular, became reflected in the attitudes of medical bodies. Unlike the British Medical Association, which, Canute-like, resisted the tide of abortion law reform, the AMA at least avoided getting salt water on its throne. In 1967 a resolution permitting termination in cases where the continuation of the pregnancy would affect the woman's life or health, as well as in cases of incest, rape or where the child might be deformed, was approved by the AMA. At the Association's Chicago meeting in 1970, after two hours of passionate debate, new conditions were laid down, which merely said that abortions should be performed by a licensed doctor, in an accredited hospital and in conformity with state law and good medical practice. An effort by the New Jersey delegation to return to a policy of only acknowledging strictly medical indications was defeated on a voice vote.

While the bulk of the medical profession slowly adjusted to the new climate of opinion, a few went on to explore their new-found freedom. A new point of view began to be canvassed. One psychologist wrote: 'The male physician won't let the woman decide' and compared this attitude with 'the moralist attitude about pain relief in childbirth before Queen Victoria demanded it for herself. The pregnant woman symbolises proof of male potency, and if the male loosens his rule over women and grants them the right to dispose of that proof when they want to, the men feel terribly threatened.'[35] To many it appeared an extreme view, but probably no more so than those which had preceded it for over a century, and it did have the novel merit of attempting to analyse the reactions of doctors, as well as of patients, in what is clearly a two-way exchange of attitudes.

Practical experience and changes of opinion were linked. By 1970, 92 per cent of New York gynaecologists had performed *D & C*s and 58 per cent vacuum aspiration. Eighty three per cent of Catholics had used the former technique and 34 per cent the latter. Jewish, Board-certified, physicians affiliated with municipal hospitals had most experience of all. By 1971 New York gynaecologists were performing, on average, three to four abortions a week.[36]

Nurses' attitudes also changed. In 1970, 93 per cent of a sample of nurses approved of abortion in cases of rape, but still only 22 per cent tolerated it for the 'convenience' of the mother. Interestingly, younger nurses were most restrictive: 83 per cent of the 20–29 year age group were *against* unrestricted abortion, while among nurses aged 50 and over, this figure fell to 73 per cent.[37]

Public opinion

Most systems of legislation favour the status quo. In the USA, as in several other countries, individual opinion has been more strongly in favour of liberal abortion than public institutions and group attitudes would suggest.[38] In 1968 a Gallup survey showed that 15 per cent of the public approved of liberalised abortion laws; in November 1969 a similar survey found 40 per cent approved. In June 1972, 64 per cent of a 1574 sample of Americans over 18 years of age and drawn from 300 localities believed that the decision to have an abortion should be made solely by the woman and her doctor. Six months earlier it had only been 57 per cent,[39] while ten years earlier, in 1962, 74 per cent of Americans in a Gallup sample had *disapproved* of abortion for economic reasons.[40]

Qualitative measures of changing public attitudes can be more vivid than quantitative ones. *Maud* is a popular situation comedy presented on television by the Columbia Broadcasting Corporation. Maud herself is a slightly earthy realist, and the programme deals with the whole spectrum of possible domestic events. When Maud had a legally induced abortion, late in 1972, it took two episodes for her to think through the situation. The programmes produced more public comment than any other event in this widely watched programme. That it could take place is a measure of changing attitudes towards abortion; that only 30 seconds of the three-minute advertising space available on the rerun could be sold, demonstrated the strength of imagined opposition still present in America.

Reader's Digest represents a different marker of social perceptions. It reflects the Bible Belt rather than the west coast; setting its vision of the spiritual above the scientific and sentiment above sapience. Therefore, it represented a considerable change in outlook when *Reader's Digest* published a sober account of the beneficial effects of liberal abortion legislation from the pen of Alan Guttmacher in November 1973, shortly before his death from leukaemia.

As in Britain, changing attitudes towards abortion have been associated with important improvements in family planning services. The domestic family planning programme of the USA expanded very considerably in the late 1960s, and in December 1970 President Nixon signed the Family Planning Services and Population Research Act making $320 million available for the years 1971–73.

Despite improvements, some paradoxes remain, thrown into even sharper relief than previously by the changed abortion attitudes. State laws still limit the distribution of condoms to pharmacies in New York and, for some social groups, it may be more difficult to find a french letter than to get a legal abortion – they are certainly less well advertised. In Massachusetts, even the pharmacy sale of contraceptives was permitted only as recently as 1966. In 1971 Dr William Baird spent an uncomfortable night in an American prison for displaying an intrauterine device in public – among the people he was held to have corrupted by this immoral act was an 18-month-old infant who, as Baird commented, could not distinguish an IUD from a rattle.

Counter movements

By mid-1971, once the actions of the Supreme Court had been set in motion and when most communities were able to seek abortions in the liberal states, the pressure for reform weakened and the explosion of change died down.

At the same time, the passage of liberal abortion legislation in some states of America generated an organised opposition which shared many common features of the post-1967 situation in Britain. Often largely supported by Catholics (although, as stated previously, not expressing the feelings of all Catholics), it also included some right-wing groups and individuals from Fundamentalist sects. When draft legislation attempting to widen the Californian statutes was discussed at a hearing in the State Capital in Sacramento in 1970 it was attended by such groups as United of Life, Right to Life League, Friends of the Fetus, Voice of the Unborn, League against Neo-Fascism and the Blue Army Against Satan. By mid-1972 the National Committee for the Right to Life had 250 affiliates. All traded on the rare case of late termination when the fetus has shown signs of life and inflated the anxieties of young nurses.

Perhaps the most expensive effort was that surrounding the Washington State referendum. The Committee of the Voice of the Unborn is reported to have spent $300000 on publicity. Buses carried posters purporting to portray fully developed fetuses and bearing the slogan 'Vote for the Right to Live'. The campaign was carried into television commercials and newspapers (p. 340). Supporters of the referendum spent less than $20000 but, as noted, it succeeded. However, a similar referendum in 1972 in Michigan, to allow a doctor to 'perform an abortion at the request of the patient if the period of gestation has not exceeded 20 weeks' was defeated by two million votes to 1300000. Whether this was the result of rising opposition to abortion, or the different political complexion of the state, is difficult to say.

In addition to these set pieces, frequent minor skirmishes between pro- and anti-abortion groups occurred. In 1971, Civic Awareness of America Inc. attempted to restrain Planned Parenthood/World Population from receiving Federal grants. The group opposed 'artificial contraception, cloning, vasectomy, abortion, infanticide and euthanasia as corrosive of our civilization, of the institution of the family, of the morals of youth and of laws against murder, fornication and other crimes endangering life and public morality'.

Not all reaction, however, was extreme. In New York, official Roman Catholic diocesan guidelines forbade a doctor or nurse to enter into 'direct participation' in an abortion operation, but specifically permitted Catholic personnel to care for a woman before and after an operation, to lay out instruments in the operating theatre, to explain the operation to the patient, and to witness consent forms. Neither was it all negative. In the spring of 1971 Archbishop Terence Cardinal Cooke of New York launched a programme called *Birthright* to aid women with unwanted pregnancies to find help or seek abortion. However, it is perhaps unfortunate that steps to fill this need, which had existed for at least a century, were only taken in response to a repeal of the state abortion laws.

State and Federal Legislation

In the first year after the repeal of the New York law about 50 draft Bills were introduced into state legislatures all round the country in an effort to *restrict* abortion laws. These efforts all failed, although some minor administrative alterations were made in several states, for example, California and New York. Some degree of change was welcomed by many who had favoured repeal. The total freedom obtained in the first few months after repeal in New York City met some restriction in October 1971, when new regulations under the Health code were drawn up limiting the non-hospital practice of the operation to facilities within ten minutes' travel time of an accredited hospital. This change helped reduce the risk for the woman, but also placed an unwelcome limit on one or two pioneer clinics operating on an outpatient basis. An amendment to reduce the 24-week limit on gestational interval to 20 was introduced in 1971 and had wide support, but failed to progress. Some regulation of referral agencies was introduced both when the Attorney General took action against one service, charging it with fraud and illegal activity, and when Senator Tarky Lombardi successfully steered a Bill outlawing profit-making agencies through the state legislature. In 1972 a Bill to 'unrepeal' the New York law was sponsored by state legislators Donovan and Crawford. The former illustrated his arguments with colour enlargements of aborted fetuses. The Bill passed by 79 votes to 68 in the lower house and 39 to 27 in the Senate. It was a victory for the counter movement and undoubtedly they had mobilised public opinion more fully than on previous occasions. In fact, the repeal never became law, because Governor Rockefeller used his power of veto, saying, ' I do not believe it right for one group to impose its vision of morality on an entire society'. Unfortunately for those attempting to judge the temper of society at this time, Rockefeller's intention to veto the repeal of the repeal was known in advance of the Albany vote. It is possible that several politicians got what they believed to be the best of both worlds by voting for a repeal, with which they privately disagreed, but had the comfort of knowing it would be vetoed. Perhaps the *New York Times* was a more accurate reflection of public opinion when it claimed that the liberal abortion situation had justified itself with a 'remarkable record of humane evidence'.[41]

Following the Supreme Court ruling in January 1973, there was a burst of abortion legislation all over the USA. Some of it came out of the ruling itself, which invited legislative attention to 'protecting the health of the pregnant woman' and the 'potentiability of human life', especially as the woman approaches term. Other legislation attempted to set back the Supreme Court ruling and Bills known to be unconstitutional were nevertheless passed. This method of counteraction slowed progress at the state level on the principle that it can take a long time, and cost a lot of money, to remove obstacles, even when demonstrably unconstitutional. The same tactic has been used in relation to the Supreme Court ruling that capital punishment was unconstitutional (1972) and within 18 months 16 states had voted to restore the death penalty. In July 1974 Governor Milton I. Shapp over-ruled a Pennsylvania Bill as 'clearly' unconstitutional,[42] a veto that was in turn to be over-ridden by the legislature forcing the issue to Federal courts. Later the same year the Governor of Massachusetts, Francis W. Sargent, over-ruled a bill from his state legislature as of 'dubious constitutionability'.[43]

Nearly all of the new state laws require a licensed physician to perform first-trimester operations and regulate the type of facility appropriate for second-trimester abortions. (One state, Montana, prohibits the use of intra-amniotic saline.) Many states legislated concerning husbands' and parental consent to abortion, although several of these statutes are likely to be proved unconstitutional. More than 30 states have passed statutes that include a conscience clause concerning the physician's role in abortion. Some states have legislated concerning protection of the fetus, requiring certain types of medical care in situations where a viable fetus could be delivered.[44] The New York statute (February 1974) restricted all abortions after 12 weeks to inpatient hospital procedures and required that 'When an abortion is being performed after the twentieth week of pregnancy a physician other than the physician performing the operation shall be in attendance to take control of and provide immediate medical care for any live birth that is the result of the abortion.'

Two Federal actions concerning abortion were also significant. In December 1973 Senator Helms, from North Carolina, succeeded in passing an amendment to the Foreign Assistance Act,[45] which forbade US money to be spent on promoting abortion, or abortion services overseas. This move was particularly inappropriate at a time when many developing countries were reviewing their own abortion legislation (partly inspired by the US Supreme Court and the subsequent American experience) and when US Aid to International Development had taken a realistic role in assisting in the treatment of illegal abortion and in improving techniques of early legal abortion. Helms is a Republican. He supports capital punishment and in 1974 attempted to amend the money Bill so as to delay the desegregation of schools.[46] An amendment to retard the use of domestic family planning funds in relation to abortion has also been attempted. In June 1974,[47] Representative Angelo D. Roncallo (Republican, New York) moved an amendment in Congress that 'No part of the funds appropriated under this Act shall be used in any manner directly or indirectly to pay for abortions or abortion referral services...As used in this section, abortion means the intentional destruction of unborn human life, which life begins at the moment of fertilization.'

The amendment was a surprise one, presented to a nearly empty House after 10 o'clock at night. It did not succeed. A Democratic Representative from New York State pointed out the wording might make IUDs illegal. One Congressman said, 'I am a Catholic. I do not believe in it [*abortion*]. However, I also do not believe in this amendment.' More and more Representatives were brought back from their dinner parties and other evening engagements and, eventually, a somewhat bad-tempered Congress defeated the Roncallo Amendment by 247 to 123 votes. Amongst those voting against this over-clever move were 33 Catholics.

In April 1975 the US Civil Rights Commission urged Congress to reject all legislative riders as unconstitutional.[48]

Constitutional amendments

Within eight days of the Supreme Court ruling, Congressman Hogan of Maryland moved an amendment stating, 'Neither the United States, nor any State, shall deprive any human being, from the moment of conception, of life without due process of law; nor deny to any human being, from the moment of conception, within its jurisdiction, the equal protection of its laws.'

Helms tabled a similar amendment: 'Every human being subject to the jursidiction of the United States or any state...shall be deemed from the moment of fertilization to be a person and entitled to the right to life.'

Such 'right-to-life' amendments have various comic-opera implications: would lady visitors to the country, who are one week late in their menses, require one visa or two? How would the census be conducted? Would damages for, say, the death of a woman who might have been pregnant in a road accident be paid for one or two? Could a doctor inserting an IUD be charged with murder? As Pilpel has pointed out, US citizens might not celebrate their birth-days, but their 'fertilization days'.[49]

James Buckley sponsored an alternative amendment where the word 'person' in the US Constitution should apply 'to all human beings, including their unborn offspring at every stage of development, irrespective of age, health, function or condition of dependence'. Representative Whitehurst introduced yet another type of amendment resting the power of abortion legislation solely in the hands of the individual states. While the US Constitution guarantees certain rights, such those of peaceable assembly or trial by jury, it does not guarantee *right to life* even for the born, let alone the unborn. The Federal government for example may draft men into the armed forces. In practice such amendments, while preventing governmental abortion services, might have no effect on private services ('if a legislative body permitted, but did not *cause* the death of any fetus, it would not, under well-established legal principles, be depriving any fetus of life without due process of law'). It would be an impossible task to enforce any 'right-to-life' amendments without a wholesale invasion of the woman's right to privacy – theoretically every miscarriage would require investigation, to rule out deliberate abortion.

Amendments to the Constitution require a two-thirds majority of both houses of Congress, and subsequently need to be ratified by three-quarters of all states within seven years. By the end of 1974 no 'right-to-life' amendment had accumulated more than 40 sponsors, although a minimum of 218 is needed to raise the issue in the House. The Equal Rights Amendment, which is less controversial than those dealing with abortion, has been before the House for 49 years. Nevertheless, major issues have been fought, or are being fought, through Constitutional amendment. The Prohibition era followed a Constitutional amendment (Volstead Act, 1919), which was not repealed until 1933 (Twenty-first Amendment). It was unenforceable, against the wishes of most people, and gave rise to a great deal of crime. It was not such a profound or significant issue as abortion, but it is not a happy precedent.

The 'right-to-life' amendments would disallow truly therapeutic abortions, run counter to the thought and practice of the majority of Americans, and leave the critical question of defining a 'human being' unsolved. As the Supreme Court showed, it is a question which is insoluble in purely legal terms.[50]

The politicians who sponsored anti-abortion legislation in Congress did not benefit politically from their actions. In the 1974 elections, amongst sitting members 98 per cent of those who had a pro-abortion voting record, but only 81 per cent of those who had an anti-abortion record, were re-elected. Hogan was amongst those who lost his seat in 1974. Many politicians began to follow the example of Catholic State Senator May Ann Krupsak before her election in New York when she said 'I would not have one [*abortion*] myself but don't impose my feelings on others'.[51]

Criminal law

Americans tend to use courts of law to argue a case or chastise their opponents, in rather the way the British use the correspondence columns of *The Times*. To compound this excess of democratic action, the American District Attorney is elected and sometimes brings cases as much to placate voting groups as to further the course of justice.

In March 1974, Dr Leonard Laufe of the Western Pennsylvania Hospital in Pittsburgh performed an abortion on a 26-year-old woman who was pregnant as the result of rape, had prevaricated in telling her husband (who had had a vasectomy) and had misled her clinical advisers about the duration of the pregnancy. Termination was performed by clamping the uterine vessels, and carrying out a vaginal hysterectomy. A large fetus (1160 g, 2lb 9oz) was present and had to be delivered through the cervix.

The intention of the operation was to kill the fetus by obstructing the uterine vessels. The legality of this act was in no way questioned, but charges were brought against Laufe for failing to resuscitate the fetus. The operation was performed before observers and, as the technique was an unusual one, was filmed as part of a teaching project. Conflicting testimony was given concerning fetal gasping following delivery. The most prominent witness was described by a fellow nurse at the time of the operation as 'shouting and screaming'. She was very upset when she came in. She said, 'He's done it again. This is murder. This will be the last one he's done.'[52]

Following expert testimony and viewing of the film by the six-person jury, the inquest concluded that the fetus had been stillborn.

Laufe had long adopted a bold and compassionate policy at his hospital, had shown great leadership in family planning as well as in abortion techniques and policy, and had worked with the International Planned Parenthood Federation team terminating pregnancies of girls who had been raped during the civil war in Bangladesh. He is well known for his international work in family planning.

In Massachusetts, charges of grave-robbing and homicide were brought against doctors operating for late abortion. In October 1973, Dr Kenneth Edelin performed a hysterotomy between the twenty-second and twenty-fourth weeks of pregnancy on a 17-year-old unmarried black girl in Boston City Hospital.[53] The State Prosecutor, in the words of *The Washington Post*,[54] 'thought up the legal theory of his case – that a fetus is a live human being – and found someone to try the theory out on'. Dr Edelin, a black physician, was tried by an all-white predominantly Roman Catholic jury. The trial ended on 15 February 1975. Judge James McGuire instructed the jury that a 'fetus is not a person and therefore not subject for an indictment for manslaughter' and that, for conviction, the jury would need to be satisfied that Dr Edelin 'caused the death of a person outside the body of the mother'.

Therefore, as in the Laufe case, the act of abortion *per se* was not contested. The prosecutor in reality created a new crime, namely murdering a fetus during a legal operation by failing to take steps to keep it alive. However, the jury did not acquit, although individual jurors said afterwards they were sorry they had not persisted in a 'not guilty' vote. The politico-legal cake was kept and eaten at the same time. Having been convicted of manslaughter, Edelin was merely put on probation for one year and immediately returned to work (the maximum sentence is 20 years in prison). A Superior Court judge rejected a first appeal, but the case is now before the Supreme Judicial Court of Massachusetts. Most jurists believe it will fall at the Federal Supreme Court. Nevertheless, unless overturned in a higher court, the conviction could be a deterrent to doctors performing abortion.

The case aroused enormous interest and passion. Support for Dr

Edelin came from several quarters. The hospital administration said they considered it 'imperative to allow Dr Edelin to continue his dedication and service to the people of Boston'. Feminist groups organised a supportive demonstration outside the State Capitol.

Again *The Washington Post* commented: 'Regardless of what one thinks about abortion, it ought to be obvious that there is something fundamentally unfair about charging a man with murder without warning him in advance that what he and other doctors have been doing for years is now to be considered murder'.[54]

Cardinal Krol said: 'Some have expressed concern that the decision may inhibit abortion. We pray to God that it will.'[53]

The grave-robbing cases were brought against four Massachusetts doctors engaged in research using fetal tissue. The case had a 'chilling effect' on research, although the use of fetal tissue had been significant in such scientific advances as the prevention of poliomyelitis and this screening of drugs for potential teratological effects.

Ex-President Nixon and abortion

In April 1971 President Nixon unexpectedly threw his personal opinions on abortion into the public debate. As state laws changed, doctors in the armed forces had found themselves in a confusing position with some military hospitals in states with liberal laws, while some were in the reverse position. In 1970 a directive had been issued permitting hospitals to follow a liberal abortion policy nationwide. The President over-ruled this practice and made state laws, which normally do *not* apply to Federal property, enforceable in military hospitals. He also took the opportunity to make his personal views known:

> 'From personal and religious beliefs I consider abortion an unacceptable form of population control. Further unrestricted abortion policies, or abortion on demand, I cannot square with my personal belief in the sanctity of human life – including the life of the yet unborn. A good and generous people will not opt, in my view, for this kind of alternative to its social dilemmas. Rather it will open its hearts and homes to the unwanted children of its own, as it has done for the unwanted children of other lands'.[55]

Although the number of abortions in military hospitals had jumped, the service doctors were probably puzzled to see their performance of abortions as an aspect of 'population control'. Some commentators were quick to point out that President Nixon had also invoked his powers as Commander-in-Chief of the Armed Forces a few days previously to release Lieutenant Calley from prison after his conviction in connection with the My Lai massacre. Nixon's remarks met with a quick and forceful rejoinder from Dr Alan Guttmacher, then president of Planned Parenthood/World Population: 'I fear, Mr. President, that the expression of your personal and religious views on abortion are ill-timed. When the Constitutionality of restrictive abortion policies is under consideration by the Supreme Court, your remarks will be held by many as interfering with the due process of law.'[55]

Some sections of the armed forces responded by issuing a directive that a woman who falls pregnant may be flown by a military plane to a state with liberal law. Nevertheless, Nixon's remarks had an impact, and abortions in military hospitals fell from 400 a month to 120.

Twelve months later (17 March 1972) the President found occasion to voice the same opinions when he rejected the recommendations of the *Report of the Commission on Population Growth and the American Future*. This Commission, which he himself had set up in 1970, was chaired by Mr John D. Rockefeller. Predictably it reported that:

> The majority of the commission believes that women should be free to determine their own fertility, that the matter of abortion should be left to the conscience of the individual concerned, in consultation with her physician, and that states should be encouraged to enact affirmative statutes creating a clear and positive framework for the practice of abortion on request. Therefore, with the admonition that abortion not be considered a primary means of fertility control, the commission recommends that present state laws restricting abortion be liberalised along the lines of the New York State statute, such abortions to be performed on request by a duly licenced physician under conditions of medical safety.[56]

Among those who protested at the Report was Cardinal Terence Cooke. Buchanan, a long-standing, right-wing Nixon aide, asked Robert Haldeman to suggest that Nixon conveyed his views on abortion in a letter to Cardinal Cooke in New York. John Mitchell approved the letter, but John Erlichman was put out because the issue cut across his relationships with Nelson Rockefeller. Safire suggests Nixon's daughter Julie may have had an influential right-to-life effect on her father, but Nixon's own feelings appear also to have been strong. 'Philosophically, the President felt that unrestricted abortion was further evidence of society granting approval to irresponsibility . . . leading to moral decay and the decline of Western civilization.'[55] When the letter was finally sent it was said to have been for purely private circulation, Nixon wrote: 'I would personally like to associate myself with the convictions you deeply feel and eloquently express'. He acknowledged, 'this is a matter . . . outside federal jurisdiction', which made the implication that the letter was an exercise in recruiting votes for the forthcoming Presidential election even stronger. One political commentator remarked, 'it appears that Cardinal Cooke cashed an IOU'. Again Nixon acted on a day when he was also to intervene in the Vietnam War, stepping up the bombing. Hearing the news at a family planning conference one speaker said, he had to 'respect the President's concern for the embryos of New York State especially at a time when the lives of already born children and not yet killed adults in another land weigh so heavily on his mind'.

Nixon's clumsy political moves helped shift the complex topic of abortion from an issue of conscience into a straight political confrontation. When the 1972 vote was taken in the New York State legislature in Albany, Republicans largely voted for repeal of the liberal situation while Democrats strove to retain the free situation that had existed for two years.

Nixon's desire to use every legal and illegal channel to secure his re-election is now well understood. His opponent, Senator McGovern, strongly supported abortion law repeal. He called abortion a 'no-win issue' and said the problem should be decided at the state level. Abortion continued to be an unusually searching test of political integrity as the Watergate crisis unfolded. Nixon's true friends were those who had taken anti-abortion stands. Rev. Billy Graham attempted to defend Nixon's Watergate record by the curious somersault of describing it as the outcome of moral permissiveness gripping the whole of society. The conference of Catholic bishops meeting in Washington in November 1973, and presided over by Cardinal Krol, condemned the Supreme Court decisions on abortion and Federal aid to parochial schools, but omitted any reference to the Watergate crisis, then reaching a new intensity. On the other hand the Quakers (Nixon's own one-time denomination) and Methodists, both of whom adopted liberal abortion attitudes, condemned Watergate and in the latter case advocated impeachment. Individuals sometimes went counter to their groups, Vincent Yano, the remarkable Catholic lawyer who had played so important a role in the Hawaii repeal was, by 1973, a member of Congress and he became the first person to move the impeachment of Nixon from the floor of the House.

In July 1974, the same Justices who had heard the *Roe* and *Doe* cases on abortion heard the case of the *United States* v. *Richard M. Nixon*. The Supreme Court's ruling, invalidating Nixon's claim to Presidential privilege in relation to the Watergate conspiracy, led directly to his resignation. The nine Justices of the Federal Supreme Court of the USA – all men and with a mean age in the late 60s – changed the course of world history in more ways than one in the 1970s.

Conclusion

The almost accidental repeal of the New York abortion law in 1970 – after 142 years of restrictive legislation – created a situation where the public health and social benefits of legal abortion could be seen. Over the past five years almost one in five of New York women of reproductive age has had an abortion. The New York experience affected the rest of the USA. The judgement of the US Supreme Court in January 1973 philosophically, legally and in its administrative implications, represents a change in abortion attitudes and practices as significant as those which occurred in Japan in 1949 and in Russia in 1920. It put an end to a piecemeal reform of state legislation. It virtually eliminated illegal abortions in the USA, had a powerful public health effect by lowering maternal mortality and made a measurable effect on the birth rate. All these achievements took place in a situation of constant or improving contraceptive practice.

Yet in some quarters the Supreme Court ruling aroused passionate opposition, which has in turn been used to frustrate and harass the implementation of the Supreme Court decision.

References

Four publications have been especially useful in compiling this and the succeeding chapters and have been used extensively:

World Health Organisation (1971). Abortion laws: a survey of current world legislation. *International Digest of Health Legislation,* **21**, 437. (Also published separately by WHO in 1971.)

Lee, L. (1973). *International Status of Abortion Legislation.* Law and Population Program of the Fletcher School of Law and Diplomacy, Tufts University, Medford, Mass.

David, H. P. (ed.) (1974). *Abortion Research: International Experience.* Lexington Books, Lexington, Mass.

Institute of Medicine (1975). *Legalized Abortion and the Public Health.* National Academy of Sciences, Washington D.C.

1 Means, C. C. (1972). Does a fetus possess constitutional or other legal rights? In *Abortion Techniques and Services,* ed. S. Lewit, p. 91. Excerpta Medica, Amsterdam.

2 Lucas, R. (1970). Laws of the United States. In *Abortion in a Changing World,* ed. R. E. Hall, vol. **1**, p. 127. Columbia University Press, New York.

3 Means, C. (1970). 'Panel Discussion'. In *Abortion in a Changing World,* ed. R. E. Hall, vol. **2**, p. 138. Columbia University Press, New York.

4 Sauer, R. (1974). Attitudes to abortion in America. *Population Studies, London,* **28**, 53.

5 Supreme Court of the United States. *Roe* v. *Wade* (22 January 1973), No. 70–18.

6 *Transactions of the American Medical Association* (1871). **22**, 258.

7 Hodge, H. L. (1872). *Foeticide or Criminal Abortion.* Lindsay & Blakiston, Philadelphia.

8 Hammond, H. (1964). Therapeutic abortion. *American Journal of Obstetrics and Gynecology,* **89**, 349.

9 Robinson, W. J. (1933). *The Law Against Abortion.* Eugenics, New York.

10 Finkbine, S. (1967). The lesser of two evils. *The Case for Legalized Abortion Now,* ed. A. F. Guttmacher, p. 15. Diablo Press, Berkeley, California.

11 American Law Institute (1962). *Model Penal Code,* Article 230.

12 Anwyl, H. (1970). Personal communication.

13 Tietze, C. (1970). United States: Therapeutic abortions, 1963–1968. *Studies in Family Planning,* no. **59**, 5.

14 Guttmacher, A. F. (1973). Abortion: odyssey of an attitude. *Family Planning Perspectives,* **4**, 5. See also, Guttmacher, A. F. (1973). Abortion. In *Abortion, Society and the Law,* ed. D. F. Walbert & J. D. Butler. Case Western Reserve, Law Review, Cleveland, Ohio.

15 Redford, M. (1972). *Abortion Report*. Battelle Human Affairs Research Center, Seattle, Washington.
16 *Time*, 11 December 1972.
17 Smith, R. G., Steinhoff, P. G., Pahmore, J. A. & Diamond, M. (1973). Abortion in Hawaii: 1970–1971. *Hawaii Medical Journal*, **32**, 213.
18 Chez, R. A. & Hutchinson, D. L. (1970). Therapeutic abortion: some dilemmas associated with increased applications. *Contraception*, **2**, 127.
19 Muller, C. (1972). Insurance for abortion. In *Abortion Techniques and Services*, ed. S. Lewit, p. 129. Excerpta Medica, Amsterdam.
20 Branch, B. N. (1972). Out-patient termination of pregnancy. In *New Concepts in Contraception*, ed. M. Potts & C. Wood, p. 175. Medical & Technical Publications Co., Oxford & Lancaster.
21 Penfield, A. J. (1972). A planned parenthood abortion service. *Advances in Planned Parenthood*, **7**, 185.
22 Tietze, C. (1973). Two years' experience with a liberal abortion law: its impact on fertility trends in New York City. *Family Planning Perspectives*, **5**, 36.
23 Tietze, C., Pakter, C. J. & Berger, G. S. (1973). Mortality associated with legal abortion in New York City, 1970/72. *Journal of the American Medical Association*, **225**, 507.
24 Hall, R. E. (1971). Induced abortion in New York City. *American Journal of Obstetrics and Gynecology*, **110**, 601.
25 Kramer, M. J. (1975). Legal abortion among New York City residents: an analysis according to socioeconomic and demographic characteristics. *Family Planning Perspective*, **7**, 128.
26 Weinstock, E., Tietze, C., Jaffe, F. S. & Dryfoos, J. G. (1975). Legal abortions in the United States since the 1973 Supreme Court decisions. *Family Planning Perspectives*, **7**, 23.
27 Moore, E. C. (1971). Abortion and public policy: what are the issues? *New York Law Forum*, **17**, 411.
28 Callahan, D. (1970). *Abortion: Law, Choice and Morality*. Macmillan, New York.
29 Calderone, M. S. (ed.) (1958). *Abortion in the United States*, a conference sponsored by the Planned Parenthood Federation of America at Arden House and the New York Academy of Medicine. Hoeber-Harper, New York.
30 Tietze, C. (1968). Therapeutic abortions in the United States, *American Journal of Obstetrics and Gynecology*, **101**, 784.
31 Eliot, J. W., Hall, R. E., Willson, J. R. & Houser, C. (1970). The obstetrician's view. In *Abortion in a Changing World*, ed. R. E. Hall, vol. **1**, p. 85. Columbia University Press, New York.
32 *Modern Medicine* (1967), **35**, 216.
33 Lerner, R. C., Arnold, C. B. & Wassertheil-Smoller, S. M. (1971). New York's obstetricians' survey on abortion. *Family Planning Perspectives*, **3**, 56.

34 Wassertheil-Smoller, S. M., Lerner, R. C., Arnold, C. B. & Heimrath, S. L. (1973). New York State physicians and the social context of abortion. *American Journal of Public Health*, **63**, 144.

35 Walter, G. (1970). Psychological and emotional consequences of elective abortion: a review. *Obstetrics and Gynecology, NY*, **36**, 482.

36 Wassertheil-Smoller, S. M., Arnold, C. B. & Lerner, R. C. (1972). New York State obstetricians and the new abortion law: physician experience with abortion techniques. *American Journal of Obstetrics and Gynecology*, **113**, 979.

37 Anonymous (1970). Abortion, the lonely problem, *Nursing Magazine*, June, 34.

38 Hall, R. E. (1970). The abortion revolution, *Playboy*, **17**, 112.

39 Association for the Study of Abortion (1972). *Newsletter*, **6**(4), 1.

40 Blake, J. (1971). Abortion and public opinion: the 1960–1970 decade. *Science, Washington*, **171**, 540.

41 *New York Times*, 5 May 1972.

42 *Family Planning – Population Reporter* (1974), **3**, 65.

43 *Family Planning – Population Reporter* (1974), **3**, 85.

44 Anonymous (1974). A review of state abortion laws enacted since January 1973. *Family Planning – Population Reporter*, **3**, 88.

45 Foreign Assistance Act (Amendment 114, Limiting Use of Funds for Abortions). *Congressional Record* – Senate S 21911, 5 December 1973.

46 *Durham Morning Herald*, 20 November 1974.

47 Fiscal Year 1975 DHEW – Labor Appropriation Bill. *World Population Washington Memorandum*, 8 July 1974. Planned Parenthood/World Population.

48 US Civil Rights Commission (1975). *Constitutional Aspects of the Right to Limit Childbearing*. Washington, D.C.

49 Pilpel, H. F. (1975). Testimony to Subcommittee on Constitutional Amendments. United States Senate Subcommittee on the Judiciary, 10 March.

50 *Planned Parenthood/World Population, Washington Memorandum*. Monthly issues from January 1974 refer.

51 Rosoff, J. I. (1975). 'Is support of abortion political suicide?' *Family Planning Perspectives*, **7**, 13–22.

52 Newspaper and court records of the Laufe case were made available to the authors.

53 Review of state laws and policies (1975). *Family Planning/Population Reporter*, **4**, no. 1.

54 *The Washington Post*, 18 February 1975.

55 Safire, W. (1975). *Before the Fall: An Inside View of the Pre-Watergate White House*. Doubleday, New York.

56 Commission on Population and the American Future (1972). *Population and the American Future*. Signet Books, New York.

11
Continental Europe

Between the wars – change and experiment
USSR (1921–36)

World War I was a watershed in European social affairs. In
Russia it precipitated a revolution. The Bolshevik party under
Lenin achieved control of the country in 1918, but civil war and
foreign invasion continued until 1921 when the Treaty of Riga ended
fighting between the Russians and Poles and their allies the French.
In the same year abortion was legalised. The decree had been issued
on 18 November 1920[1] and the philosophy behind the change was
made explicit in its rather unlegalistic wording:

> During the past decades the number of women resorting to
> artificial discontinuation of pregnancy has grown both in the
> West and this country. The legislation of all countries combats
> this evil by punishing the woman who chooses to have an
> abortion and the doctor who performs it. Without leading to
> favourable results, this method of combating abortions has
> driven the operation underground... as a result, up to 50 per
> cent of such women are infected in the course of the operation,
> and up to 4 per cent of them die.
>
> The Workers and Peasants' Government is conscious of this
> serious evil to the community. It combats this evil by
> propaganda against abortions... but the moral survivals of the
> past and the difficult economic conditions of the present still
> compel many women to resort to this operation...
> [*It was decided:*]
>
> (1) To permit such operations to be performed freely and
> without charge in Soviet hospitals, where conditions are assured
> of minimising the harm of the operation.

(2) Absolutely to forbid anyone but a doctor to carry out this operation.

(3) Any nurse or midwife found guilty of making such an operation will be deprived of the right to practise, and tried by a People's Court.

(4) A doctor carrying out an abortion in his private practice with mercenary aims will be called to account by a People's Court.

It is important to note that the law was changed on the basis of female equality and in recognition of a woman's right to control her own fertility and was without demographic considerations. Lenin believed women should have the right 'of deciding for themselves a fundamentl issue of their lives'.[2] The alteration came at a time of sweeping social and economic changes and against a background of very little contraceptive use. In theory, the reform was accompanied by an educational programme about the effects of abortion and the possibilities of contraceptive use but, as is often the case in the field of human fertility, ideals and reality appear to have been far apart.

Abortion was performed without anaesthesia and initially the woman had to remain in bed for three days and off work for two weeks. No doctor could refuse a request although he was exhorted to discourage the practice, especially with women with fewer than three children.

The mortality and morbidity rates may have been moderately high, although certainly lower than in the preceding period of illegal abortions. Slowly, attitudes became restrictive. In 1924 a fee was introduced. In 1927 a conference of gynaecologists in Kiev condemned abortion and *Izvestia* began to proclaim its dangers.

While the original reform of the law had grown out of an analysis of the problem and the decree even quoted statistics (albeit of doubtful validity), the re-introduced restrictive legislation refrained from discussing any aspect of abortion *per se*. A leading article in *Pravda* (28 May 1936)[3] dwelt at length on 'strengthening the Soviet family'.

> We alone have all the conditions under which a working
> woman can fulfil her duties as a citizen and a mother
> responsible for the birth and early upbringing of her children.
> A woman without children merits our pity, for she does not
> know the full joy of life. Our Soviet women, full-blooded

citizens of the freest country of the world, have been given the
bliss of motherhood. We must safeguard our family and raise
and rear healthy Soviet heroes.

Some letter writers to *Pravda* raised problems that the mushy prose
of the editorial had avoided, 'The projected law is premature
because the housing problem in our towns is a painful one'; 'A
pregnant woman who is nursing a baby and has again become
pregnant should be allowed to have an abortion'; 'The prohibition
of abortion means the compulsory birth of a child to a woman who
does not want children.' 'It must not be thought,' wrote Professor
K. Bogolepov from Leningrad, 'that the majority of abortions are
the result of irresponsible behaviour. Experience shows that a
woman resorts to abortion as a last resort when other methods of
safeguard against pregnancy have failed and the birth of a child
threatens to make life more difficult.'

Izvestia reported (4 June 1936) receiving 3713 letters on abortion
(and the other changes in family legislation including divorce). One
professor wrote that 'performing an abortion is an operation
undoubtedly involving great risks. There are few operations so
dangerous as cleaning out the womb', but he went on to say that
'our surgeons have brought the technique of performing abortions
to perfection. The foreign doctors who have watched operations in
our gynaecological hospitals have unanimously testified that their
technique is irreproachable.'

The debate revealed the same range of attitudes found in Western
countries today. Termination of a first pregnancy was forbidden in
1935, and on 27 June 1936 the Council of the People's Commissars
decided:

> In view of the proven harm of abortions, to forbid the
> performance of abortions whether in hospitals and special
> institutions, or in the homes of doctors and the private homes of
> pregnant women. The performance of abortions shall be
> allowed exclusively in those cases when the continuation of the
> pregnancy endangers the life of or threatens serious injury to
> the health of the pregnant woman and likewise when a serious
> disease of the parents may be inherited, and only under
> hospital or maternity home conditions.

Violations of the law were to be punished by two or three years'
imprisonment. Maternity homes and kindergartens were made more
numerous and alimony regulations stricter.

The Russian experience had little influence outside the country and it seems to have been the events leading up to the re-introduction of a restrictive law which were reported abroad, rather than any analysis of the social, medical or demographic effects of the period of liberalisation.

Within Russia, liberalisation, restriction and subsequent re-liberalisation had different degrees of significance in different localities. In 1936 Stalin introduced the present constitution of the country, which, on paper but not in practice, gave considerable rights to each of the 15 republics. With varying degrees of severity Stalin, and those who followed him, have enforced a 'coming together' of the ethnic and linguistic groups that make up Russia, but no ruler has ironed out the marked variation in the use of abortion and therefore of birth rates in the different republics.

Western Europe

World War I produced some of the most profound social changes of all time: women entered employment in unprecedented numbers, in some countries they won the struggle for the vote, churchgoing declined dramatically and many nations abandoned the gold standard. People began to whisper about birth control. A famous soldier, back from the war, wrote 'When I left England in 1911 contraceptives were hard to buy outside London and the other large cities. By 1919 every village chemist was selling them.'[4] In Britain Marie Stopes published *Married Love*; in France Victor Margueritte wrote *La garçonne* telling women 'their body was theirs'. However, for all but the most radical, acceptance of abortion was unthinkable. What did occur was a dawning appreciation of the inadequacies of many existing abortion laws.

At the end of the war, France and Belgium had laws dating from 1810, founded on the *Code Napoléon* (paragraph 317) prescribing five to ten years' penal servitude for the operator as well as the woman. The severity of the punishment necessitated trial by jury. Prosecutions were rare and convictions even rarer, because in the majority of convicted cases juries found there to be extenuating circumstances. Between 1881 and 1910 in France, there were less than 30 prosecutions annually; in Belgium there were more cases (3323 between 1919 and 1923 but only 283 sentences). It was partly in recognition of the fact that the old law was unworkable that lesser sentences of fines and imprisonment, which no longer necessitated jury decisions, were introduced by France in 1923. In Belgium *tribunaux correctionnels* (magistrate courts) also came to deal with abortions as misdemeanours, and between 1926 and 1935 only five people were tried by jury and 809 sentenced by these courts.[5] Still the spirit of the law remained highly restrictive and a failure to induce an abortion was no defence. Abortions continued at a very high rate, although prosecutions were still extremely rare.

The pattern of ineffectual legislation characterised developed countries as a whole. In one series of prosecutions in Denmark, where women came before juries, 14 out of 15 cases were acquitted. However, the response to the situation varied. In Italy several desperate efforts were made between the wars to make restrictive legislation work. Anti-contraceptive legislation was passed in 1931, and in 1927 and 1934 steps were taken to enforce abortion legislation more strictly. Under a Royal Decree of 27 July 1934 (No. 1265) doctors were obliged to notify medical officers of every case of abortion coming to their notice, within two days and in full detail. Illegal abortions continued nevertheless and even the death certificates of women who had died from abortion came to be falsified – a practice which continues to the present day.

In 1926 Germany also modified her nineteenth-century abortion laws. Under the 1872 Penal Code, abortion had been punishable by up to five years' imprisonment for the woman and up to life imprisonment for the operator, with various extra terms in the case of maternal death, but some alleviation if there were extenuating circumstances. Abortion where the woman's life was endangered by the pregnancy appears to have been possible. The 1926 alteration led to a simpler and slightly less harsh law with imprisonment for the woman of from one day to five years and for the operator of from one to 15 years. These changes were the result of left-wing political pressure and had the support of the medical profession, which, as in Britain, thought limited modification of the law desirable; for example, 96 per cent of the doctors approached by the Hamburg Medical Board in 1930 held opinions more liberal than the existing law.[6]

After the Nazis came to power, abortion on eugenic grounds was permitted, but the main trend was to attempt to enforce the existing legislation more strictly. The reasoning was that of promoting the Master Race. In 1938 a Jewish couple were acquitted of attempting to procure an abortion on the grounds that the relevant section of the criminal code could not be used for the protection of Jewish embryos.[7] German doctors were supposed to report every abortion they attended. Prosecutions doubled after 1936. The large number of deaths due to illegal abortion were said to be exaggerations put about by Jews and Communists. (It is revealing of the emotive nature of abortion that discussion of the reported *low* death rates from legal abortion in post-war eastern Europe was said in England to be 'politically adjusted').

In 1943 the law was extended to include the death penalty as those guilty of abortion 'continually impaired the vitality of the German people by such deeds'. In private, Hitler was partly realistic about abortion. In 1941, in one of his numerous rambling, after-dinner talks, the Führer told his guests how he himself had been imprisoned in Landsberg jail with a man sentenced to eight months' imprisonment for sending his girl-friend to an abortionist. Hitler used the case to illustrate the virtues of corporal punishment. 'Of course, some punishment was necessary,' he said, 'but if he'd been given a sound licking, and then let go, he'd have had his lesson. He was a nice boy.'[8] In public, Hitler was intolerant of abortion. 'The use of contraceptives means a violation of nature, a degradation of womanhood, motherhood and love,' he wrote, 'Nazi ideals. . . demand that the practice of abortion. . .shall be exterminated with a strong hand. Women inflamed by Marxist propaganda, claim the right to bear children only when they desire, first furs, radio, new furniture, then perhaps one child.'[7]

It was claimed that the stricter law caused a marked drop in the induced abortion rate, although it seems equally likely that it merely led to a reluctance by doctors to register what they took to be criminal abortions.

A trend of increasing restrictiveness also characterised France immediately prior to World War II and was continued and entrenched under German domination during the war. In 1939, the *Code de la Famille* was enacted, with one to five years imprisonment, together with heavy fines for abortionists (which could be doubled in the case of recidivists). Members of the medical profession who were involved in abortion were automatically debarred from practice for a minimum of five years and, to make the procurement of abortion a harder task for the woman, pregnancy tests had to be registered and countersigned by the local mayor. At first sight, it is strange that, beside these desperate attempts to tighten up the law, an exception was allowed for therapeutic abortion. However, the wording is circumspect: 'Where the necessity of saving the life of the mother, gravely threatened, demands either a surgical intervention or the use of a therapeutic medium likely to cause interruption of pregnancy'. It could be interpreted merely to cover those procedures of hysterectomy and operation for ectopic pregnancy, seen as licit by Catholic theologians.

Within a few months of signing an armistice with Hitler, Marshal Pétain and the Vichy Government of France found time to make the aborton laws even more stringent. Even the non-pregnant woman who attempted an abortion could be prosecuted.

Vichy France ranked abortion with treason and sabotage. Penalties which included solitary confinement and hard labour for life were imposed. The regime has the distinction of witnessing the last-known occasion in world history when an individual was executed for a crime relating to abortion. Madame Giraud was a laundress who had performed 26 abortions. She was executed in February 1942.[9,10]

Scandinavia

Iceland has a tradition of independent and far-sighted social legislation. In 1802 it was the first country in the world to make vaccination compulsory and in 1934 the Icelandic parliament led the way in abortion reform amongst northern European legislatures. The country had become politically independent of Denmark in 1918, although it acknowledged the sovereignty of the Danish king until 1944. Law No. 38 of 28 January 1935 was without precedent, dealing with the social as well as the medical indications for abortion,

> When estimating how far childbirth may be likely to damage the health of a pregnant woman...it may...be taken into consideration whether the woman has already borne many children at short intervals and a short time has passed since her last confinement, also whether her domestic conditions are difficult, either on account of a large flock of children, poverty or serious ill-health or other members of the family.[11]

Any two doctors are permitted to certify the need for abortion, which must be carried out in a registered place. Social indications are only valid until eight weeks of pregnancy (although in practice they are taken into account up to 12 weeks), while strictly medical reasons are allowed until 28 weeks. Eugenic considerations are not included in the law, but a commission of doctors and a judge consider requests for termination. The same commission also decides on requests for sterilisation and, as in other Scandinavian countries, vasectomy remains practically unknown and tubal ligation difficult to obtain.

The law has remained unchanged, and the abortion rate relatively constant, since 1935. In 1968 there were 66 abortions and, in 15 of these, social as well as medical considerations were taken into account.[12] In 1971 a commission was set up to advise on possible changes which may include a further liberalisation during the first trimester.

Most Scandinavian countries enacted strict anti-abortion legislation in the nineteenth century. For example, a Swedish law of 1864 involved anything from six years' penal servitude to capital punishment for abortionists. Interestingly, however, the law was modified as early as 1890 to permit termination on genuine medical grounds. Scandinavia, like the rest of Europe, had also enacted anti-contraception laws, but they began to repeal or overlook them at an early stage. Public family planning clinics were set up in Norway in 1924 and in Sweden in 1933. The ineffectual, unenforceable nature of anti-abortion legislation was also recognised. As in post-war eastern Europe, these changes occurred against an awareness and concern about *falling* birth rates and sometimes at a time when legislation to increase the financial incentives for having children was being passed.

In Norway, the medical community sought reform in 1930, the Church in 1934 and, backed by a public petition, an official committee was set up and recommended law reform in 1935, but legislation failed to progress in parliament and a law of 1902, punishing abortion by two- to six-year prison sentences, remained operative.

In 1935 the Swedish Riksdag set up a Royal Population Commission to consider the falling birth rate and two years later a subcommittee of this same Commission recommended limited reform of abortion laws to permit termination for medical, eugenic and ethical reasons, but excluding social indications. The Commission expressed the pious hope that social reforms would eliminate the need for abortion. In 1938, the Riksdag passed the first reform law and it came into force on 1 January 1939.

The evolution of Danish thinking was similar. In 1929, a delegation of working women sought to bring about changes in the then existing punitive legislation. In 1932, the government set up a commission on abortion legislation which recommended a law embodying medical, socio-humanitarian and eugenic principles in 1936.[13] While the commission was deliberating the trial, initial acquittal and subsequent imprisonment of Dr Leunbach became a *cause célèbre* in the Danish movement for reform. Leunbach openly performed abortions in a working-class area. At his trial he claimed 'many medical men refused poverty as an indication for abortion but readily accepted wealth'.[14] Following Sweden's example, Denmark passed reform legislation in 1939.

Post-war liberalisation
Scandinavia

For almost two decades, amongst those who sought a liberalisation of attitudes towards abortion in Europe and America, the experience of Scandinavia appeared to be exemplary. However, in retrospect these countries may have taught more by systematic errors than precept. Basically, the evolution of abortion attitudes and services in Scandinavia in general, and in Sweden in particular, was by a process of erosion, as traditional attitudes and myths slowly disappeared in the face of practical experience. At no time was there an effort to devise solutions to complex problems by rational building upon a total analysis of the situation.

In practice, the Scandinavian experience can be split into two phases: a traditional and an innovatory. The number of legal abortions was low until the late 1960s, decisions were made in the framework of illness and not as part of the pattern of preventive medicine, conclusions were reached laboriously and the operation performed late and by conservative procedures. Slowly, familiarity led to a softening of attitudes, doctors became confident and willing to take greater responsibilities (Fig. 15, p. 73). The turning point in Sweden came about 1967. Prior to this date, abortion rates had run at less than one per 1000 of the population, the average duration of gestation at operation was well over 12 weeks (Table 27),[15] the hospital stay was generally over a week, and two to three weeks were devoted to the investigation of the problem. The mortality rate was always over 40 and sometimes over 100 per 100000 operations. The reasons registered for termination were predominantly 'weakness'

Table 27. *Medically induced delay in granting legal abortion in Umea Hospital, Sweden*

	Number of abortions	Days of investi-gation	Days in hospital	Medium duration of preg-nancy at operation (weeks)
1963–64	45	25.8	10.1	16.0
1967	127	11.6	5.6	12.6

and 'illness'. After 1967 the rate passed the one in a 1000 mark, the median duration of gestation fell to 12 weeks, techniques improved, mortality began to approach the eastern European level (although it still remains above it) and that delightful euphemism 'anticipated weakness' began to appear more frequently on the registration forms as a reason for operation – indicating that the doctor was listening to his patients rather than recalling the words of his teachers.[16]

As recently as 1966 in one Stockholm hospital, there were as many terminations at 22 weeks as at 11. Reviewing 30 years' experience of abortion in Sweden, Ottensen-Jensen[16, 17] has commented, 'Women who have applied for an abortion have borne witness to the strain of an investigation lasting three or four weeks or more. At hospitals and centres where close collaboration has been established around problems of abortion, it has been shown that an investigation need not take more than a fortnight at the most from the first contact to the operation.' He adds, with unintentional irony, 'This means that the abortion can be performed at an early stage, which is very desirable' – apparently unaware that in parts of Yugoslavia and the USA the operation is done within 24 to 48 hours of first contact (see also Fig. 21, p. 107). More recently, doctors came to bypass the rather complex decision-making procedures in order to avoid second-trimester operations. The law had always allowed decisions to be made either by the National Board of Health (which represented a group decision after detailed enquiry and clinical assessment), or on the opinion of two doctors. In 1965 approximately 3000 abortions were decided by the National Board of Health and less than 500 by two doctors; in 1969 over 4000 were decided by two doctors, and the National Board of Health, which had in the interim greatly increased the percentage of requests accepted, granted 11 000 operations, Over the years 1955–59, when the percentage of requests granted by the National Board of Health and the total number of abortions both fell, the mortality rate for the operation was more than twice that for the next quinquennium, when these two trends were reversed.

The experiences of the other Scandinavian countries have been similar to that of Sweden, although some have telescoped the evolution of law and practice, beginning later than Sweden but reaching a comparable point by the 1970s (Fig. 16, p. 73). Denmark and Finland both enacted liberal laws, in March 1970, but Norway lagged behind with a law of December 1963, which, although recognising socio-economic grounds, is somewhat more restrictive.

Switzerland

Abortion legislation in Switzerland, like the country itself, is subject to ethnic and religious variation in interpretation.

Abortion was first legalised just after World War I and current legislation is based on a revision enacted in 1939. The only ground for termination is a 'very serious' threat to the health or life of the mother. In cantons such as Geneva and Vaud, the law has allowed a liberal practice to grow up and many doctors take into account the social background of the mother, whether it be a large family or an unmarried girl. For Swiss residents it is not a case of a few doctors stretching the law for their own purposes, but a genuine interpretation of the law that has grown up over the years, and in Geneva 90 per cent of applications are accepted. In public hospitals the fee is 400–2000 Swiss francs ($194–968) . The cantons appoint a panel of experts to decide on abortions. In the Catholic cantons such as St Gall or Basle a different atmosphere exists and abortions are rarely performed. The Swiss appear largely satisfied with the schizophrenic working of their law. Efforts have to be made to arrest the influx of foreigners seeking to escape from the unreality of their own national laws and only 50 per cent of non-resident applications are accepted.

A Swiss society for the legalisation of abortion was founded in 1973, but in March 1975 the parliament rejected a Bill to legalise first-trimester abortion on request.

Socialist countries of eastern Europe and USSR

The nations of eastern Europe, like Poland, have predominantly Roman Catholic populations and had restrictive abortion laws until the redistribution of political power after World War II. The German Democratic Republic altered its law in 1947. In November 1955, the USSR repealed the 1936 legislation restricting abortion to purely medical causes. The official commentary on the legislation summarised the thinking of the Supreme Soviet,

> The decree points out that the measures taken by the Soviet state to encourage motherhood and protect children, together with the increasing growth in the awareness of cultural level of women actively participating in all spheres of the country's national economic, cultural and social life, make it possible to dispense at the present time with the prohibition of abortion carried out according to law, and states that the prevention of abortion can be ensured by extending further the state measures for the encouragement of motherhood and measures of an education and explanatory nature.
>
> The repeal of the prohibition of abortion will also make it possible to avert the harm caused to the health of women by abortions performed outside medical establishments.[18]

Between 1956 and 1960 Poland, Czechoslovakia, Bulgaria, Hungary, Romania and Yugoslavia, all altered their laws and included social grounds amongst the reasons for abortion.[19,20] As in the USSR, the overall intention of the eastern European laws was seen as a public health measure. Thus, the preamble to the Polish law of 27 April 1956 defines its intentions as providing abortion in order to protect the health of the woman against the ill effects of abortion done in all conditions and not by a doctor'. Usually abortion is a committee decision, but in Hungary it must be granted, 'if the applicant insists on interruption of pregnancy'.

On the whole, the experience in eastern Europe, as in Scandinavia and Japan, has been of a moving towards progressively liberal legislations – a theme most consistently developed in Yugoslavia. Termination was allowed on strict medical grounds in 1951. In January 1952 the law was altered to permit termination on medical and eugenic grounds in cases of rape, incest and carnal knowledge and 'in exceptional cases, the interruption of a pregnancy may be authorised where there is good reason to believe that the birth of a child may be injurious to the health of the pregnant woman because her living, personal or family conditions are particularly difficult'.[21] These exceptional circumstances appear to have been common and in 1960 the law was altered again. The key clause permitting termination for social reasons now reads, 'when it can be reasonably expected that the woman will find herself placed, as a result of the birth of a child, in difficult personal, family or material conditions which cannot be remedied by other means'.[22] As Yugoslavian law is interpreted by a commission, the law may be more directly related to the number of terminations performed than in many other countries. It is to be noted that the number of terminations per 1000 fertile women doubled between 1959 and 1961. In 1969 the Yugoslavian Federal Assembly passed a resolution on family planning that stated, 'It is one of the basic human rights and duties of parents to be able to plan the size of their families,' and noted that 'society should make it possible for married couples to get informaion about modern methods of birth control'. The Federal Assembly also drafted a new law which accomplished the last step in the path trodden by its predecessors. After dealing with medical eugenic and humanitarian grounds, the draft law of 1969 states, 'The interruption of pregnancy will be done on demand of the woman if during the pregnancy and after birth she could fall into serious personal, material and other troubles'. The draft became law in June 1974.

The German Democratic Republic was the first of the socialist countries of eastern Europe to reform its abortion law, doing so in 1947. The law was amended in 1950, but remained more restrictive than in some neighbouring countries. Termination required a commission decision, it was allowed automatically for women over 40 years of age or under 16, for those with five children and in certain circumstances for those with four, and the medical examination allowed consideration of the 'total life situation of the pregnant woman'.

Hungary and Romania arrived at the position of total freedom earlier and more precipitously. In addition to specifying medical, eugenic and social reasons, the Hungarian law directed that termination was legal 'if the personal or family circumstances of the applicant justify interruption of pregnancy or if the applicant maintains her application despite the explanations given by the Board,'[23] i.e. the Board should inform the woman about the advisability of keeping her child and of the dangers of termination. The Romanian law[24] simply did away with all legal requirements for the woman under 12 weeks of pregnancy and allowed her to go directly to a centre without the hurdle of a commission.

Hungary subsequently withdrew from this position and the commissions were empowered to delay the operation so that the woman can think over the problem, but the final choice still rests with the mother. In addition, there have been significant increases in family allowances. The Romanians have retreated much further and the violent reversal of their law in 1966 provides one of the most dramatic illustrations of the effect of abortion legislation on birth rates ever recorded or ever likely to be recorded (p. 145). A similar change took place in Bulgaria in March 1968,[25] but its results are less well documented. It must be noted that in both countries socio-economic grounds explicitly remain in the revised laws.

The magnitude of the demographic changes in post-war eastern and central Europe, which have been partially achieved through induced abortion, is such that it is reasonable to ask if they have had any influence on the post-war economic progress of these countries. It is well known that the certain changes in the age structure of the population, particularly those associated with a decline in the dependency burden, can be economically advantageous and are the goal of many family planning programmes in developing countries. But birth rates were also falling in western Europe and any differential effect would be very small; if it does exist, it is buried among other, more important, variables in economic development that have characterised the two sides of the Iron Curtain.[26] For instance, it is interesting to compare East and West Germany. Before World War II they had comparable industrial and agricultural development. After the war, East German recovery was much slower and less complete. West Germany regained its pre-war level of production in the early 1950s, East Germany in the late 1950s. By 1967 West Germany's industrial product had grown to 380 per cent of the 1936 level; that of East Germany to only 213 per cent. In quality of food consumption, or use of consumer goods, or most other indices, it remains behind West Germany. In 1967 64 per cent of houses in East Germany had neither inside toilet, bath nor central heating; in West Germany the comparable figure was 25 per cent. There are several reasons for the differences. War between Germany and the USSR had been more vicious and more costly

than in the West, and the Russians exacted a heavier toll in repara-
tions, dismantling much of the industry and even taking one set
of all double-tracked railway lines. A fundamental reorientation of
trade towards the East took place. The centralisation of industry
acted adversely on expansion; it took twice as long to complete a
building in the East as in West Germany. Some two million people
emigrated to the West, mostly educated young males, and this
represented an economic loss to East Germany, although it took
some of the strain off limited resources such as housing.

Current changes

Despite a decade's experience of liberal abortion in Scandinavia and eastern Europe, it was the enactment of the 1967 British
law and the revolution of attitude in the USA which seem to have
been major factors releasing the avalanche of changes that has
overwhelmed Europe in the 1970s.

Abortion has become a significant public issue in all western
European countries, except Spain and Portugal. Change has continued in Scandinavia, liberal legislation has been enacted in the
German Federal Republic, France and Austria, and a remarkable
alteration in practice, without law reform, has occurred in Holland.
Meanwhile, eastern Europe has moved to a more homogeneous
situation than it was in previously, with some restriction of the
previously ultra-liberal situation in Hungary and some liberalisation
in East Germany (which had long been more restrictive than its
neighbours).

The situation in western Europe in the 1970s is somewhat similar
to that in the USA in the late 60s. There is a general movement
towards liberal abortion but an increasingly noisy opposition; there
are a variety of local laws varying from restrictive to very liberal
reform; yet some of the most innovative services have evolved
outside the law and there is a considerable passage of women in need
across frontiers of legislation and medical practice (Table 28).
However, the only analogous authority to Washington D.C. is Stras-
burg. The Human Rights Commission is very much weaker than
the US Supreme Court and its authority in the realm of fertility
regulation is untested. In 1971 a draft calling for free sale of contraceptives and abortion for medical and 'serious social' indications
came before the 17-nation Council of Europe. It received an equally

Table 28. *Legal abortions, registered in Britain, on women from other European countries*

	Abortions				Number of abortions obtained in Britain per 100 live births in country of residence			
	1969	1971	1973	1975	1969	1971	1973	1975
German Federal Republic	1559	13315	11326	3417	0.2	1.7	0.3	0.4
Belgium	150	2073	1462	390	0.1	1.5	1.0	0.2
France	471	11529	35293	14809	0.1	1.3	4.0	1.7
Ireland	218	1225	1193	1562	0.2	1.2	1.2	1.5
Netherlands	137	843	101	—	0.1	0.4	0.0	—
Switzerland	45	381	719	422	0.0	0.4	0.8	0.3
Denmark	38	228	27	—	0.1	0.3	0.0	—
Austria	7	158	291	—	0.0	0.1	0.2	—
Spain	21	191	1765	4230	0.0	0.0	0.3	0.6
Italy	19	184	1171	5304	0.0	0.0	0.1	0.4
Other countries	54	376	4428	3379	—	—	—	—
Total	2719	30503	57776	33513	—	—	—	—
Britain	53600	94600	110568	106648	6.0	11.7	13.6	13.2

divided vote, 45:45. A two-thirds majority was necessary and Piet Dankert of Holland, who introduced the measure, withdrew it.

The legal reform in Britain has ended up somewhat like the 1967 reform in Colorado – an important pioneer step, but one that has been unassociated with any important development in the human or social aspects of services. Some countries that undertook legal change later than the pioneers have gone further. Austria, like Washington State, now has a more liberal abortion law than Britain. Some of the most exciting services, as well as some of the best and cheapest, have evolved in Holland, where the law has never been reformed or repealed, just as Washington D.C. became the home of one of the most rational services in the USA.

Scandinavia

In the 1960s the Nordic Council began examining legislation in all Scandinavian countries and recommended harmonisation of the abortion laws. Basically, the several countries involved have all moved towards a very liberal situation, but some differences remain.

Denmark introduced legislation to permit elective abortion at the request of any woman over 38 years of age, or with four or more children, in April 1970. In 1973 it legislated to permit abortion at the request of any woman within the first trimester of pregnancy.[27] Finland revised her law in 1970 to allow abortion on wide socio-economic grounds.[28] Among other indications abortion is permitted, 'if delivery and care of the child would place a notable strain on [*the woman*] in relation to her living conditions and those of her family and other circumstances'. Abortion on request was granted to women under 17 and over 40. In 1969 there were 8179 legal abortions (12.1 per 100 births); in 1970 14525 (22.5 per 100 births.)[29] But Norway felt unable to accept the Nordic Council's recommendations because of insurmountable 'Christian and ethical objections', and in January 1975 rejected a Bill to permit abortion on request in the first three months of pregnancy. However, in May 1975 some degree of liberalisation did take place and 90 per cent of requests are now granted.

Sweden, characteristically, took several years to move from the position of reasonable liberality obtaining in the late 1960s, to abortion at the request of the woman. A committee on abortion had begun work in 1965 and reported in September 1971. It recommended that abortion, including self-induced abortion, should be removed from the Penal Code, although abortion by lay persons should remain illegal. It also recommended that all abortions should be done in public hospitals free of charge, and by the least traumatic procedure, as early as possible in pregnancy.

Eventually, a non-restrictive law was passed and implemented from 1 January 1975. It permitted abortion on request during the first 18 weeks of pregnancy (less than 19 weeks from the last menstrual period). Indeed refusal to carry out an abortion carries a penalty of up to one year in prison. After 12 weeks, discussion with a social worker is obligatory. The law is limited to Swedish residents.

The Common Market

The greater part of the enlarged Common Market behaves as a homogeneous block in its pattern of fertility, as well as in trade, although certain areas present problems in demography as well as in regional economic planning. Scotland has a higher birth rate than England and Wales, Ulster a higher rate still and some southern Italian provinces have birth rates double that obtaining in the north.

The desired and achieved family size in Common Market countries is similar, but the public provision of contraceptive services and the legality of abortion differ greatly. There is some variation in the emphasis on individual methods: for example, there are 50 per cent more oral contraceptive users in the German Federal Republic than in the UK.[30] This is probably the effect of availability, for in Britain women are restricted to particular general practitioners, who may also exercise a veto if a woman attends one of the thousand-odd family planning clinics in the country, while in West Germany the woman has a wider choice of options from which to seek a prescription for oral contraceptives. However, the overall use of contraceptives is broadly similar and it seems reasonable to suggest that induced abortion plays a comparable role in fertility control in each country, even though the laws have been very different.

GERMAN FEDERAL REPUBLIC

West Germany, the most populous and also one of the most prosperous nations of the Common Market, has a low birth rate (1971, 15 per 1000). Forty-four per cent of the population are Roman Catholic. It is thought about 200 000 illegal abortions occurred annually in the 1960s and early 70s.

After World War II, the Allied Control Council reinstated the 1926 legislation. The immediate post-war period was a time of great social stress in Europe and it is interesting that the Control Council considered altering the law to permit abortion on certain social grounds. It is possible that such legislation, once instituted, would not have been revised after the occupation. The history of fertility control on the western side of the Iron Curtain might have been somewhat different if this action had been taken.

The 1926 legislation had only been a minor modification of a law of 1871 which forbade abortion except where the continuance of the pregnancy would result 'in severe consequences for the mother'. In 1970 the Minister of Justice asked the West German Gynaecological Society to give an opinion on abortion law reform. Some lawyers had advised that abortion should be available on request up to six weeks after the last menstrual period, but the Gynaecological Society recommended that there should be no time limit on the operation and that it should be available if pregnancy involves a risk for the woman's health – health being defined within the WHO meaning of 'a state of physical, mental and social well being'. However, when the Government put a Bill up for discussion in 1972 the main body of medical opinion was against the liberal reform. In a poll, gynaecologists were shown to be opposed to legalised abortion. In the debate within the medical profession, which was fought more on impressions than firm statistics, the views of British doctors opposed to the 1967 legislation were quoted widely.

Further draft legislation was tabled early in 1973 by the SPD (Social Democrats), who dominated the government coalition at that time. The proposal was a radical one, permitting abortion on request up to 12 weeks, and was one item in a group of proposed reforms including the free advice and prescription of contraceptives as well as changes in divorce legislation. However, a minority of SPD Deputies opposed change (including the Justice Minister, Gerhard Jahn). The Christian Democrats and most of the opposition parties had serious reservations, and the gynaecologists, although shifting slightly, remained opposed to abortion on other than medical indications.

Wealthy West German women had long obtained safe abortions, as a group of prominent women 'confessed' in 1971.[31] It was estimated that about 10000 a year obtained hospital abortions in West Germany. In 1972 17531 West German women were recorded as having obtained legal abortions in Britain, while others went to Scandinavia, Holland and Switzerland. The demand for social justice was strong.

A group of West German parliamentarians, both favouring and opposing reform, travelled overseas in 1973 to learn from the experience of other countries. An increasingly passionate debate, with a well-organised opposition, was generated. Cardinal Döpfner of Munich, head of the Conference of Roman Catholic Bishops, was prepared to see legislation permitting abortion for strictly medical reasons, but remained adamantly opposed to any other change. Some lower-echelon Catholic writers, however, forgot their history and one newspaper likened abortion law reformers to the Nazis (p. 381).

In April 1974, four Bills were presented to the Bundestag at the same time. One permitted abortion on request, one abortion for mixed medical and social reasons, one in cases of 'grave emergency' and one strictly limited to cases where the continuation of the pregnancy endangered the woman's life. The Bills were debated for

18 hours over two days, much of it televised directly. Chancellor Herr Willy Brandt said of the most liberal Bill that it was 'a reform to remove intolerable social injustices dating from the past centuries'. The most liberal Bill, passed by a narrow margin (247, to 233, with nine abstentions), included not only abortion on request but provisions for social security institutions to cover costs. Voting was much more strictly along party political lines than had been the case in Britain or in most American states.

In June 1974, a few hours before the law was due to be implemented, the Christian Democrat-governed state of Baden-Württemberg successfully obtained an injunction in the Constitutional Court to suspend the law and decide on its constitutional validity. In February 1975 the Court ruled that abortion on request was unconstitutional. It stated, however, that abortion would be permitted on grounds of rape, danger to the mother's health, in cases of suspected fetal defect and 'when a birth could cause a grave hardship'. The Court accepted the argument that conception should be defined as occurring after fertilisation.

AUSTRIA

Austria is a more staunchly Catholic country than West Germany but it passed legislation permitting abortion on request a few months earlier. The pre-1974 law was among the most restrictive in western Europe, recognising only a threat to the woman's life as justification for legal abortion. At the end of 1973, a new criminal code passed through the Parliamentary Criminal Justice Committee allowing abortion in the first three months of gestation on the approval of a single doctor and without any statutory indications. Within a few days a massive public protest, headed by Cardinal Koenig, Archbishop of Vienna, was organised, and a pastoral letter condemning the change was read in the Austrian churches. However, the new code passed the lower House by a margin of five votes on 29 November 1973. It was blocked by the upper House on 9 December, but, the power of the upper House is limited and in March 1974 the new criminal code, including the option of first-trimester abortion on request, received parliamentary approval. It became operative on 1 January 1975. The husband's consent for the operation is not mandatory. Second-trimester abortion is permitted when the woman's life is in danger, if pregnancy involves a child under age 14 at the time of conception, or there is serious risk of fetal abnormality.

The implementation of the new law by the largely conservative Austrian medical establishment has been slow. But at least one free-standing abortion clinic has been established.

FRANCE

Legislative change through democratic means was a more difficult goal in France, where many religious and political forces are ranged to maintain the status quo in favour of restrictive abortion legislation, even though opinion polls show that a majority of French people favour a change to legislation of the British type. A passionate campaign was fought, with individual and group acts of great courage.

In 1971, 300 prominent French women, including the actress Jeanne Moreau, signed a manifesto admitting that they had broken the law against abortion. In February 1973, 345 French doctors signed a manifesto confessing that they had practised or aided abortions and advocating abortion on request. Theoretically they were liable to prosecution, with up to 10 years' imprisonment, but no action has been taken against them. The furthest that the Council of the Order of Doctors went was to reprimand one Dean of a Medical School for giving· evidence at a trial for abortion. The National Association for the Study of Abortion also issued a manifesto with 240 signatures, including four medical Nobel Prize winners, which asked for abortion to be permitted in cases of grave risk to the health of the mother, serious risk of congenital malformation, mental illness, rape or incest, pregnancies in girls under 15, and for pressing social reasons.

As in West Germany, many women with means or lucky connections obtained abortions by travelling outside the frontiers, especially to England (25 189 in 1972) and Holland, often by the bus or plane load. Such women were harassed by custom officials when *returning* to France and perhaps the ultimate injustice was that some, who had been given oral contraceptives post-abortion, were fined £100 ($200) and had the contraceptives confiscated. Such peripatetic abortions cost £80–£100 ($160–$220) inclusive.

Several reform pressure groups arose. The National Association for the Study of Abortion, rather like the American Association for the Study of Abortion, maintained high scholastic standards, and moved moderate legislation of a sort most likely to appeal widely. The French Movement for Family Planning, Group for Health Information, Choice (founded by Mme Simone de Beauvoir), and

Movement for Freedom of Abortion and Contraception were involved in more direct action.

A small but growing group of physicians began to perform abortions relatively openly, especially using Karman techniques; Harvey Karman himself visited Paris and Grenoble, training some doctors, while others visited centres in England to learn appropriate techniques. The clinic in Grenoble performed operations free of charge and was closely linked to Choice and the local family planning association. It was well known to everybody, except the local police. In May 1973, they traced a 17-year-old girl, one of a family of seven, who had been made pregnant by a 42-year-old married man, but was given an abortion at the clinic. The police immediately arrested a local doctor, Dr Ferrey-Martin (at 6.0 a.m.). But she had not performed the operation, although she freely admitted being one of a group of well-known citizens involved in running a high-standard service and had indeed performed many abortions. Within a few days 3000 Grenoble people demonstrated at a public meeting on behalf of Dr Ferrey-Martin, helping to discredit the implementation as well the letter, of the French law. The Grenoble group threatened to carry out an abortion in public, but later called a day of protest in support of legislative change.

One of the interesting facets of humane abortion services operating outside the law is that there are no artificial and unnecessary political restraints on rational medical practice. Some operations were delegated to paramedical workers, some performed by medical students, some carried out actually in the woman's home.

The first serious attempt to move new legislation was made in December 1973, with a Bill to legalise abortion where the woman's health is in danger, in cases of pregnancy following rape or incest, or where there is risk of fetal defect. The draft included parental consent for girls under 18, written application, seven days delay for reflection and two-doctor decision-making. In the parliamentary debate the Minister of Justice, M. Jean Taittinger claimed the existing law was 'archaic, unsuitable, inefficient and unjust'. He estimated that 1000 illegal abortions occurred daily and perhaps one woman a day died as a result. He remarked that if the 1920 law had been strictly applied 15 million French women would have been imprisoned since it was introduced. The Right wing of the Gaullist party opposed the Bill as too liberal, and the opposition opposed it for not going far enough. The Bill was shunted into a committee.

A scientific conference of the French Society for the Study of Fertility and Sterility held in Paris in June 1974, heard a report on samples of early abortions performed by a gynaecologist, in a free-standing clinic and in a family planning service in Paris.[32] At the latter, 50 to 100 women were seeking an abortion daily. The women were all counselled in the way Karman had taught and most operations did not require any anaesthesia. Half the women were married. There was a marked improvement in contraceptive use after the procedure.

A year after the failure of the 1973 Reform Bill a more liberal measure was introduced. The Minister of Health, Mme Simme Veil, fought vigorously for the measure. By late 1974, public opinion had shifted sufficiently to ensure its support. Finally, on 17 January 1975 the French parliament promulgated a law permitting abortion on request in the first 10 weeks after conception (12 weeks from the last menstrual period). Later in pregnancy, termination was limited to cases involving a serious threat to the life of the woman, or a strong probability of a serious, incurable fetal malformation.

Having been philosophically liberal the legislators were technically restrictive. The law[33] extended normal conscientious objection in such a way that a whole institution can opt out of providing abortions on the decision of the senior medical leadership. Girls under 18 require the consent of one parent or legal guardian. The doctor to whom the application for abortion is made must

(*a*) provide information to the woman concerning the medical risks involved;

(*b*) give her a booklet containing a description of the laws relating to her rights and the available aid she can seek if she is unmarried;

(*c*) send her to a counselling service when the question of whether or not to have the abortion will be discussed with her, after which she will be given an attendance certificate by the counsellor.

The woman for her part is required to give the doctor written confirmation, together with her counselling certificate, of her desire to have an abortion, not earlier than one week following her first application. Finally, and most important of all, the number of induced abortions performed in a hospital or clinic is not supposed to exceed 25 per cent of the 'total number of surgical or obstetric acts performed'.[34] Infringement of the regulations concerning numbers 'will constitute grounds for closing the establishment for one year. In case of a repeated offence the closure will be permanent.'

The law is limited to French nationals, but also applies to Réunion, Guadeloupe and Martinique, which are Départements of France.

The implementation of the law is proving a little more liberal than some of its own fine print might be expected to have allowed. The '25 per cent' rule has not been strictly enforced. At the same time, many institutions have refused abortion cases. Already there have been clashes, and in March 1975 militant doctors forcibly took over the operating theatre in a hospital where the head of the surgical department adamantly opposed abortion for any reason.[35]

BELGIUM

The current Belgium law forbids abortion even to save the woman's life. In a survey of fertility practices in Belgium in 1972, Cliquet[36] wrote, 'Considering the incidence of ineffective contraceptive practices, it may be wondered how [this] can be reconciled with the demographic reality of the low mean family size. The main explanation must be sought in the corrective effect of abortion, of which even the lowest estimates lead to quite impressive figures.' The birth rate in 1972 was 13.8 per 1000.

As in France, activity to alter the law has been spearheaded by acts of individual bravery. In 1973 Dr Wilby Peers, a member of the Belgian Association for the Liberalisation of Abortion was imprisoned for allegedly aborting a 16-year-old mentally retarded girl who, it was claimed, had been raped by her father. Dr Peers' release was recommended by a higher court, but refused by the Public Prosecutor. Hundreds of thousands of people signed a petition on his behalf and eventually he was released on the orders of the examining magistrate. The case was partly instrumental in persuading the Minister of Justice, Mr Van der Poorten, of the Liberal Party, to draft a Bill that would allow abortions when the woman's mental or physical health was in danger. In 1974 a feminist party made abortion on request one of the planks of its political reform.

Some leading Belgian doctors, like Professor P. Hubinot, have supported legal change. Bourg has argued reform in the *Bulletin de l'Academie royale de médicine de Belgique*,[37] but it seems that change will be slow. Meanwhile, many women travel the short journey into Holland to solve their problems.

ITALY

In 1971 Professor Luigi de Marchi reversed the Italian anti-contraceptive laws by an appeal to the Constitutional Court. In August 1971 a parliamentary representative, Signor Antonio Brizioli, introduced a draft Bill to permit abortion in cases of rape and incest, where the physical health of the child or mother was threatened, or where the woman had five children and was unable to care for more. The legislation made little progress.

In January 1973 Signor Loris Fortuna, a Socialist Deputy, who had achieved success in changing the Italian divorce laws, announced a Bill to permit abortion in hospitals when approved for medical reasons by two doctors. A campaign was launched to collect the half million signatures necessary under the Italian Constitution for a public referendum. Debates on changing abortion laws followed the same lines as in most Western industrialised nations, although in Italy the pro- and anti-abortion groups are particularly far apart. Both sides used questionable data in their discussions and the Vatican newspaper *L'Osservatore Romano* not unreasonably pointed out that the claim that 20000 women died each year from abortion in Italy (which had been put forward by a reform group) was twice the number of registered deaths from all causes amongst women of the fertile years. Many bitter episodes took place. In December 1973 the State Prosecutor in Trento filed criminal charges against 263 women whose names were found by the police in the records of one gynaecologist.

The strength of the vote in the 1974 referendum to keep the divorce legislation encouraged further attempts at abortion reform. The tide in favour of abortion rose and one survey by the magazine *Panorama* in 1974 surprised politicians by showing that 75 per cent of Italians favoured legal abortion.

Abortion referral agencies became bolder. The Radical Party gave particular support to CISA (Centre of Information on Sterilisation and Abortion). During 15 months they referred 6000 women for abortion working, among other places, with Dr Giorgio Conciani's clinic in Florence. The clinic charged the equivalent of $50 for first-trimester abortions and vacuum aspiration operations were openly performed until January 1975 when Dr Conciani, four nurses, a sociologist and Signor Gianfranco Spadaccia (Secretary of the Radical Party) were all arrested. Senator Pisano, a member of the neo-fascist Italian Social Movement (MSI) had been particularly vigorous in denouncing the clinic.

In January 1975 the editor of *L'Espresso* was charged with contempt of the religion of the state for publishing a cover picture of a naked, pregnant woman nailed to a cross, with the caption 'Aborto: una tragedia italiana'. The main parliamentary parties were forced to draft abortion laws and the feminists and Radicals were not averse to launching, in a Holy Year, the most massive abortion reform campaign in Italian history. The opening round in the fight went to the abortion reformers when in February 1975 the Constitutional Court declared the existing Article 54 of the Penal Code (restricting abortion) to be unconstitutional, forcing legislation to be introduced at least to permit abortion where the woman's health was strongly endangered.

Next, the reformers set a referendum in motion. More than half a million signatures were collected, as required by the Italian Constitution. The threat of a referendum, in turn lead to more political activity. Both the Christian Democrats and the Communists wanted to avoid a referendum. By the end of 1975 a draft Bill had progressed to the stage of detailed discussion of possible grounds for termination. Threats to the mental and physical health of the woman, her socio-economic environment, as well as pregnancy associated with rape or the risk of congenital defect, were all accepted as grounds for abortion. Although such legislation did not meet the demands for abortion on request made by the Radical Party and the feminists, it might have been accepted but for forceful intervention by the Church. In December 1975 the bishops, apparently with the approval of the Pope, condemned 'the slaying of the innocents' in one of the most vehement outbursts the hierarchy had ever made. Individual members of parliament were stimulated to denounce the Concordat. Views were further polarised and the fragile alliance between the Communists and some of the right-wing liberals broken. Eventually, at the end of April 1976, the inability to solve the abortion issue brought down the Christian Democrat government of Signor Aldo Moro. This event, at a time of economic collapse and increasing political violence, was judged by many political commentators as contributing to the possibility of a Communist victory in the succeeding elections. On 19 January 1977 the Italian parliament approved abortion in the first 90 days of pregnancy for mental and physical health indications.

REPUBLIC OF IRELAND

Ireland is unique in the practice and sociology of family planning. Alone among the nations of the world it is consumed with a debate concerning the legalisation of contraceptives. Although the Supreme Court, in the case of Mary McGee (December 1973) upheld the basic human right to use contraceptives, it did not overthrow the right of the Irish Customs to confiscate them. Oral contraceptives are prescribed to regulate epidemics of menstrual irregularity, but action is taken against the import of condoms, spermicides and intra-uterine devices. By a farcical oversight, sterilisation has never been made illegal and, although tubal ligation is unobtainable because of hospital restrictions, some doctors perform outpatient vasectomies.[38]

Abortion is almost unmentionable, except in hushed tones of condemnation. Ironically, it is illegal under the 1861 Offences Against the Person Act, passed long before partition and one of the influences from Westminster that has not been overthrown. Reform of the law has not been seriously contemplated by any individual or group. Nevertheless, anti-abortion rallies are held. Father Marx, who illustrates his lectures with a 14-week fetus in a jar, has said of the Irish Family Planning Association, 'I give you my word of honour that these people promote abortion – soon if not already'.[39] There is no evidence to substantiate his claim. Indeed, the large number of Irish girls who travel to England for abortions use more direct channels.

The attitude of the majority of the Irish Medical Association is simple and was summed up at the 1973 meeting by the Honorary Secretary who said there had been a lot of loose talk in recent times on the subject of abortion, 'but in the eyes of most members of the IMA it was still murder'. A member, Mr Colin Galvin, was quoted as saying, 'You are either for or against abortion and I am against it.'[40]

HOLLAND

Unlike the other continental Common Market countries, the Dutch have begun to perform significant numbers of terminations by doctors, in good facilities, without any change in the law. By 1973 seven non-profit-making abortion clinics were active in the Netherlands, three accepting women from outside the country (mainly from Belgium, France and the German Federal Republic).

It was estimated that they were performing about 25 000 abortions a year. By 1974, 13 clinics were operating and were carrying out 80 000 abortions a year, 60 per cent on non-resident women.

Nearly all the operations are performed as outpatient procedures and there is a wise reluctance to undertake any termination after 12 weeks. Prices are moderate (£55 ($110) or less). One clinic run by the Nederlandse Vereniging voor Seksueel Hervorming (NVSH); (Dutch family planning association) performs abortions free, if the woman cannot pay, and integrates the service into wider aspects of family planning, offering vasectomy, laproscopic sterilisation and the reversible methods of contraception (some French women visit the clinic twice a year to obtain oral contraceptives). Women come from Austria and West Germany, as well as France and Belgium. Sixty per cent of the women are married and 75 per cent have a stable relationship.[41]

The best of the Dutch clinics have become the most innovative in Europe, using vacuum aspiration outpatient techniques. The doctors in the NVSH clinic are general practitioners. At least one Dutch university now uses such clinics in its routine clinical training. The Dutch clinics contrast interestingly with those in Britain, which are more expensive, often use overqualified surgeons and sometimes continue to use less than optimal techniques. There can be real advantages to operating outside, rather than within, the law.

The Dutch clinics originated when groups organising abortions to be performed in England for Dutch women began to see how ridiculous it was to send a plane load of women every day for an operation that was relatively simple and that they themselves had the skill to do – so they did it. After more than three years, and well over 100 000 abortions, Dutch clinics know that they have public support and are in very little danger of closure.

Eastern Europe

The revolution in abortion attitudes that took place in eastern Europe in the two decades after the war has come to rest, with certain adjustments, at the liberal end of the spectrum.

The German Democratic Republic, which was the first country in the area to change its law after World War II, had by the 1960s been overtaken by its neighbours in liberality. In 1972 a radically different law was passed.[42] The preamble states, 'equality of the woman in education and occupation, as well as in marriage and the family, demands that the woman have the right to decide about pregnancy and carry that pregnancy to term'. And the law itself states, 'the pregnant woman has the right for medical interruption of pregnancy, within the first 12 weeks of onset, in an obstetrical gynaecological institution'. The law makes the physician responsible for explaining the procedure and its possible consequences. After 12 weeks, termination can only be performed when there are real dangers to the woman's life. Interruption is not permitted if a previous abortion has taken place within the last six months. Prescription of contraceptives is free.

The passage of the legislation was unusual in that, for practically the first time within a Communist parliament, a number of delegates abstained. Opposition was led by both Roman Catholic and Protestant churches in East Germany and Cardinal Benesch condemned the legislation.

Two eastern European countries followed the example of Romania (1966, p. 145) and passed new and more restrictive laws in the 1970s. By previous standards the new laws were a considerable reverse, but by a global yardstick they remain liberal statutes. Bulgaria in 1973[43] limited the availability of abortion at the request of the woman to those with two or more children and to unmarried girls under 18 years of age. Change began in Hungary in October 1973 when the Council of Ministers agreed a new abortion law, which came into force on 1 January 1974. Abortion is available on request to mothers with three children and to women over 40. It is permitted in cases of rape and suspected fetal defect. Consideration is given to applicants whose request 'is seriously motivated by social reasons', and abortion is permitted for single girls, wives who have been separated for more than six months and for those without a home of their own. Both Bulgaria and Hungary obviously permit abortion in cases of maternal illness.

As is usual in eastern Europe the new abortion law in Hungary was introduced along with further massive increases in maternity and other benefits. The legal abortion rate is thought to have declined by 40 per cent (July 1974),[44] but it is impossible to partition this effect between the alterations in abortion legislation and the other pro-natalist policies.

The conservative core

Spain, Portugal and Greece have been outside the democratic traditions of the rest of Europe for much of this century. As in Italy, abortion is common, prosecutions few, and political condemnation heavy. In contrast with Italy, the topic is rarely voiced in public. In 1971 one popular Athens daily paper *Apoyevmatini* reported that in an admittedly small and biased survey 97 per cent of women favoured liberalisation of the abortion laws. Among those opposing the idea, a spokesman commented, 'Men will become completely immune . . . as soon as they get a woman pregnant they will rush her to a doctor for an abortion.'[45]

But such sentiments may be short lived. The return to free parliamentary elections in Portugal in 1975 and the death of Franco in Spain are both events which are likely to permit the issue of abortion reform to surface in these two countries. As in Greece, there is probably already a mute, but majority, public opinion in favour of liberalisation.

Conclusion

The attitudes of European countries towards abortion can be envisaged as hares and tortoises. Sweden is a typical hare: starting early, giving every appearance of rushing forward and yet either sleeping on the way or becoming too busy in self-analysis that it finds the tortoises, such as France or Austria, arriving at the winning post of abortion on request at almost the same time. Indeed, in this particular race, even the Italian body politic, which any reasonable observer would have pronounced dead to the problem of abortion as recently as the 1960s, has had an unpredictable ability to be aroused and to leap forward.

Abortion which was such an uncertain political topic ten years ago that it had to fight merely for time for debate in the British parliament, and would have been untouchable in most of the rest of western Europe, became the final issue to topple the government of Italy at a critically important moment in its history.

The early reforms in eastern Europe, Britain, South Australia, many US states and Scandinavia were sincere efforts to deal with a problem containing many sociological and clinical unknowns. The laws that were created gave detailed indications so that a second party (the involved doctors, or a committee) might know if an abortion was to be granted. Often subsidiary regulations controlled not only the specific diagnosis of maternal illness that might justify an abortion (as in Czechoslovakia) but the details of operative procedure (as in Britain).

This degree of state regulation had never been applied in any other aspect of medicine. It had several origins. Those who wanted reform and those who opposed it were equally uncertain about the possible consequences. How dangerous would legal abortion prove to be? Would its availability change the profile of contraceptive use inside the community? We now know the answers to these problems and the age of such detailed regulation must now be passed. New laws will need to offer abortion on request (as has happened in Austria) or medical practice will merely bypass out-of-date legislation (as in Holland).

References

1 Decree on the Legalisation of Abortion of 18 November 1920.
2 *Works of Vladimir Ilich Lenin*, vol. **19**, pp. 206–7. Quoted in David (1970); see note 19.
3 Schesinger, R. (1949). *The Family in the USSR*. Routledge & Kegan Paul, London.
4 Lockhart, R. B. (1955). *Your England*. Quoted by Marwick, A. (1965). *The Deluge*. Bodley Head, Oxford.
5 Glass, D. V. (1940). *Population Policies and Movement in Europe*. Clarendon Press. Oxford.
6 *Sexus*, April 1931, p. 46.
7 Davis, D. (1938). The law of abortion and necessity. *Modern Law Review*, **2**, 126.
8 Trevor-Roper, H. R. (1953). *Hitler's Table Talk 1941–44*. Weidenfeld & Nicolson, London.
9 Fedou, G. (1946). L'avortment. *De sa répréssion et de sa prévention dans le Code de la Famille det lois postérieurs*. Margues, Villeurbanne.
10 Watson, C. (1952). Birth control and abortion in France since 1937. *Population Studies, London*, **5**, 261.
11 Jóhsson, V. (1937). The Icelandic Birth Control and Feticide Act. *Journal of Contraception*, **2**, 219.
12 *Heilbrigdisskyrslur (Public Health in Iceland)* (1968). Samdar af Skrifstofu Landlaeknis, Reykjavik.
13 Guyon, R. (1936). *Etudes d'éthique sexuelle*: vol. **4**, *Politique rationnelle*

de sexualité. La réproduction humaine. Dardaillon & Dagniaux, St Denis.

14 Hodann, M. (1937). A prosecution for abortion in Denmark. *Marriage Hygiene*, **3**, 202.

15 Arwidsson, L. *et al.* (1968). A liberal abortion practice. *Lakartidningen Svensk Skotidning*, **65**, 4027.

16 Ottensen-Jensen, O. (1971). Legal abortion in Sweden: thirty years' experience. *Journal of Biosocial Science*, **3**, 173.

17 Hutlin, M. & Ottensen-Jensen, O. (1962). In-patient observation of abortion applicants. *Lakartidningen Svensk Skotidning*, **59**, 1365.

18 *Current Digest of the Soviet Press* (1956), **48**, 25.

19 David, H. P. (1970). *Family Planning and Abortion in the Socialist Countries of Central and Eastern Europe.* Population Council, New York.

20 Potts, M. (1967). Legal abortion in Eastern Europe. *Eugenics Review*, **59**, 232.

21 Decree No. 27 of 11 January 1952. (Yugoslavia).

22 Decree No. 33 of 16 February 1960. (Yugoslavia).

23 Ordinance No. 2 of 24 June 1956. (Hungary).

24 Decree No. 463 of 25 September 1957. (Romania).

25 Decree No. 220 of 16 March 1968, Section 126. (Bulgaria).

26 Snell, E. M. & Harper, M. (1970). Postwar economic growth in East Germany: a comparison with West Germany. In *Economic Developments in Countries of Eastern Europe*, a compendium of papers submitted to the Subcommittee on foreign economic policy of the Joint Economic Committee Congress of the United States, p. 558. US Government Printing Office, Washington D.C.

27 Law No. 350 of 13 June 1973. (Denmark).

28 Law No. 239. of 24 March 1970. (Finland).

29 Turpeinen, K. (1971). Legal abortion in Finland. *IPPF Medical Bulletin*, **5** (3), 3.

30 International Health Foundation (1971). *Family Planning.* IHF, Geneva.

31 *Daily Express* (London), 23 June 1971.

32 Anonymous (1974). Les interruptions précoces de grossesse par la méthode Karman: l'expérience Française. In *Avortement et Parturition Provoqués*, ed. M. J. Bosc. R. Palmer & C. I. Sureau, p. 427. Masson et Cie, Paris.

33 Article L 178–1, Public Health Code.

34 Wanstall-Sautz, M. & Cook, R. (1975). Liberalized abortion in four countries. *IPPF Medical Bulletin*, **9**(2), 4.

35 *The Times*, 8 March 1975.

36 Cliquet, R. L. (1972). Knowledge, practice and effectiveness of contraceptive practice in Belgium. *Journal of Biosocial Science*, **4**, 41.

37 Bourg, R. (1973). Dans quel sens faut-il modifier notre législation sur les avortements? *Bulletin de l'Academie royale de médicine de Belgique*, **128**, 189.

38 Deys, C. (1975). Personal communication.
39 Bishops set up protest. *Guardian*, 18 October 1976.
40 Nowlan, D. (1973). *Irish Times*, 24 April.
41 Smit, C. (1974). Personal communication.
42 Law of 9 March 1972. (German Democratic Republic).
43 Instruction No. 0–27 of 20 April 1973. (Bulgaria).
44 Szabady, E. Personal communication.
45 *Manchester Evening News*, 29 May 1971.

12

The experience of other countries

In the opening decade of this century abortion was illegal throughout the world. By 1975, 60 per cent of the world's population lived in countries permitting abortion on request or for social indications (Fig. 45). As a result of rapid population growth, more people now live under liberal abortion statutes than there were people living in the whole world at the turn of the century.

The revolution that has taken place is one of great social significance, for the health and happiness of individuals and, now that the population explosion has been detonated, for the welfare of all mankind.

All the nations of Christendom ended the nineteenth century with restrictive abortion laws. The Western countries were at the height of their colonial expansion. Many millions of Europeans migrated overseas and, even when they remained a minority in their new land, they imposed their laws and attitudes on abortion on a great many alien cultures. By 1900 Ethiopia, Liberia and the two Boer republics were the only independent areas of Africa, the rest of the continent being divided between the Netherlands, Germany, Portugal and Britain. When Spain began to lose control of her Far East possessions, after the end of the Spanish–American War in 1898, the Philippines and numerous other Pacific islands passed to the jurisdiction of USA. On the mainland of Asia, British rule on the Indian subcontinent was at its height and extended into Burma, where it met with French influence in what are now North and South Vietnam, Laos and Cambodia, with only Thailand withstanding colonial pressure. Latin America was an exception. The former Spanish and Portuguese colonies had been independent, if somewhat unstable, nations since the 1820s and 30s. However, the native

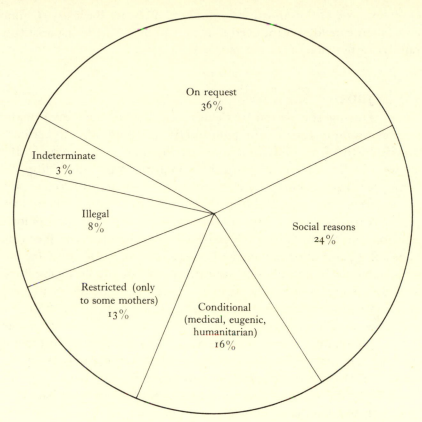

Fig. 45. Percentage of the world's population living in countries where abortion is illegal, restricted, conditional, allowed for social reasons, available on request or undetermined.

American Indian cultures had been so thoroughly transformed that from the point of view of public laws and attitudes on abortion, they were more Western than the West.

Two great nations – Japan and China – remained uncolonised, although they each became deeply affected by Western culture. As the Manchu Empire in China crumbled, Russia, Japan, Britain, France and the USA all strove to break in and extend their influence in military and economic terms. Japan sought to bring some aspects of Western influence into the country, yet Western ways did not always penetrate deeply and perhaps it is no accident that Japan and China were among the first nations to pass liberal abortion laws after World War II. And they have continued to attempt to deal with the complex problem of abortion on their own terms. Basically, China and Japan considered induced abortion to be a 'crime' against the family, rather than a 'crime' against the state.

Japan

During the period of Seclusion, abortion and infanticide were common in Japan. The Samurai did not congratulate a friend on the birth of a child until it was clear that it was going to be allowed to live. In 1754 one commentator wrote 'up to fifty or sixty years ago a couple on the farm used to bring up five or six or even seven or eight children [but] it has become the custom in recent years among farmers for each married couple to rear no more than one or two children'. However, with contact with Western civilisation, anti-abortion legislation was introduced in 1873. Infanticide came to be treated with the full rigour of the homicide laws and, by the first half of this century, Japanese public policy treated abortion and contraception in much the same way as the West. In the 1920s at a time when the Japanese population was growing rapidly, Madam Shidzve Kato invited Margaret Sanger to Japan. The pro-nationalist Japanese government refused her permission to land until she signed an affidavit promising not to speak on birth control – an event which created more public interest than any lecture tour. In 1940, following the Nazi example, the law was tightened up with the passage of the National Eugenic Law. But, basically perhaps, the Japanese culture had not become so fully a child of the West as it seemed and by 1948 the law was to be radically altered.

The same Madam Kato became a member of the House of Representatives during the Occupation and she and Dr Tenly Ota (who pioneered intrauterine devices in Japan) drafted the Eugenic Protection Bill aimed mainly at improving contraceptive services.[1] Although condoms had been manufactured in Japan (and distributed free to the troops) contraceptives were, in theory, illegal. Unfortunately, the draft Bill was presented shortly after a public mention of birth control which had resulted in General MacArthur, Supreme Commander of the Allied Powers, receiving a great many protests from the USA. The Bill was presented to a silent assembly on two occasions, not a single question was asked, and it lapsed. Shortly afterwards, however, in 1948 a group of doctors in the upper

Chamber headed by Dr Paniguchi and backed by the powerful Japanese Medical Association, presented another Bill. It was solely concerned with abortion and it reached the statute book. It was amended in 1949 to include economic indications for termination. The present law permits abortion in the case of genetic disease, rape and when 'there is danger that, if the pregnancy continues or childbirth ensues, the mother's health will be impaired for physical or economic reasons'. This clause is invoked in more than two-thirds of all cases. The Japanese Medical Association is vested with the responsibility of designating doctors who have the experience to perform the operation and with setting fees. Currently about 13000 Japanese doctors are so designated and perform at least 800000 abortions a year. Legally, abortion is possible up to 28 weeks of gestation, but nearly all are performed in the first trimester.

When the law was first introduced, authorisation to operate was in the hands of a committee, but after four years this system was seen to be counter-productive and the decision to operate was transferred to a single doctor. Now it is not unusual for abortion to be done on the day the decision is taken and nearly always it is within a very few days.

In 1949, after the passing of the Eugenics Protection Law, the original intention of the Kato–Ota Bill was achieved and contraception legalised. So, as in Britain in 1967, liberal abortion legislation was *succeeded* by changes in the law relating to contraception – a paradox which underlies the key role played by abortion in public attitudes on birth control, which in the absence of external stimulus rarely seem to establish rational priorities.

The law has remained unaltered for more than a quarter of a century. During that time, contraceptive practice has improved and the peak of legal abortion has come and gone (Fig. 12, p. 69). Japan has transformed itself into the third richest nation in the world. It is suggested elsewhere (p. 137) that, if the abortion law had not been changed, illegal abortions would have risen to play the same demographic role. If, on purely theoretical grounds, there had been no induced abortions at all, what would have happened? Assuming 85 per cent of the fetuses of recorded abortions had gone to term, the rate of population increase in Japan would have nearly doubled (1961–65, 18.6 rather than the observed 10.3 per 1000 of the population).[2] Therefore, in the absence of induced abortion (legal or illegal), the rate of population growth would have swallowed up much of the wealth that went to make the investment on which Japan's economic strength was built. Additionally, an already over-crowded country, with massive and visible problems of pollution, would have been faced with even more formidable environmental problems.

In the early months of 1973 information was leaked to the Japanese press, suggesting that the Eugenics Protection Law might be revised during the session of the Diet due to end in mid-June. Minority religious/military groups were pressing for authorisations that would omit economic grounds for abortion. The Minister of Health and Welfare belonged to such a party and appeared to be in favour of the changes. The Japanese Family Planning Association responded rapidly and aroused press and media concern for maintaining the law in its existing form. There were very considerable discussion and coverage of the whole problem of abortion in Japan. The majority opinion remains that the law should remain unaltered, but further political fighting is likely.

People's Republic of China

In a famous speech before the Supreme State Conference in Peking on 27 February 1957, the late Chairman Mao, commenting on the 30 million births which take place every year in China, is reported to have said,

> These figures must also be of great concern to us all. I will quote two other figures. The increase in grain harvest for the last two years has been 10 million tons a year. This is barely sufficient to cover the needs of our growing population. The second figure concerns the problem of education. It is estimated that at present 40 per cent of our youth have not been placed in primary schools. Steps must, therefore, be taken to keep our population for a long time at a stable level, say of 600 million. A wide campaign of explanation and proper help must be undertaken to achieve this aim.[3]

The speech lasted four hours and has never been fully released in the West, but was widely reported at the time.

In one sense, Chairman Mao was the only national leader ever to advocate a policy of zero population growth. In another sense, the Maoist interpretation of Communism can be regarded as analogous to a religion, and it may be said that Mao was the only

Father of a church to speak out in favour of birth control. Of course, in practice, the population of Mainland China cannot be stabilised for many decades, and there are difficulties common to all developing nations as Mao recognised in an interview in 1971. The American author Edgar Snow commented that there had been great changes in family planning in the previous five or ten years. 'No, I have been taken in,' Mao is reported to have answered. 'In the countryside a woman still wanted to have boy children. If the first and second were girls, she would make another try. If the third one came and was still a girl, the mother would try again. Pretty soon there would be nine of them, the mother was already 45 or so, and she would finally decide to leave it at that. The attitude must be changed but it is taking time. Perhaps the same thing is true in the United States?'[4] In 1964, the late Chou En-lai had expressed the real goal of the country which is to reduce the current growth rate to one per cent by A.D. 2000.

Governmental zeal for family planning has waxed and waned with the political changes that have taken place.

Birth control has been discussed by Shao Li-tzu in 1954, was spurred on by food shortages and became Ministry of Public Health policy in 1956, prior to Mao's speech already quoted.[3,5] The programme was organized by the Party, involved the press, which reported numerous case histories of the beneficial effects of family planning, and was initially concentrated 'first in the cities and towns, then the rural areas; first the cadres then the masses'. Family planning went into partial eclipse in the period of 'one hundred flowers' in 1956–57.

In 1958 the country embarked on the 'great leap forward'. National statistics for everything from steel and grain production to birth rates were interpreted 'creatively'[6] and problems of population appeared to pale beside the rising tables of production. There was even talk of allowing much of the land to lie fallow, but by 1961–62 food shortages had reappeared. Statistics were interpreted less 'creatively' and items on family planning returned to the press. During the years 1958–62 some condom factories closed for lack of use.

The unique aspect of the Chinse programme is that, from a very early stage, it has encouraged all methods of fertility limitation, from endeavouring to raise the age of marriage, through the commercial distribution of contraceptives, to induced abortion, and it has ensured that they are available in a culturally acceptable way. There has not been the emphasis on a particular method, or group of methods, that has often marred family planning programmes in other Asian countries. In the late 1950s a real effort was made to encourage the use of traditional, cottage techniques of contraception.[3] The swallowing of live tadpoles was a bizarre example of a sensible trend, but unfortunately no indigenous method was found to be useful. The rhythm method has received publicity and the commercial distribution of contraceptives was very much encouraged. Forty-five million condoms were produced in 1957. It is the law that pharmacies, departmental stores, co-operatives and trading companies must 'maintain reasonable stocks'. Machinery for the manufacture of condoms was imported from Japan in the 1950s. Foams, diaphragms and gels are available. An intrauterine device programme began in 1957, a 22-tablet combined oral contraceptive was issued in 1970 and may now be being used by 15 million women. In the rural communes near Peking it is claimed that 40 per cent of fertile women are using this method, but the extent of its distribution in the country as a whole is unknown. Pioneer work has been done in developing 'paper pills', which, like vacuum aspiration in the field of abortion, appear to be a genuine leap forward.[7] Vasectomy and tubal ligation are performed; vasectomy, because of its clinical simplicity, is the more common and has had a high priority since 1962. It is offered after the birth of one or two children. There are reports of vasectomies being performed in the homes of peasants. There is a monetary incentive for vasectomy, equivalent to 20 per cent of the man's monthly salary.

China is the only nation that, as a political principle, has made a genuine effort to raise the age of marriage with the overt intention of reducing the population growth rate.[8] The minimum age of marriage was set at 20 for men and 18 for women soon after the Revolution. Proposals of 23 and 20, respectively, from the National People's Consultative Conference were rejected in 1956, but an optional marriage age of 30 for men and 22 for women was recommended by the Party in 1963. Propaganda to this effect has been strong and practical provisions have been made, such as separate dormitories for the unmarried to live in.

The structure of society in Mainland China, with the commune as the basic unit of social organisation, lends itself to enthusiastic family planning. Young men can only achieve status in leadership positions if they have small families.[8] In many ways, the Cultural

Revolution, by reaching society and especially by weakening traditional bonds between the generations will further the changes necessary to achieve small families.

Chinese legislation concerning abortion dates back to about 1890 and was introduced as a response to Western pressures, rather than as an expression of intrinsic Chinese beliefs. Indeed abortion had for centuries been considered merely a crime against the family. The only historical precedent for abortion legislation in Chinese culture goes back to a single episode in the T'ang dynasty (A.D. 618–906) when abortion was classified with a number of other offences against the person, such as biting off the penis. In modern China, abortion has become an integral part of the Chinese family planning, but the evolution of its acceptability was irregular. In 1956 Shao Li-tzu pointed out that health regulations only allowed abortion on strictly medical grounds, or where a mother became pregnant within four months of delivery and it required approval by a doctor, and the organisation to which the women belonged. But, in March 1957, the Health Minister of the Chinese People's Political Consultative Conference, Li Teh-ch'uan, said that, with 'the greatest reluctance', the regulations on abortion would be changed so that decisions would be made 'mainly on the basis of the wish of the individuals'.[9] The philosophy was the same as that motivating the US Supreme Court 16 years later; reaction of the medical profession was also that which many Western countries were to experience in the next decade. Nineteen members of the health committee immediately expressed their dissent, the physical danger of abortion was emphasised and the Ministerial regulations implemented very unevenly, although some hospitals were swamped with requests. It was said that easy abortion would discourage contraception, that there were insufficient facilities in rural areas, that women should pay the costs of the operation and that the operation should be forbidden to the nulliparous. One Communist paper[10] said it was hypocritical to permit abortions but object to infanticide – a philosophy that right-to-life groups were to echo in other countries in the 1970s.

The regulations were changed a month later to require a doctor's certificate that (1) the woman was in the first trimester, (2) no complications would result for the operation, and (3) there had been no operation in the preceding year. The government had partially backed down, and the medical profession, through the second caveat, re-established its control of the situation.

However, experience changed attitudes in China as elsewhere.

In addition, the medical profession was going through a unique marriage of Western and traditional practices.[11] The barefoot doctor evolved as someone taken from the community he was to serve and trained in simple techniques, in particular concerned with antenatal care, obstetrics and family planning. The Western-trained physician was encouraged and cajoled to work in the villages. Nearly all those who know the health problems of developing countries agree that the Chinese solution to rural health care is bold, humane and appears to be successful.

By 1963 the press had replaced its previous statements about the horrors and dangers of legal abortion with pieces that pointed out that the procedure was safer than delivery.

At least in the cities, abortion now appears to be readily available and widely used. In Peking in 1964, a visitor observed a poster 'in praise of artificial termination of pregnancy'.[12] The operation can cost $2, or may be paid for by the husband's commune, or performed free for those who cannot afford it. Payment for an item of medical service is common in China. In the first trimester, outpatient techniques are often used; after three months of gestation the women may stay in hospital three to five days.

China is the home of the vacuum aspiration method of terminating pregnancy. As has been noted, the vacuum aspiration method has been carried to the rural areas by the ingenious use of both a large bottle, in which alcohol is burnt to create a partial vacuum, and hand-operated pumps and hand-operated suction syringes. As was remarked in the *Chinese Journal of Gynaecology and Obstetrics* in 1966, 'this method of performing an abortion is simple, convenient and easy to control, it has the additional advantage – it can be taught quickly to lower level health personnel'.[13] Abortion is now said to be available in the 20000 commune hospitals. It seems that the implementation of the family planning programmes at the rural level cannot be less, and may be much greater, than in India, Pakistan or Indonesia.

Edgar Snow saw two typical abortions performed in 1971. Acupuncture is used as anaesthesia, but perhaps the effect was partly similar to the counselling used in some clinics in the USA. Although the women claimed to be eligible for two weeks' paid leave, they went back to work the same afternoon. Except that one patient cheered herself with Mao's thought 'Fear neither hardship nor death', the similarity in clinical procedure in Peking and New York is remarkable.

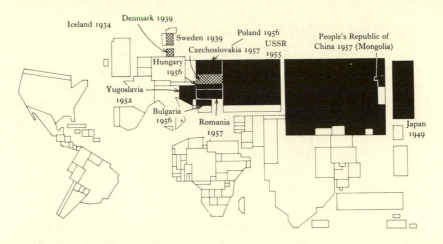

Iceland 1934
Denmark 1939
Sweden 1939
Czechoslovakia 1957
Poland 1956
USSR 1955
People's Republic of China 1957 (Mongolia)
Hungary 1956
Yugoslavia 1952
Bulgaria 1956
Romania 1957
Japan 1949

■ Elective abortions (*de jure* or *de facto*, first-trimester abortion on request)

▨ Abortion available for social as well as medical indications (law reform under discussion)

Fig. 46. Legal status of abortion, 1964. The area of each country is proportional to the population in 1964. USSR, Asia and the Middle East have been artificially separated for clarity.

The population growth rate is now believed to be under two per cent per annum, although the evidence is shaky. If it is true, then China has the distinction of being the first really large nation to achieve a demonstrable impact on fertility with a national family planning programme. Serious problems remain, of which food is the greatest. In the 1950s China imported hardly any fertiliser, by 1970 she imported over eight million tons or 20 per cent of the world's international trade in fertilisers. However, even to scrape by in the race away from starvation and towards some small degree of economic development is an achievement. Politically, the future of Asia may well be determined by which of the two largest nations brings down its birth rate first – on the present showing, China is further ahead than India.

Very little is known about the availability of legal abortion in North Korea and North Vietnam. One observer suggests the North Vietnamese situation is rather like the Chinese.[14]

The British Commonwealth

A quarter of the world's population lives in the British Commonwealth, and nearly every member nation, when it gained independence, inherited an abortion law based on the British legislation of 1861. The 1861 law had been passed shortly before the British Empire reached its zenith. Even more important than the political influences of Great Britain, the British pattern of medicine, with its antagonism to abortion and its uncertainty about contraception, became a model for a sizeable portion of the world's population. Today it seems strange that, as countries became independent and eager to assert their right to self-determination, a Victorian legal imperialism and moral colonialism on the subject of abortion persisted long after most other traditions were cast off.

Singapore

The wind of change first stirred in Singapore in the wake of the 1967 British legislation. When draft legislation was introduced into parliament, comment was invited from many groups in the community and it is notable that no serious opposition was received. The law passed in 1969 is broadly similar to the British one in the legal conditions required for termination, but the administrative procedures are more complex. The Ministry of Health is empowered to appoint a Termination of Pregnancy Authorisation Board with 11 members, and the decision to operate is not legally invested in individual practitioners. In Singapore, the situation is one of the few where a complicated law works well in practice. A tight rein was kept on all aspects of initial experience. Only well-qualified obstetricians at the Kerdang Kabu Hospital were licensed to perform the operation. Rigid restrictions are imposed on private operations, although illegal doctor-performed abortions do occur, usually because a woman seeks privacy. At least one death due to illegal abortion occurred in 1974.

Vacuum aspiration is widely used, but saline inductions and sometimes hysterectomies also take place. Initially, vaginal terminations were performed under general anaesthesia and the woman brought in the night prior to the operation and discharged later the same day, but since 1971 outpatient terminations have become more common. Approximately 25 operations a day are performed at the Kerdang Kabu Hospital. The women are mostly married, relatively few come late and the menstrual regulation service is the most advanced in the world. By 1975, 4000 procedures had been performed, with a minimum of complications.[15] The law operates against a background of efficient contraceptive and sterilisation services. Recidivism is rare.

Every year the law and its regulations are interpreted a little more liberally. By 1972 a ratio of seven abortions to 100 live births had been reached. In the spring of 1974, parliament in the Republic of Singapore passed a second piece of abortion legislation: abortion became available on request. The physician can refuse a request, but is obliged to refer the woman to another doctor. A girl of any age can request an abortion, if necessary, without the consent of her husband or parents. In 1974, 6600 abortions were performed, a rate of 12.3 per 1000 women aged 15–44 years (cf. 11.5 in England and Wales in the same year.)

India

Since independence, India has added 250 million to her population – equivalent to the entire population of the USSR, which has six times the land area of India. The government family planning programme, while being the first in the world, has tended to do today what could and should have been done a decade earlier. The problem of abortion first found lucid and persuasive expression in a committee under the chairmanship of Shantilal H. Shah, which reported in 1966.[16] The committee was sensitive to the debate then taking place in Britain and quoted the text on the draft British Bill, which accounts for much of the wording of the Bill finally passed by the Rajya Sabha in 1971. The Indian Medical Association (IMA) was represented on the Shantilal Shah Committee. The IMA supported law reform, with much less caution than its British counterparts. Among other groups supporting the change was the UN Expert Team on family planning which visited India in May 1969.

The Medical Termination of Pregnancy Bill entered the Rajya Sabha in 1969. A draft Bill proposed that, prior to 12 weeks, one registered medical practitioner and, after 12 weeks, two practitioners should be involved in determining if an abortion is necessary. The first clause is an abbreviated form of that found in the 1967 British Act and permits termination if the medical practitioner(s) is of the opinion, formed in good faith, that 'The continuance of the pregnancy would involve risk to the life of the pregnant woman or of injury to her physical or mental health.' The second clause is a eugenic one and identical to that found in the British Act. In the explanations put forward with the proposed legislation, rape was mentioned as a threat to mental health. More important, when a pregnancy 'occurs as the result of failure of any device used by any married woman or her husband for the purpose of limiting the number of children, the anguish caused by such unwanted pregnancy may be presumed to constitute a grave injury to the mental health of the pregnant woman'. The operation should be performed only in registered places and must be certified. There are some additional items which are relevant to the Indian scene, such as consent from a second party in the case of widows and unmarried girls.

A survey of approximately 100 doctors[17] in India in 1971 (60 per cent women) showed more than half were prepared to do abortions and another 21 per cent would refer women to other doctors. The majority accepted the need for abortion on grounds of health, but only 30 per cent accepted it as a population control measure. Most agreed some point after fertilisation as the time when human life begins. Christian and Jain doctors were more restrictive than Hindu and Zoroastrian.

It is greatly to the credit of Indian legislators that they tackled the difficult and unpleasant topic of abortion realistically. The administrators, charged with drafting regulations to help implement the law in a vast and diverse country, were sometimes pragmatic but mostly too complex. The original rules governing the Act extended to 21 typed pages and covered all probable and many improbable eventualities. Rule 2f defined the 'place' where the operation is performed as meaning a 'building, tent, vehicle or vessel'. The crucial rules governing the training of personnel needed to perform the abortion were drawn too cautiously and the 'building, tent, vehicle, or vessel' must have full facilities for a laporotomy and a trained anaesthetist (Rules 6(2)a and 6(2)d, i, ii, iii). However, Rule 9(1) required members of the Board who inspected operating doctors to report on any who, 'by reason of any defect or deficiency in his training or experience, rashness or negligence, caused the death of, or injury to, *more than one* pregnant woman' (italics added).

As the law neared implementation, so the langour that has characterised so much of the Indian family planning effort grew. A team of Indian gynaecologists had visited England and Yugoslavia in 1970 at the invitation of the International Planned Parenthood Federation and gained useful insight into the problems of large-scale abortion, but when the Sixteenth All Indian Obstetric and Gynaecological Congress discussed the implementaton of the law in April 1972 the informed minority could not argue away the mythology of danger and difficulty that has surrounded the abortion operation for so long in the English-speaking world and hospital, inpatient operations became the general rule. A further setback was the decision to vest the responsibility for implementing the law in the Ministry of Health and not the Family Planning Ministry.

However, in 1975 the regulations and reporting procedures were simplified. Outpatient abortions have become more acceptable and in Calcutta C. S. Dawn (Professor of Gynaecology) has set up an efficient, simple and much used menstrual regulation service.[18]

Even in a country with a high birth rate, abortion can be a problem of some magnitude and the official guess at the time of the debate in the Rajya Sabha was of a possible need for over one million abortions annually. Between the law coming into force and November 1972, fewer than 10000 abortions were registered in the whole of India. In 1973 possibly 70000 were performed. The original complexity of registering the 'place' and the surgeon deterred many operators, some of whom no doubt performed unregistered abortions.

The 1969 legislation omitted the states of Jamma and Kashmir, but subsequently local legislation has been passed permitting abortion in cases of 'grave risk' to the mother's health.

Canada

Canada, with its strong Catholic influence and French tradition, is not at first sight a likely candidate for abortion law reform. However, in the Criminal Law Amendment Act 1968–69 (Section 251) Mr Trudeau's government, not only did away with some very archaic anti-contraceptive legislation, but made important modifications in the abortion law. The Criminal Law Amendment Act is a curious hodgepodge of legislation from road traffic to abortion Acts. The abortion law was modified to permit termination when there is a majority approval by the hospital therapeutic abortion committee (consisting of three or more medically qualified persons) or a certified request from a doctor. The doctor must state that in his 'opinion the continuation of the pregnancy for such female person would or would be likely to endanger her life or health'.

Hospitals must be approved by the Provincial Health Minister, to whom the operation must also be reported.

While the impetus to reform the Canadian law has been an important one, many observers feel the 1968–69 Amendment has not achieved its purpose. Regional inequalities have been even more extreme in Canada than in England. In some provinces, liberal doctors claim that it has been more and not less difficult to perform operations. In the province of Quebec by late 1970 only 14 out of 250 hospitals had chosen to register as places where abortions might be performed. Between them, in the first few months of the operation of the new law, these hospitals performed only 85 operations and 67 of these were in a single Jewish hospital. In the first 10 months of the law, Quebec performed 181 operations or slightly over 4 per cent of the national total although the province contains 30 per cent of the population.

Whatever its defects, the law has been responsible for an important change. In 1970, 11 000 legal abortions were performed; in 1971 30 000; nearly 39 000 in 1972; and more than 43 000 in 1973. The three-man hospital committees have been criticised by the Canadian Medical Association and the Canadian Psychiatric Association.[19,20] There is no appeal against a committee's decisions and moral views may become 'rationalised into the medical level'. However, by 1971 the psychiatrist was 'dropped from the game' at least in British Columbia. By 1972 the family physician was permitted to perform the operation in hospitals. Hospital Committees still meet but often they now 'rubber-stamp' operations.

As in England, techniques evolved somewhat more slowly than in the USA. In 1972, throughout Canada, 30 per cent of operations were still performed by dilatation and curettage and 12 per cent by hysterotomy or hysterectomy. The restrictive nature of the Canadian law still leads to an average delay of one to three weeks between the decision to seek an abortion and the operation being performed.

Prior to the 1968–69 changes, a significant number of women travelled to Britain, Japan or Scandinavia. From British Columbia they used to travel down to Seattle and then, for $600, they could travel by jet airline to Japan leaving on Friday evening and they could return in time for work on Monday morning. This trek westwards to seek the freedom to control fertility came to be known as the 'D & C 8'.

Dissatisfaction with the Canadian situation has led to a variety of responses. In May 1970 a group of 30 young women demonstrated in the Canadian House of Commons in support of 'free abortion on demand'. They gained access to the press gallery with forged passes, chained themselves to the chairs and, for the first time in its history, forced the Canadian House to adjourn the sitting. It is not quite clear what effect this unusual procedure had on the members of the Canadian parliament but, as is often the case in abortion law reform, it drew attention to the need for family planning. The Family Planning Federation of Canada, while unconnected with the demonstration, followed it up by seeking, and obtaining, the support of many of the members for easier access to the knowledge and means of family planning.

Early in 1973, Mr Stuart Leggatt introduced a Bill to permit abortion on request in the first 12 weeks of pregnancy, and for medical reasons in the second trimester. The first reading of the Bill – normally an automatic process – was resisted and only taken after a vote (179 for, 56 against). It was the first time in a century that Ottawa had seen a division so early in the life of a piece of legislation. Subsequently, the Bill was dropped and in legislation Canada seems currently to have rested at a British-type reform, rather than proceeding to a US-style repeal.

Later, in 1973 a new trend emerged. The reformed abortion law was challenged and at least temporarily over-ridden by the trial and acquittal of Dr Henry Morgentaler. The case involved a unique interpretation of statute law. Morgentaler had a private outpatient, mainly vacuum aspiration, abortion service in Montreal.[21] He was fully qualified and on his own admission had done 5000 abortions (without a death); he charged moderate fees, which he was willing to reduce in difficult social circumstances, and was respected by his fellow doctors. The reason for his trial had been referred to him by two major Montreal hospitals. She was a 26-year-old black, unmarried, postgraduate student from Sierra Leone and the father of the child was a student and unable to support her. She spoke only English in a French-speaking community. In fact, the police prosecution seem to have been unable to get any other of Morgentaler's patients to testify against him, even though they took away close on 800 record cards. The girl from overseas was probably frightened that she would be expelled from the country if she did not assist the police.

Before a French-speaking jury of 11 men and one woman, the prosecution case turned more and more into a recital of the inequalities in the application of the Canadian Abortion Law. Those in the Quebec court were aware that only 11 out of the 199 French-speaking hospitals in the Province perform abortions. The defence produced local testimony of Dr Morgentaler's skill, while the prosecution had to import expert witnesses from the USA. At the time of the police raid, the woman in question had been rapidly removed and transferred to a Montreal hospital, but a senior official from that hospital pointed out that admission had been unnecessary.

The defence lawyers were Charles Flan and Claude Armand Sheppard, and with the consent of the Associate Chief Justice, James K. Hugessen, pleaded article 45 of the Criminal Code in Dr Morgentaler's defence: 'Everyone is protected from criminal responsibility for performing a surgical operation on any person for the benefit of that person if (a) the operation is performed with reasonable care and skill and (b) it is reasonable to perform the operation, having regard to the state of health of the person at the time the operation and all the circumstances of the case'.

Morgentaler was acquitted. One lawyer commented, 'Twelve ordinary Quebecers did what the legislators of this country were reluctant to do – change the abortion law a great deal'.

However, the prosecution appealed against the verdict and the judgement was struck down in a higher court. He was imprisoned for 18 months and the case came to the Canadian Supreme Court. In a six to three ruling in March 1975, Morgentaler was convicted of not applying the 1969 Act. As with the original acquittal, the Supreme Court ruling raised unusual legal issues: in this case a superior court condemned a person who had *not* been committed by a jury, challenging a legal tradition that can be traced back to the Magna Carta. An opinion poll showed 56 per cent of Canadians wanted Morgentaler freed.

Morgentaler's case embarrassed the government. In 1974 the Federal Minister of Justice sent round a memorandum stating that 'social and economic considerations are not to be taken into account in determining whether a pregnancy can be lawfully terminated'. A few months later he said 'health is a broad word and a medical term that can include mental and other factors'. Canada, like

Britain, was made to face the problem that statutory 'indications' for abortion can mean whatever lawyers and doctors choose to make them mean at any moment.

Morgentaler was then tried on a second case, this time of aborting a 17-year-old unmarried girl. Again he based his case not on any interpretation of the abortion law but on the common law principle of 'necessity'. Judge Bisson said to the jury, 'In law you must not consider the defence of 'necessity' and you would be seriously remiss in your duty if you did so'.[21]

But again the jury acquitted. And the Quebec Court of Appeal upheld the acquittal, even though at this time (January 1976) Morgentaler was still in prison on the first case where he had also been acquitted by a jury but the same Appeal Court had over-ruled the verdict. (During imprisonment he suffered a heart attack but a request for parole was refused.) The case can still go to the Canadian Supreme Court but it 'opens', in the words of Crown Prosecutor Domique, 'the door to abortion on demand'.

Several criminal codes contain clauses similar to Article 45 of the Canadian one and it will be interesting to see if the Morgentaler precedent will be used in other countries.

Australia

Australia, like the USA before the Supreme Court ruling, decides its abortion laws state by state. On the 8 January 1970 South Australia amended its abortion law to allow termination when two doctors are of the opinion 'that continuance of the pregnancy would involve greater risk to the life of the pregnant woman or greater risk of injury to the physical or mental health of the pregnant woman than if the pregnancy were terminated', and in cases where there is a 'substantial risk' that 'the child would suffer from such physical or mental abnormalities as to be seriously handicapped'. In deciding to perform the operation the doctor may take into account the pregnant woman's actual or reasonably foreseeable environment. Reporting of the operation and registration of hospitals where the operation may be performed is required. The law also allows for emergency operations and contains a clause permitting conscientious objections. The law is limited to women who have been resident in the state for two months, but a drafting error appears to allow for legal termination in the case of a woman who spent *any* two months of her life in South Australia, and not necessarily in relation to the unplanned pregnancy.

The influence of the British law is plainly evident and, as in Britain, the passing of the new legislation brought in its wake the first state initiative in contraceptive services. The change required a Private Members' Debate over 11 parliamentary weeks and, although it was a non-party Bill the government aided progress by granting time. (It is said that it was a 'toss up' between whether to grant time to legislate on late-night shopping or abortion.)

The ratio of abortions to births and the division between the married and the unmarried has been broadly similar to that of the British experience (see p. 321). The Australians are proud of their regional differences and the geographical dimensions of the country add to their sense of local loyalty. Abortion law reform has been canvassed in other states, but has made little progress. However, several very important legal precedents exist. In the acquittal of a Dr Davidson (1969) in Melbourne, Victoria, Mr Justice Menhennitt ruled that termination of pregnancy was licit if the woman's physical or mental health was in danger: 'The accused must have honestly believed on reasonable grounds that the act done by him was (a) necessary to preserve the woman from a worse danger to her life or her physical or mental health, not being the normal dangers of pregnancy and child birth which the continuance of pregnancy would entail and (b) in the circumstances not out of proportion to the dangers to be averted'.[22]

Melbourne has had a particularly dramatic series of incidents in which the police came into conflict with doctors performing abortions. For many years Dr Bertram Wainer[23] publicly challenged the law, until he came to the conclusion as he puts it, 'I felt I could have done an abortion in the middle of the main street and all the police would do, would be to hold up the trams until I was finished'. The Fertility Control Clinic in Melbourne now carries out about 3000 terminations annually for A\$80 (US \$100) a case. In Sydney, case precedents similar to those set in the Menhennitt ruling were created in 1969 and 1971 (Levine ruling) although harassment of doctors by police continued. However, the precedents were used, although initially almost unnoticed by the public or the medical profession: in 1972 the numbers of induced abortions in large obstetric hospitals in Adelaide (South Australia) and Melbourne were comparable. Medical attitudes are becoming more liberal. The majority of a sample of Sydney doctors in 1970 favoured reform.[24] A free-standing Preterm Inc. clinic was opened in Sydney (April 1975) but burnt down nine months after it opened. Population Services International now provides two clinics performing 200–300 abortions a week between them.

While some degree of abortion reform was proceeding in several states, in Queensland in 1971, steps were taken not only to entrench restrictive abortion legislation, but to obstruct male sterilisation operations. However, it is easy to cross state borders and by late 1975 Children by Choice in Brisbane had referred 5000 women for terminations in New South Wales.[25]

The Australian Labour Party contains a strong Catholic element. A Labour government was returned to power towards the end of 1972. One of the first actions in the new parliament was a Private Members Bill to move new abortion legislation. The draft could have permitted abortions on request up to 12 weeks and abortion on the signature of two doctors between 12 and 14 weeks. The campaign was a symbolic one because of the Federal structure of Australian government. (If passed, the legislation would have applied only to Canberra and the Northern Territory). In the event, Australia, like Canada soundly rejected the proposed liberal legislation (by 98 votes to 23), although reform on the British lines may continue to spread from state to state, or be established in the courts. Mr Gough Whitlam, the former Prime Minister, was among those voting for the Bill.

The trend in Australia has been for medical practice and the interpretation of the law to become more liberal. The Federally funded Medibank system pays for abortion in all states.[26] Yet in 1974 the Perth Abortion Information Service and a clinic performing outpatient abortions were raided by 45 policemen at 6 a.m. and patients' records impounded. Those involved never at any time denied their involvement in abortion. They did point out that the service was listed in the telephone directory, that every woman had been seen by two doctors, that they had a letter of advice from the State Attorney General and that state and Federal agencies had reimbursed most of the cost to the women. Many doctors, including Roman Catholics not involved in the Service, were affronted by the invasion of medical privacy and after two days the patient records were returned and the threatened charges of conspiracy were never brought. However, the publicity given to the raid by the media spread news of the Service as far away as New Zealand.[27]

New Zealand

As in Britain, nineteenth-century restrictive abortion legislation (Offences Against the Person Act, 1866) passed through New Zealand parliament without debate.[28] When the law was rewritten in 1893 it was not in a spirit of humane concern for the weak and helpless but as part of a harsh criminal code, clause after clause of which specified the punishments of flogging and whipping.[29] The current law dates from 1961 and Section 183 specifies up to 14 years imprisonment for anyone 'who, with intent to procure a miscarriage of any woman or girl, whether she is with child or not, unlawfully administers to or causes to be taken' any poison or instrument. Changing law and practice of abortion in Britain and Australia in the 1960s has affected New Zealand in two ways: in some institutions medical attitudes have eased and doctors have begun to perform abortions and a political pro-abortion lobby has gained strength.

In 1969 public hospitals in New Zealand performed 212 therapeutic abortions, but by 1973 the number exceeded 1000. A freestanding clinic – the Auckland Medical Aid Centre[30] – was set up as attitudes eased. In 1975 Dr Gerald Walls introduced a Private Member's Bill (Hospital Amendment Act) in an attempt to destroy private clinics that perform abortions, but when the Auckland Medical Aid Centre appealed to the Supreme Court Mr Justice Speight, in a declaratory judgement, described the legislation both as 'ill drafted' and likely to encompass circumstances not foreseen in the Act, as well as failing to deal with others that it should have covered. The Auckland clinic continues to function charging NZ$80 (US $87) for a termination, and the state is now obliged to pay it a subsidy.

A second legal event in 1975 was the acquittal of Dr Woolnough, also of the Medical Aid Centre, who had been charged with the 'unlawful' use of a suction curette with intent to procure an abortion under Section 182 of the 1961 Act. Mr Justice Chilwell, instructed the jury on the use of the word 'unlawful' in the Act: 'The test of whether or not the use of an instrument is unlawful is whether it is necessary to preserve the woman from serious danger to her life or to her physical or mental health, not being normal dangers of pregnancy and childbirth.' An acquittal was achieved.

In New Zealand as in Canada, Australia, the USA and Britain, juries and appeal court judges have grappled with the problem of abortion more straightforwardly than politicians. The passions released by the New Zealand cases and the development of powerful lobby groups, for and against abortion reform, has forced the government to set up a Royal Commission on Contraception, Sterilisation and Abortion, which is now (1976) sitting.

Other Commonwealth countries

The Indian and Singaporian precedents are having widespread effects. A public call to reform the abortion laws in Ghana was made shortly after the government adopted a national population policy in 1969. There has been discussion of reform in Nigeria and Kenya. For example, Colonel Ogbemvdia, a Nigerian State Governor, called for reform in 1971. In Zambia, a law based on the British legislation was passed on 13 October 1972 allowing abortion in situations that threaten the mother's health, that of her existing children, or where congenital defect is likely. It takes into account 'the pregnant woman's actual or reasonably foreseeable environment *or her age*'. The law makes provision for termination by a registered doctor if 'he and *two* other registered medical practitioners, one of whom has specialised in the branch of medicine in which the patient is specifically required to be examined,' agree on the desirability of termination. Conscientious objection is permitted; the operation is limited to hospitals, and must be notified. The law produced a violent reaction from Roman Catholics and has not been realistically implemented.

A survey of medical opinion in Nigeria in 1973 showed the majority of doctors felt reform would cut the abortion death rate. Most wanted the law to be liberalised, and they believed abortion was 'more common than any other disease' and that doctors commonly operated, usually for a fee of about $25.[31] In August 1974 the Nigerian Medical Association urged the Federal Commissioner for Health to review and liberalise the abortion law.[32] A few months later the Nigerian Medical Association and the Society of Obstetricians and Gynaecologists sent a memorandum to the government that strongly argued the case for abortion repeal or reform. It reviewed the present law: in the six southern states, all abortions are illegal, but, in the six northern states, abortion is not illegal 'if caused on good faith for the purpose of saving the life of the woman'. The Bourne precedent of 1938 (see p. 288) is thought to apply to the whole country. The Society of Obstetricians and Gynaecologists had questioned 1000 doctors in the country and 80 per cent thought the abortion law ought to be liberalised. Other opinion polls show that 79 per cent of obstetric specialists, 76 per cent of nurses, and 69 per cent of the total public favour reform. The memorandum stated, 'It can therefore be said that the majority opinion of both medical and law people in this country is that the law is harmful and out of date and requires to be modernised so as to allow therapeutic termination of undesirable pregnancies'.

In neighbouring Ghana a movement for reform, spearheaded by professional groups, is also gaining momentum. In 1974 the Ghana Law Reform Commission circulated three possible draft laws: (1) along the English lines with the exception that one gynaecologist or two general practitioners should make the decision, (2) a total repeal situation, and (3) a law which would allow termination for social indications and in cases of failed family planning. In November 1975 the Government said it was considering liberalisation.

Dahomey, under a Government Ordinance in 1973, permitted abortion where the mother's life was compromised. Two consultant physicians must certify the operation. (There are 30000 people for every physician in Dahomey.)

Uganda and Botswana have no specific legislation on abortion, but inherited the old British code of practice. President Amin of Uganda, along with Hitler and President Nixon, as a head of state, has publicly condemned induced abortion. He has threatened women with dire punishments and presumably regrets that the laws of Queen Victoria were not adopted and strictly applied to his nation in the past.

With the exception of Uganda it seems reasonable to suppose that other countries will follow the Zambian example. An International Planned Parenthood Federation conference on the medical and social aspects of abortion held in Accra in December 1973 focused attention on the abortion problem in the African continent. One of its suggestions was that the Karman curette should be routine equipment for paramedical workers and traditional midwives.

The Republic of South Africa is no longer a member of the British Commonwealth but British medical practice tends to remain influential, even when other ties are strained. 'The repercussions of these drastic changes [in attitudes to abortion in Britain] have reached South Africa', proclaimed the editorial of a South African medical journal in 1971, 'where the problem of extending the legal basis for performing abortions has become a topic of concern and discussion.'[33] In March 1975 the law was modified to permit abortion in limited circumstances if three doctors sign the relevant certificates.[34] Parliament had set up an all-male Commission to review the problem and Helen Suzman, the only Progressive Party member of parliament called the law 'totally inadequate'. She also claimed that a woman should be 'mistress of her soul and body' which stimulated another member to comment, 'That is the opinion of a very small group in this country, I am happy to say'. Those few doctors who have performed abortions find the new law restricting.

Law reform has also been discussed in Rhodesia. But in both Rhodesia and South Africa, abortion presents an unusually tortuous political problem. The economic advancement of the black population and the possibility of reforming, or overthrowing, existing political discrimination is partly dependent upon a falling birth rate. If the availability of legal abortion were to accelerate any trend to smaller families and greater income *per capita* for the black community, it would also bring nearer the peaceful (or violent) end of apartheid. However, the extreme Right of the white community is likely to view abortion law reform merely as a weapon against rising numbers of black Africans, which the black community might, not unreasonably, interpret as genocide. An argument against the present restrictive laws put forward by the medical community in South Africa concerns the difficulty that arises 'in a multiracial society, especially in cases of rape involving White and non-White persons'.[33] In short, whatever, decision is made, it will, in political terms, be wrong, although in social and health terms it is likely to be beneficial.

Sri Lanka is the only Asian country still enforcing nineteenth-century British abortion legislation. The Medico-Legal Society of the Law and Population Committee is pressing for change.

Public and medical opinion in the Caribbean is also beginning to crystallise in favour of law reform, although paradoxically the only changes that have taken place have been in Guadeloupe and Martinique, which (as Départements of France) acquired the new 1975 liberal French law, and Cuba.

Public discussion and sometimes parliamentary debate have

begun in Barbados, Trinidad and Jamaica. A meeting of family planning leaders in Trinidad in December 1970 voted to invite family planning associations to urge their government to review abortion legislation, pointing out that such legislation was governed 'by statute enacted during the nineteenth century'. They recommended that laws should be brought 'more into line with present day scientific thought and development'. A conference sponsored by the Jamaica Family Planning Association, the University of The West Indies, and the National Family Planning Board of Jamaica, held in Kingston in December 1972, recommended that governments enact legislation permitting abortion on request up to 20 weeks of pregnancy.[35] The right-to-life group, supported the more than usually liberal reform suggestion to permit termination in cases where continuance of the pregnancy presented 'a substantial risk to the woman's mental or physical health'.

The abortion law in Jamaica dates from 1864, and that in Trinidad is part of the Offences Against the Person Act (1925), based on the British 1861 Act. A review of illegal abortion methods in Jamaica found that doctors would perform operations in a hopsital for between $100 and $1000 (average $300), but those who could not afford this service sought the help of unqualified abortionists at fees from $5 to $50 (average $30). Many of the unqualified practitioners worked under assumed names and a member of the Family Planning Association of Jamaica visited a clinic in 1972 that was held in a shop every afternoon of the week and he found upwards of 30 women waiting for the operation.[36] One of the senior gynaecologists in the island, Dr James Burrowes, risked a prison sentence in 1973 by confessing that he had carried out abortions. He called attention for the need to change the law and abortion practice. In Trinidad those illegal abortions that require medical treatment find their way to one of two main hospitals serving an island population of just over one million. At the General Hospital, Port of Spain, there is a 23-bed ward and 10 to 15 admissions daily for incomplete abortion.

Barbados set up a committee representing all sections of the community to review abortion legislation in May 1974.

Puerto Rico falls under the decisions of the US Supreme Court, but the medical community has resisted implementing them.

Hong Kong is a British colony, which has been left with restrictive legislation while Britain has reformed her own laws – an interesting example of the inertia characteristic of abortion law. However, the

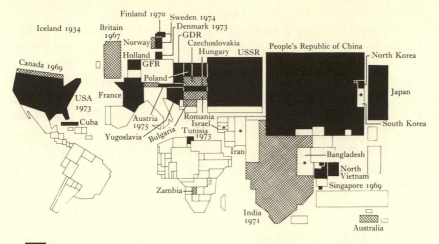

■ Elective abortions (*de jure* or *de facto*, abortions available on request)
▨ Abortions available for social as well as medical indications (law reform under discussion)

Fig. 47. Legal status of abortion, 1974. See also Fig. 46.
* Doctor-performed abortions are widely available in South Korea, Taiwan and Israel, although services are not as developed as in the Netherlands and Cuba, where the de facto availability of abortion is greater than in some countries with a de-jure liberal abortion situation. In South-East Asia, South Vietnam and Laos are assumed to be implementing a liberal abortion policy. In Bangladesh a permissive policy is adopted towards early abortion, but services are limited.

abortion law was amended in 1973 to permit therapeutic abortion for specified indications when two doctors sign the appropriate papers and if the operation is performed in one of the 11 government hospitals. It is estimated that perhaps 600 legal abortions were performed in 1974. The most were carried out in the Church Missionary Society Hospital. Illegal abortion is widely practised. A small number of Western-trained doctors carry out the operation for modest to high fees. The bulk of illegal abortions are performed on the poorest Chinese at a cost of HK$200–HK$400 (US$50–$100), often by the thousand or so physicians who come from the People's Republic of China and who are commonly illegal immigrants into the colony. The illegal services are easily accessible and clinically competent, with a few incomplete abortions being admitted for treatment at the Government hospitals. One illegal practice is

situated opposite the neighbourhood police headquarters. An unknown, but probably significant number of women, pay the HK$2
(US $0.5) train fare into the People's Republic of China for a legal
operation.

Following the 1974 war between Turks and Greeks in Cyprus,
a number of pregnancies resulting from rape were terminated. As
in Bangladesh, this dramatic and unhappy episode led to a review
of the existing restrictive legislation and in 1975 the Cypriot abortion
law was amended to permit legal abortion on socio-economic and
psychological grounds, making it one of the most liberal in the
Commonwealth.

Islam

Occasionally, Islamic culture has been as opposed to abortion as that of Christendom. At one time, in Tunisia, abortion was
punished by crucifixion. Early in the nineteenth century Islamic
traditions were reinforced by cultural influences consequent upon
the military expansion of western European nations. The *Code
Napoléon* was adopted as the foundaton of statute law by many
nations of the Near East and, in the case of Iran, the nineteenth
century abortion law was modelled on that of nearby British India.
Jordan obtained her anti-abortion laws as a Mandated British Territory, and Indonesia was influenced by Dutch legislation. The end
of World War II found abortion illegal, except to save the mother's
life, in all the Moslem countries from Morocco to Indonesia.

A meeting, organised by the Near East Region of the International
Planned Parenthood Federation, in 1971 on *Induced Abortion: A
Hazard to Public Health?*[37] was a landmark in the collection of
factual data on abortion and their objective evaluation.

The first Moslem country to allow termination on other than
strictly medical grounds was Tunisia, which altered its legislation
in July 1965 so that any mother with five or more children, or any
woman who became pregnant after an IUD insertion, might request
an abortion. Health administrators were formally reminded of this
change and asked to perform terminations free of charge three years
later.[38]

In Morocco the law was revised in 1967 to allow termination when
the survival of the mother was in jeopardy, or when the mental or
physical health would be endangered by the continuation of the

pregnancy. The latter is a provision of some latitude, which in future years may become more important as professional health care is extended to the community, but between 1964 and 1971 in one busy hospital there were 60000 deliveries and only 110 legal abortions. As might be expected in an Islamic culture, the husband must consent to the operation or, in default of the woman's partner being available, the local Health Officer can give consent.[39]

With the exception of Tunisia and Morocco, the laws of the other North African countries are universally conservative. For example, in Algeria, 'physicians, midwives, dentists, pharmacists, students of medicine and dentistry, pharmacy employees, herbalists, truss makers, sellers of surgical instruments, male and female nurses and masseurs who show, assist, or use the means to bring about abortion shall receive a heavy fine or imprisonment with hard labour from ten to twenty years'.

In Iran, Egypt, Turkey, Iraq, and the Sudan, termination is limited to medical indications (in the Sudan three doctors must agree on termination). In Jordan there has been some leniency of interpretation in recent years, and when termination is performed in the presence of mitigating circumstances, such as family honour and reputation, it is not usually prosecuted. In the Jerusalem area of West Jordan, no prosecutions took place in the 15 years prior to the June 1967 war. Although there has been no change in the law, a movement to change attitudes can be recognised. In Turkey and parts of Egypt, pregnancy with an intrauterine device in place is sometimes a *de facto* reason for a hospital termination. The Turkish law permits abortion in the case of certain stated diseases and it will be easy for a more liberal practice to arise. The Sudanese Medical Council and Society of Obstetricians and Gynaecologists are preparing a memorandum on abortion, and a new legal code is in preparation, although any change is expected to be slight.

Indonesia, Bangladesh, and the Moslem minorities in India and Pakistan constitute the four biggest groups of Moslems in the world. Indian Moslems live under the reformed law of the country. Possibly, they resort to abortion slightly less frequently than the Hindus and considerably less than the Christians.[40] Indonesia, Bangladesh and Pakistan, where Islam is the state religion, still retain laws from colonial times, but an increasingly active debate is taking place and liberalisation of abortion practices may be anticipated in the coming five or ten years.

During early 1972 in Bangladesh, the abortion law was waived in cases of girls who were pregnant following rape at the time of the civil war. A team of Bangladesh, Indian, British and America doctors set up a clinic in Dacca and visited all the district hospitals in the country. Rape had been very common during the war; some army camps had hundreds of girls corralled within them at any one time; reports of rapes from villages amounted to 200000, and refugees fleeing into India were sometimes ransomed and the daughters of families who could not pay were raped.[41] Some girls were raped many times, some died, most were young and some very young.

The emotional trauma of rape in a rural traditional society is even greater than in the West. Wives were cast out by their husbands, daughters became unmarriageable (surgeons were asked to repair the hymen) and totally destroyed emotionally and socially.

Few babies were delivered and practically none survived. The village abortionists solved many problems using sharpened sticks, or plant infusions. Some women committed suicide and others killed the babies they delivered. Decisions were made privately within the close-knit family, and often by parents rather than the girl, who was a helpless pawn at every stage of the tragedy. The medical teams believe they may have been responsible for terminating about 2000 pregnancies. They arrived when many of the problems had already been solved and all the remaining pregnancies were very advanced. They suffered from an almost insuperable problem of communication as the official statements sometimes masked the intention of the surgeons a little too well and, if they were understood, the village community did not believe the law had been altered. Even when they were believed, the social pressures still made it very difficult for a girl to be brought outside the family, as to do this meant some degree of public recognition of a literally insupportable shame.

Nevertheless, tragic and unusual as were the circumstances, the episode did something to ease attitudes towards abortion in a strict society. A liberal law was drafted in 1976 and awaits ratification.

In 1612 the first Dutch Governor-General of the East Indies advised the East India Company in the Netherlands that there were many European women leading scandalous lives and advocated intermarriage with indigenous women, although he noted that Moslem women would not make suitable brides since they deliberately aborted any babies conceived by Christian fathers.[42] However, during Dutch colonial times the land that is now Indonesia adopted laws totally prohibiting abortion. It has taken almost 30 years of independence for less traditional attitudes to surface. In 1973 a National Seminar on the Status of Women and Family Planning in Jakarta discussed abortion and concluded that the Indonesian Penal Code was too restrictive.[43] A seminar on *Law and Population* in 1974 unanimously identified the need to legalise abortion on medical grounds and a majority saw the need to alter it for socio-economic reasons.[44] Medical practice is becoming more liberal, and termination to avoid danger to life or health is acceptable, although Article 299 of the Penal Code makes abortion of any type a violation of morals. Menstrual regulation is becoming an accepted practice in some hospitals. The use of menstrual regulation is also commencing in Malaysia, although the abortion law remains restrictive.

The Malaysia Medical Association has set up a select committee on abortion and the majority of doctors want reform and believe the Association should take a lead.

In 1974–75 Tunisia and Iran became the first two Islamic countries to move out of a phase of modest reform into an abortion-on-request situation. Iran achieved this by the virtual repeal of its anti-abortion laws and so became legislatively one of the most innovative nations in the world.

The National Congress of Obstetrics and Gynaecologists in Iran passed a unanimous resolution in 1970 setting up a joint medical and legal committee to examine the country's abortion law. The Shah and the Queen showed a personal interest in the social problems posed by abortion. In 1973 the Penal Code was rewritten and the restrictive clauses dealing with abortion and sterilisation were replaced by a single item, specifying that any operation that is internationally recognised and carried out by a registered physician, 'with the consent of the parties legally involved', shall be licit. This is an exceptional and original method of dealing with abortion. (The only parallel is a partial one: in Canada the Morgentaler case represents a precedent with the same flavour as the Iranian statute.) Regulations governing the operation will be drawn up. Mohit[45] has reviewed the practice of illegal abortion in Iran (among family planning acceptors in 1969–70, 15 per cent had had one to seven induced abortions) and the implementation of the new law, when it occurs, can be expected to add credibility to the family planning programme.

The restriction of abortion to women of specified parity in Tunisia became visibly inappropriate as the 1965 reform was applied in practice. Further liberalisation was suggested in 1971. On 26 September 1973 a new law was passed (ratified 19 November 1973) permitting abortion on request in the first three months of pregnancy. After this time abortion is available on medical and psychological indications. The operation can only be performed by a registered medical practitioner and must be carried out in an authorised place. It is notable that the consent of the spouse is not obligatory. As the Minister of Health pointed out in the parliamentary debate on the law, it is a logical extension of a series of legislative changes related to the status of women (for example, in divorce), which President Habib Bourguiba began within a few months of independence in 1956.

The pace of change in Islamic nations is rapid. In seven years Tunisia ran through an experience of abortion legislation and practice, from modest reform to total liberality, which took 25 years to achieve in Sweden. In a single step, Iran passed from conservatism to a change as profound as that achieved by the US Supreme Court ruling, and it did it calmly and rationally. These changes are taking place at the very time when induced-abortion rates are beginning to rise, early in the demographic transition. It is possible that Islam will avoid the painful experience of making changes too late, which has characterised the history of Christendom.

Latin America

In many parts of Central and South America, strong religious influences combine with pro-natalist, military-dominated political systems to outlaw abortion. Yet in the urban centres of the continent, induced abortion is remarkably frequent and some of the best surveys of the incidence of abortion have come from this area.

Legislation on abortion is not subject to much attention and, with few exceptions, changes are unlikely in the near future. Nevertheless, when examined in detail there is an interesting range in the legislative spectrum. Some countries such as the Dominican Republic[46] rigorously exclude any possibility of therapeutic abortion, but several countries make an exception where the woman's life is in danger. Costa Rica,[47] Peru,[48] Honduras,[49] Chile[50] and

Brazil[51] demand incontrovertible evidence – furnished by two, three or a whole committee of doctors – that the woman's life is at risk if the pregnancy continues. Colombia[52] and Uruguay[53] maintain that all abortion is illegal, but recommend reduced penalties when the mother's life is at risk. Argentina,[54] Ecuador,[55] Mexico[56] and Paraguay[57] exclude any penalty when the women's life is in danger. In Uruguay the penalty for abortion may be reduced in cases of serious economic difficulty and in Costa Rica future health as well as life can be a reason for termination if no other treatment is available to avert the danger. In many countries pregnancies following rape are treated with some leniency. In 1973, Guatemala and El Salvador revised their Penal Codes to permit therapeutic abortion in cases of suspected fetal defect, rape and to save the life of the mother. The laws are wider in their implications than the medical professions appreciate.

These therapeutic exceptions are the hairline cracks into which liberal thought, sooner or later, is likely to drive its wedges. But, to date, only the slightest splits have appeared in the apparently monolithic rejection of legal abortion found in Central and South America. However, the fact that Latin American legislation requires *proof* of pregnancy to convict an abortionist (as opposed to the *intention* in British-influenced legislation) is of profound significance, and menstrual regulation offers an important and immediate escape from traditional Latin American abortion attitudes and practices.

The pre-revolutionary abortion law in Cuba was unusually liberal, permitting abortion in order to save the woman's life, preserve her health from serious damage, as well as in cases of rape and possible fetal abnormality,[58] although few abortions were performed. The same law appears to be in force today but has been set aside in practice and the rate of physician-induced abortions has risen from 117 per 1000 deliveries in 1968 to 403 in 1972. Ninety-eight per cent of terminations are performed in hospitals, but *D & C* remains in almost universal use.[59] In 1973, 112107 abortions were performed, a rate of 500 per 1000 deliveries.[60] The rate in urban areas is more than twice as high as that in rural areas. Contraceptive information is available in all polyclinics and hospitals,[61,62] although restrictions on trade with Cuba have made it difficult to obtain intrauterine devices or oral contraceptives. Data from the 1970 census show that, unlike other developing countries, the number of children under five is less than those aged five to nine.[63] It is claimed there are 20000 fewer children aged one to two years, and the population growth rate is estimated to have fallen from 2.6 to 1.9 per cent in the past five years. Castro has said, 'Population is one of the world's greatest problems', although he has denounced US aid to family planning.

In Chile a draft abortion law reform Bill permitting abortion on socio-economic grounds was presented to the legislature in 1969.[64] Although it made no significant progress it was important as the first exercise of this type in any Latin American country. When Dr Allende, a physician and a Communist, was elected as president he expressed his concern about illegal abortions, noting that they were responsible for half the female deaths in the country. Within one month of Allende taking office the government announced its intention of introducing legislation to permit abortion. It proposed to change the abortion law as part of a package 'to protect the family' and included such measures as maternity and child allowances. In February 1973 a conference of journalists went so far as to resolve that the Chilean abortion law should be amended to permit abortion at the request of the woman. The momentum for change was such that it persisted after the overthrow of Allende. When the military government took over, the Ministry of Health, Dr Spoerer took expert advice on several aspects of family planning in Chile. A committee of five recommended a relaxation of attitudes toward sterilisation. This was approved. Shortly afterwards, the same committee recommended that legal abortion should be available in cases of contraceptive failure and again the Minister supported this recommendation. However, within 24 hours, he had been relieved of his job. The present regime has legislated against women wearing slacks, can send children who play truant to prison, and recently sent two sailors to jail for showing a pornographic film. It appears to have an individualistic interpretation of what affects public morality and seems unlikely to do anything to put down the high toll of illegal abortion in Chile, or to create a situation where termination of pregnancy can be part of a rational interlocking of fertility regulation methods.

Those who believe in Communism and those who believe in Catholicism see the two systems as in real, or potential, conflict. The economic and social progress of Latin American nations is linked, among other factors, to their demographic evolution. It is perhaps piquant that, on the same day as the Allende Government announced its intention to reform the abortion law, the Pope, visiting the Food and Agriculture Organisation of the United Nations in Rome, reiterated his intense opposition to artificial contraception.[65] It may be that in the all-important race for economic and social progress one side is unwittingly handing the baton to its competitor.

Other countries

Some of the remaining countries of the world, like Thailand and Ethiopia, are characterised by never having been colonies, yet in the area of abortion legislation, they usually came under the influence of the dominant powers of the nineteenth and early twentieth centuries. They are relatively slow in finding their own national, culturally appropriate, solution to the abortion problem, but some changes are occurring.

Asia

The rising incidence of induced abortion in Korea and Taiwan has been noted (p. 102). In the Republic of Korea anti-abortion and anti-contraceptive legislation was introduced in the 1930s, during the period of Japanese influence. As has been the case in the British Commonwealth, outside influence persisted long after the dominant power had changed its own law.

The family planning programme in South Korea, while it can claim more successful results than most, is still disappointing. It was initially thought that the annual population growth rate had fallen to 1.9 per cent for the years 1966–71, but re-analysis reveals that it fell to only 2.2 per cent. Induced abortion, although illegal, made a significant contribution to the modest results achieved (p. 103).

The Ministry of Health and Social Affairs submitted draft reform laws to the National Assembly in 1965 and 1966, but they were shelved. In 1970 and 1971 it resubmitted alternative legislation as a Maternal and Child Health Bill. The draft was accepted by the Ministry of Legislature and the Executive Committee, but failed in parliament. One of the reasons for failure was a desire for excessive political caution. The law had been framed under the heading of a maternal and child health statute. Predictably, it was opposed by the small Catholic minority in Korea, and by certain Protestant groups. It was supported by obstetricians and the majority of the medical profession, but the pediatric specialists said they felt constrained to oppose the legislation because it really had nothing to do with child health. It seems wise always to call an abortion an abortion.

The National Council of Women, the Planned Parenthood Federation of Korea and a regional seminar organised by the International Planned Parenthood Federation;[66] all publicly discussed abortion in 1972. At the woman's meeting 90 per cent of those present were in favour of liberalising the law.[67] Eventually, on 30 January 1973 the Extraordinary State Council (the marital law authority) passed the Maternal and Child Health Law[68] 'to protect the life and health of the mother, to assist in normal delivery, and to help parents in raising children thereby contributing to the promotion of the health of the people'.

Article 8 of this law permits a single physician to perform an abortion, with the consent of the woman and her spouse, in cases of hereditary defect, certain infectious diseases, when the pregnancy results from rape or when marriage cannot take place because of kinship ties and, 'when from a health and medical point of view the continuation of pregnancy is severely damaging the health of the mother, or is likely to damage the health of the mother'. The law came into effect on 9 May 1973. In practice, it hardly validates the very liberal medical tradition in the country.

The law and practice in North Korea is not known for certain, but is thought to be liberal, as in China.

Taiwan is moving along the road South Korea has trodden, but even more haltingly. In 1971 the Taiwan Public Health and Demonstration Center held a seminar on 'Should abortion Be legalized?' A number of doctors and Protestant church leaders supported abortion reform and at this time a draft Bill went to the Ministry of the Interior for consideration.[69] It would have permitted abortion in cases of suspected congenital defect, rape and incest, or mental and physical disease and for the unmarried. The law has not progressed. The elderly military élite in Taiwan are opposed to abortion on mixed demographic and moral grounds. It is also felt that the effort to change the law was too public and too enthusiastic and that it generated a counter-movement.

All abortions in Taiwan are illegal, with the paradoxical exception that the woman may perform an abortion on herself if the pregnancy endangers her life, although such a therapeutic procedure remains illegal for a doctor – it is not clear if the woman is also expected to be the best judge of the dangers of the pregnancy, or if she should take professional advice before embarking on the operation!

Much of South-east Asia is strongly influenced by the French colonial legal tradition. For example, in 1933 Vietnam modelled its abortion laws on the then current French laws.[70] The code remained in force until the end of the war and prescribed two to ten years' imprisonment for performing, or merely recommending, abortions, and it even contrived to contain anti-contraception legislation, although France herself had repealed this aspect of her law. A move to repeal the anti-contraceptive laws in 1973 failed.[71] The Khmer Republic (Cambodia)[72] and Laos also had French anti-abortion legislation. Today, it seems certain that South Vietnam will follow the liberal practices of the North. The course of events in the Khmer Republic is much more difficult to predict.

Thailand is a predominantly Buddhist country, which has been subject to French and English influence, but never colonised. The most recent revision of abortion legislation was in 1956[73] and abortion is prohibited, except to preserve the woman's life or in pregnancies following rape. A number of academic studies on illegally induced abortion have been completed and a public debate on abortion is slowly building up. In 1973 the Public Health Legislation Promotion Division suggested legalising abortion. In the public debate which followed, Aree Somburanasuk of the Chulalongkorn Hospital said, 'Abortion ought to be legalised in view of the fact most people wanting abortions are poor who have used contraceptives unsuccessfully, so their children will not get the same chance in life as other children might'. But there was also a vociferous opposition. Mr Prayoon Chanyawongse said, 'Abortion is murder. If we legalise abortions we might as well give up believing in Buddhism.'[74] Whether the law is changed or not, medical practice *de facto* is becoming increasingly liberal.

Nepal, like Thailand, is a Buddhist country, although there are many Hindus and Moslems along the Indian border. It has been heavily influenced by British India, has had treaties of friendship with Britain and her troops fought beside Britain in two world wars, yet she always retained her independence. Induced abortion is probably not a serious problem, but the country has a national family planning programme and the existing anti-abortion legislation is likely to have an adverse effect if, or when, the community begins to control its fertility more rigorously. Preliminary discussion of abortion reform took place in 1969, and in 1971, probably influenced by the fact that India was about to implement her new law, there was a brief discussion of reform in the National Panchayat introduced by Mrs Sushila Thapa. The Assistant Minister of Health, Mr Jaya Trakash, stressed the need to adopt suitable legislation on abortion 'in order to promote an effective family planning campaign'. Proposals for 'relaxing penal provisions for abortions' were introduced in 1975 and reform seems likely in the forseeable future.

The Philippines is the only Roman Catholic country in Asia. Abortion is illegal, without any exceptions.[75] President Marcos was one of the 30 heads of state who signed a declaration on population in 1967, and two years later the government declared a national population policy, although it specifically excluded sterilisation and abortion as options open to couples. The population growth rate is one of the highest in the world, and the nation of just under 40 million, already burdened by a great deal of unemployment, gross underemployment and the need to import rice, increases at the rate of a million a year. Until 1969 contraceptives were banned. Female and male sterilisation have become more common in the 1970s, but abortion remains strictly condemned. Like condoms in the years of prohibition, it is available illegally. Early in 1976, in an interview in the *Stars and Stripes* (which is a newspaper not yet in general circulation) the First Lady, Imalda Marcos, referred to abortion as 'a dirty word – like martial law' and saw extreme situations where it might be necessary. This was probably a very cautious attempt to test public opinion and following this statement the first public discussion of abortion has begun – albeit restrained.

The birth rate in Manila fell from 46 per 1000 of the population in 1962 to 32.9 in 1968 and, no doubt, induced abortion played a significant role in this change. If the government-sponsored programme succeeds in accelerating family planning acceptance in the Philippines, then it seems likely that the criminal abortion rate will rise further among certain sections of the community. No doubt it will be many years before abortion is legalised but the revolution in thought about contraception has been rapid. Already there are Jesuit priests who feel that it is not the role of state law to enforce Catholic teaching, even in a field as contentious as that of induced abortion, and individual doctors with an interest in family planning are discussing the role of abortion and especially of 'menstrual regulation' in fertility control.

Africa and the Middle East

The Moslem and Commonwealth countries of this area have been discussed above.

Among the remaining nations of the Middle East, Lebanon, with its mixed Moslem and Maronite Christian (a sect dating back to the seventeenth century, partially autonomous, but subject to Vatican discipline) population, is probably the least likely to modify its anti-abortion laws.[76] It is a country with a strict code of sexual behaviour and the unmarried village girl who loses her virginity still risks having her throat cut by her brother, who, even if brought to justice at all, is likely to receive only a nominal prison sentence.

The Christian groups are probably the most antagonistic to legal abortion, but the common paradox applies that the most vociferous opposition comes from those who probably resort to induced abortion with above average frequency (p. 120).

It has recently been pointed out[77] that in cases like the Lebanon, where strict anti-abortion laws are deeply entrenched a legal argument (apart from specific abortion legislation) might be set up to defend the performance of the operation for *bona fide* medical or social reasons. The Lebanese Penal Code, like that of many other countries, has a clause which says, 'No doer of an action is punishable under this Code if his action is aimed at defending himself or his property; or defending the life of others or their property from the threat of imminent danger.' It is felt a case could be made that the continuation of a pregnancy in, say, a sick woman constituted such an 'imminent danger'.

Israel, like Jordan (p. 437) was a British Mandated Territory. The two countries have similar anti-abortion laws ultimately deriving from Victorian Britain and serving as an unexpected cultural link between politically opposed nations. The British Mandate law in Palestine specified up to 14 years' imprisonment for abortion. In 1952, four years after the end of the Mandate, the District of Haifa court declared abortion for genuine medical indications permissible and Israeli practice, at least for certain social and ethnic groups, is liberal. Ten years later the then Prime Minister, Mr Ben Gurion, appointed a Population Committee. When it reported in 1966, various recommendations of a pro-natalist character were made concerning the Jewish population of the country, one of them being that induced abortion (which was recognised to be common) should be more vigorously controlled. An attempt was made to limit induced abortions to approved places, and it was suggested that committees should screen requests and that money should be available to support women whose requests were rejected. In practice, little has been done along these lines and estimates suggest that almost 50 per cent of Jewish women over the age of 40 have had at least one abortion.[78,79] Like all other communities the resort to induced abortion appears to be determined by socio-economic factors and uninfluenced by religion.*

Ethiopia is an ethnically mixed country, where Moslems make up two-thirds of the population, but are dominated by the Amhara (Coptic Christians) The country successfully resisted attempts at colonisation by Italy. The most recent revision of the abortion law, partially derived from the Swiss Penal Code, presumably on the principle of comrades in neutrality, reads, 'Termination of pregnancy is not punishable where it is done to save the pregnant woman from grave and permanent damage to life or health which it is impossible to avert in any other way.' The woman's consent, the opinion of a second doctor and written confirmation are required. The health services of the country are unusually weak and any interpretation of the law is irrelevant to the rural serfs. On the whole, the country adopts a conservative stance in public attitudes to fertility regulation, although prostitution is a major factor in the economy – and in the national balance of payments, as most Sudanese prostitutes are Ethiopian.

The remaining countries of continental Africa, outside the Anglophone and Moslem group, are dominated by the French (or Belgian) legal system, are conservative in medical attitudes towards abortion and seem likely to see any important changes in law or practice in the next five years or so. Senegal[80] and the Ivory Coast,[81] for example, follow the French anti-abortion law of 1920. Even Liberia, the oldest independent black African nation (established 1847) finds itself, by a process of legal osmosis, with a law based on the French statute of 1810.

* The Knesset passed a reform law in January 1977.

One world

The inconsistency, on the one hand, of twentieth-century nationalism where, with good reason, countries asserted their independence and own proud cultural heritages with, on the other, continued submission to the Western anti-abortion laws and moral colonialism of the nineteenth century has been noted many times in this chapter and elsewhere. It is all the more surprising since such laws were probably always inappropriate in the country of origin and have been, or are being, revised themselves. With the exceptions of the People's Republic of China and Japan, the Third World has followed the precedent of Western nations with respect to abortion laws and attitudes. And in the cases of Japan and China many of the details of the debate on the topic have been reminiscent of similar discussions in Europe and North America.

Asian countries, such as Singapore and India, even when they had adopted liberal legislation seemed compelled to go through the painful experience of countries like Sweden and Britain of exercising extreme caution, delaying the setting up of liberal services only then to discover that abortion was not the frightening and dangerous monster it had been perceived to be. Admittedly the acceptance of liberal attitudes in the developing world has been more rapid than the corresponding evolution in the West and the switch from caution to realism, once a law has been changed has been quicker. But the problems of poverty and population facing the developing world are also more acute than they were in the West. Is the evolution in abortion attitudes rapid enough? Almost certainly not.

In 1976 four states in India passed legislation *compelling* sterilisation after a specified number of children. 'It is clear that public opinion is now ready to accept more stringent measures than before,' said Karan Singh, Minister of Health and Family Planning, in a National Policy Statement. He went on to say there was no intention 'to bring in central legislation for this purpose at least for the time being.' There are many who may feel the vicious circle of population and poverty in India curtails many more human freedoms than the state threatens to do in introducing compulsory sterilisation and it is not difficult to understand and sympathise with the changes that are taking place. Nevertheless, there may be cause for thought in the fact that a bureaucracy that a few years ago did a great deal to frustrate the practical implementation of a liberal abortion law now finds itself encouraging compulsory sterilisation.

But the Indian paradox is not likely to be unique. In five to seven years most African states will probably permit free abortion and in 10 to 15, Latin America will follow suit – but by then Lagos may be another Calcutta and Brazil's dream of greatness may have floundered on the inability to close the gap between rich and poor. And if these socio-economic guesses concerning the effect of postponing abortion choices that must ultimately be made prove too pessimistic, it still seems reasonable to conclude that that postponement will lead to a great deal of otherwise avoidable human suffering.

References

1 Madam Kato (1972). Personal communication.
2 Burnhill, M. S. (1971). The effect of induced abortion policies on maternal health, birth rate and natural increase. Unpublished paper, quoted by van der Tak, J. (1971). *The Impact of Abortion Legislation on Fertility.* Lexington Books, Lexington, Mass.
3 Aird, J. (1972). Population policy and demographic prospects of the People's Republic of China. In Joint Economic Committee of United States Congress. *People's Republic of China: An Economic Assessment,* p. 220. US Government Printing Office, Washington D.C.
4 Snow, E. (1971). Chairman Mao: Why I welcome Mr Nixon. *Sunday Times,* 2 May.
5 Pi-Chao Chen (1970). China's birth control action programme (1956–64). *Population Studies, London,* **24,** 141.
6 Two ways of doing statistical work. *People's Daily Editorial,* 2 April 1958.
7 Djerassi, C. (1974). Fertility limitation through contraceptive steroids in the People's Republic of China. *Studies in Family Planning,* **5,** 13.
8 Salaff, J. W. (1972). Institutionalised motivation for the family limitation in China. *Population Studies, London,* **26,** 233.
9 Health Minister on Birth Control (1957). *New China News Agency,* 7 March.
10 *Hangchow,* 12 May 1957.
11 Horn, J. S. (1969). '*Away with all Pests...an English Surgeon in People's China.* Paul Hamlyn, London.
12 Snow, E. (1971). Population care and control. *New Republic,* 1 May, p. 20.
13 Orleans, L. A. (1969). Evidence from Chinese medical journals on current population policy. *China Quarterly,* 15 December.

14 Moskin, J. R. (1970). The hard-line demand victory. *Look*, 29 December.

15 Lean, H. (1975). Personal communication.

16 *Report of The Committee to Study the Question of Legislation of Abortion* (1966). Ministry of Health and Family Planning; chairman Shantilal H. Shah.

17 Israel, S. (1971). A study of doctors' attitudes to abortion. *Journal of Obstetrics and Gynaecology of India*, **21**, 187.

18 Dawn, C. S. (1975). *Menstrual Regulation: A New Procedure for Fertility Control*. Dawn Books, Calcutta.

19 Boyce, R. M. & Osman, R. W. (1970). Therapeutic abortion in a Canadian city. *Canadian Medical Association Journal*, **103**, 461.

20 Wilson, E. (1971). The organisation and function of therapeutic abortion communities. *Canadian Hospital*, **48**, 38.

21 Morgentaler, H. (1970). Outpatient abortions. *Canadian Medical Association Journal*, **106**, 218.

22 Woolnough, J. (1971). The New South Wales abortion trials. *Australian Humanist*, p. 18.

23 Wainer, B. (1972). *It Is'nt Nice*. Alpha Books, Sydney.

24 Sussman, W. & Adams, A. I. (1970). General practitioners' views of pregnancy termination. *Medical Journal of Australia*, **2**, 169.

25 Sauer, T. (1975). Personal communication.

26 McMichael, T. (ed.) (1972). *Abortion: the Unenforceable Law*. ALRA, Melbourne, Victoria.

27 Short, R. (1975). Personal communication.

28 Facer, W. A. P. (1972). Criminal abortion in New Zealand. *New Zealand Law Journal*, **15**, 337.

29 Littlewood, B. (1975). Abortion in perspective. II. *New Zealand Law Journal*, **x**, 102.

30 Facer, W. A. P. (1974). Therapeutic abortion in N.Z. Public Hospitals. *Nursing Forum*, September/October, 12.

31 Bakare, C. G. M. (1977). A Nigerian survey of medical opinion on abortion. In *Proceedings of the Accra Conference on Medical and Surgical Aspects of Abortion, 1973*. IPPF. (In press.)

32 Nigerian Medical Association (1974). *Nigeria and her Abortion Law: A Case for Urgent Review*. Memorandum to Federal Commissioner of Health, Lagos.

33 Editorial (1971). *Medical Proceedings*, **17**, 221.

34 Abortion and Sterilization Act, Act No. 2. 1975. (South Africa).

35 UJIN Conference (1971). University of the West Indies. (Duplicated document.)

36 *Family Planning News, Jamaica*, **4**, 6.

37 Nazer, I. R. (ed.) (1971). *Induced Abortion: a Hazard to Public Health*. IPPF, Beirut.

38 Nazer, I. R. (1970). Abortion in the Near East. In *Abortion in a Changing World*, ed. R. E. Hall, vol. **1**, p. 267. Columbia University Press, New York.

39 Laraqui, A. (1971). Report on Morocco. In *Induced Abortion: A Hazard to Public Health?* ed. I. R. Nazer, p. 225. IPPF, Beirut.

40 Kulkarni, S. P. & Purandare, B. N. (1974). Patient profile of 800 first trimester abortions by vacuum aspiration. In *Medical Termination of Pregnancy and Sterilization*, p. 20. N.W. Maternity Hospital & Institute for Postgraduate Training and Research in Obstetrics, Gynaecology & Family Planning, Bombay.

41 Davis, G. (1973). The changing face of genocide, Bangladesh 1971–72. In *Proceedings of the Medical Association for the Prevention of War*, vol. **2**, p. 173.

42 Boxer, C. R. (1965). *The Dutch Seaborne Empire 1600–1800.* Hutchinson, London.

43 Soewondo, N. (1974). Social and economic change and planned parenthood. In *Planning for the Future*. IPPF, London.

44 Soewondo, N. (ed.) (1974). *Seminar on Law and Population.* Maternal Training and Research Centre, Indonesian Planned Parenthood Federation, Jakarta.

45 Mohit, B. (1974). The abortion situation in Iran. In *Induced Abortion: A Hazard to Public Health*, ed. I. R. Nazer. IPPF, Beirut.

46 Law No. 1690, 19 April 1948. (Dominican Republic)

47 Section 199 of the Penal Code No. 21, 1 August 1971. (Costa Rica)

48 Law, 18 March 1969. (Peru)

49 Decree, 25 June 1954. (Honduras)

50 Decree, 11 December 1967. (Chile)

51 Decree Law No. 2848, 7 December 1940. (Brazil)

52 Decree, 24 September 1936. (Colombia)

53 Section 328 of the Penal Code, amended 26 January 1938. (Uruguay)

54 Section 86 Penal Code, amended 6 December 1967. (Argentina)

55 Section 423 of the Penal Code, 22 March 1938. (Ecuador)

56 Section 333 of the Penal Code, 13 August 1931. (Mexico)

57 Section 352 of the Penal Code, 18 June 1914. (Paraguay)

58 Social Defence Code, 10 October 1938. (Cuba)

59 Kaiser, I. (1975). Alan Guttmacher, and family planning in Cuba, 1966 to 1974. *Mount Sinai Journal of Medicine*, **42**, 300.

60 Ministry of Public Health Statistics. Quoted in *Abortion Research Notes* (1975), **4**(2), 1.

61 Aurdius, J. & Borell, U. (1969). *Family Planning in Latin America.* Swedish International Development Association, Stockholm.

62 Isaaca, S. & Sanhueza, H. (1976). Abortion in Latin America: the legal perspective. In *Epidemiology of Abortion and Practices of Fertility Regulation in Latin America: Selected Studies*. Pan American Health Organization, Washington D.C.

63 Stamper, B. M. (1971). Some demographic consequences of the Cuban evolution. *Concerned Demography*, **2**(4), 19.

64 *Boletin Asociación Chilena de Protección de la Familia*, **9** (1–2).

65 *The Times*, 17 November 1970.

66 IPPF (1973). *Family Planning and Maternal and Child Health,*

Proceedings of the Seminar of the Western Pacific Region of the IPPF. IPPF, Tokyo.

67 Planned Parenthood Federation of Korea (1972). *Activity Report*, **14**, 1.

68 Maternal and Child Health Law. Providential Decree no. 6713, 30 January 1973. (South Korea).

69 *China News*, 13 June 1971.

70 Decree No. 2163, 18 December 1963, reinstated the Decree of 30 May 1933. (France)

71 Senator Ton-That Niem (1974). Personal communication.

72 Crown Ordinance No. 103, 23 July 1934. Penal Code Sections 455–460. (Khymer Republic)

73 Penal Code, Section 305, 13 November 1956. (Thailand)

74 *Bankok Post*, 22 March 1973.

75 Revised Penal Code, Book 2, Articles 256–259: 5th edition 1963. (Phillippines)

76 Penal Code, Articles 539–546. (Lebanon)

77 Dibb, G. (1974). Personal communication.

78 Bachi, R. (1970). Induced abortions in Israel. In *Abortion in a Changing World*, ed. R. E. Hall, vol. **1**, p. 274. Columbia University Press, New York.

79 Friedlander, D. & Sabatello, E. (1972). *Country Profiles: Israel*. Population Council, New York.

80 Decree No. 67–147, Section 35, 10 February 1967. (Senegal)

81 Law No. 62–248, Section 36, 31 July 1962. (Ivory Coast)

13
Contraception and abortion

Those interested in family planning have often been at great pains to distinguish between abortion and contraception as birth control methods. Contraception is usually advocated as a remedy for abortion. The unpalatable fact that resort to abortion and the use of contraceptives are often positively related has been slow to emerge. Perhaps the first academic recognition of such a relationship occurred in Raymond Pearl's studies of family limitation carried out in the USA in the 1930s. In *Natural History of Population*,[1] he wrote of a 'not exactly pleasant working partnership between criminal abortion and birth control, regardless of religion'. In a sample of nearly 20000 obstetric case histories of

> respectable white married women, those who practice contraception as part of their sex life, by their own admission, resort to criminally induced abortion about *three times* as often proportionately as do their comparable non-contraceptor contemporaries. It requires no elaborate analysis or documentation as to why this is so. It is because criminal abortion is the last desperate remedy to correct failures of contraceptive techniques. A cynic might suggest that the best evidence of real improvement in contraceptive methodology will be afforded if and when the proportionate part of total reproductive wastage due to criminal abortion begins to decline among the contraceptor moiety of the population. In the meantime, a not unreasonable deduction would be that for something like three-quarters of that part of the professional abortionist's business that derives from urban American married women he can thank the birth controllers and the current imperfections in the technique of their art.

This crucial observation was largely overlooked. In 1940 Glass,[2] commenting upon the incidence of abortion in England early in the twentieth century, appends a footnote remarking, 'the propagandist campaigns of Charles Bradlaugh and Mrs Besant seem, in many areas, to have focused attention on the possibilities of family limitation'. And two years later in the USA Beebe,[3] discussing fertility control, in the southern Appalachians of the USA, wrote: 'Desire to practice birth control should correlate with resort to induced abortion, since both are means to limit family size'. But, to those working in family planning, a partnership between abortion and contraception aroused the possibility of inflaming an opposition that was just beginning to die down; the facts could not be tolerated and were passionately rejected.

A copy of Pearl's book found its way to the library of the Society for Constructive Birth Control and Racial Progress. On the fly sheet, Marie Stopes wrote in her characteristic large round hand, 'Pearl is both nasty-minded and quite *un*scientific in much of what he says', and then she refers to the passage quoted above. She attempted to interpret the available facts in other ways and claimed, 'What is obvious to anyone of scientific acumen, that the "non-contraceptors" as he calls them are mainly women who are physiologically less fertile'. Contraceptive methods, she protests, fail in the USA because it is the 'technique which is bad and commercially corrupt'. For Marie Stopes, as no doubt for many others, emotion wins and she rejects Pearl's observation that those who use contraceptive devices have most abortions, with the note 'so his fine-jaw talk about it is all rather revolting'.

The 'revolting' picture Pearl drew has now much more evidence to support it. At the community level, several types of experience can be recognised. First, there are situations where the abortion rate and the use of contraception both increase. Secondly, there are areas where contraceptive practice appears to be gaining on, and replacing, induced abortion. In other communities, however, induced abortion appears to have remained the primary method of birth control, with contraception playing a relatively unimportant role.

At the individual level, abortion among contraceptive users and among those who do not attempt to postpone pregnancies makes a revealing comparison. The possibility of public family planning programmes accelerating the shift from abortion to contraception needs to be assessed. Finally, the clinical implications of the relation between contraception and abortion are reviewed.

Situations where the use of contraception and the resort to induced abortion are increasing

Epidemiological evidence that the induced abortion rate rises in many (or possibly all) communities at the beginning of the demographic transition has been produced earlier. For most developed countries there are no quantitative data on contraceptive use at the time when birth rates began to fall, although there is some useful qualitative information Chapter 5. Contemporary, developing countries have been subject to numerous – perhaps even an excess of – knowledge, attitude and practice (KAP) surveys on contraception. Unfortunately, many such surveys omit questions on abortion, but in a few important studies statistics on both abortion and contraceptive usage have been collected.

Korea

In Korea a national family planning programme began in 1962, at a time of social change and rapid population growth following the Korean War (1950–53). Education became widespread, universal military service continued, the age of marriage rose significantly and, despite some aspects of the culture which favour fertility (such as a strong desire for sons), there was increasing pressure to control family size, especially in urban areas. Government programmes really got under way in 1965 and in the next year almost 30 per cent of the total health budget was devoted to family planning. During the 1960s, $14 million was spent on family planning.[4] Intrauterine devices (IUDs) have been more widely used than in any other country, and among women in the 35–39 age group over half have had an IUD inserted at some time.[5,6] The birth rate is thought to have fallen 10 points to around 32 per 1000; although with a death rate of 9–10 per 1000, formidable demographic problems remain. Unemployment will remain until A.D. 2000, even if fertility continues to decline.

Material for analysis comes from the KAP surveys that have been a regular feature of the family planning programme since 1964, from

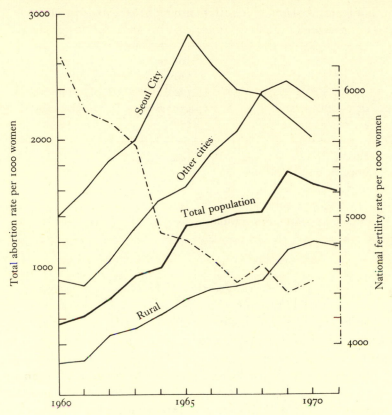

Fig. 48. National fertility (– · –) and abortion (——) rates per 1000 women in Korea (1960–71), by residence.

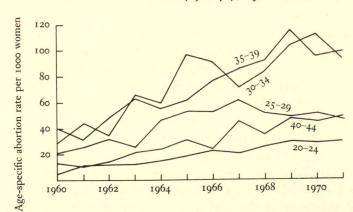

Fig. 49. Age-specific abortion rates of the total population of Korea (1960–71).

Table 29. *Impact of family planning programme on abortion rate in Korea*

Birth control method 1963–64	Intensive family planning programme (%)	National family planning programme only (%)
None	44	64
Abortion only	—	3
Abortion and contraception	9	7
Contraception only	47	26
Number of women in sample	356	315

detailed pre- and post-insertion studies of IUD users and from the excellent surveys of Hong[7] already cited in other chapters.

Age-specific fertility fell most rapidly in young age groups in urban areas. Much of this particular fall is attributed to the rise in the age of marriage. Nationwide data collected by the Ministry of Health and Social Affairs (1968)[8] suggest that the number of Korean women in the 20–44 age group reporting that they have ever experienced one or more induced abortions doubled between 1964 and 1968, exactly parallelling the use of contraceptives. The rise in rural areas was the same as in urban areas, although the absolute rates were lower and peak rates were reached some years later (Fig. 48). When broken down into cohort groups, women currently in a given age group have a very much higher induced abortion rate (Fig. 49) than women of a corresponding age at an earlier point in time. In Hong's studies of Seoul the number of induced abortions per 100 pregnancies rose throughout the decade of the 1960s from 5.2 in 1961 to 17.6 in 1969.[9,10] It must be noted that the abortion ratio dramatises the changes that have occurred, because the number of births has fallen.

There are slight discrepancies between the data from retrospective surveys and KAP studies. The 1970 survey reported a higher incidence of induced abortion for the years prior to 1964 than the 1964 survey itself, perhaps reflecting a loosening in attitudes in the intervening years, leading to a greater honesty. However, a pilot

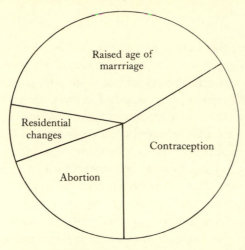

Fig. 50. Decline in fertility in Korea (1960–68). The total fall was 30 per cent.

	Age-specific fertility		Mean age of marriage	% pregnancies reported ending in abortion	% women who have had an IUD inserted
	15–24	25–49			
1960	297	917	21.8	5.2	—
1968	1153	694	23.0	21.3	16

re-survey 12 months after the 1964 survey showed that at that time a third of all abortions had occurred in the preceding year and the changes recorded all seem recent and accelerating. In summary the trends shown are all consistent and should be accepted and the absolute rates recorded in Korea appear to be closer to reality than for most other countries.

Several authors[11-14] have attempted to look at the overall picture and attribute 63 per cent of the fertility decline to contraception and 37 per cent to illegal abortion. They partition the decline in marital fertility as approximately two-thirds due to contraception and one-third to illegal abortion. The rising age of marriage (which is partly the result of universal military service for men) has proved as important in the fertility decline as the adoption of family planning (Fig. 50).

Taiwan

In Taiwan there has been a 28 per cent decline in the crude birth rate between 1961 (37.7 per 1000) and 1970 (27.2 per 1000). Like Korea, there has been a rise in the age of marriage, and the number of women married in the 15–19 age group has fallen by over a third. It has been computed that 21 per cent of the decline that has occurred in the birth rate can be attributed to changing marriage patterns, a further 12 per cent to a changing structure of the population pyramid and 6 per cent to an interaction of these two factors. Put the other way about, approximately 60 per cent of the fall in the birth rate can be attributed to contraception and abortion.[15] There has been a two- to three-fold increase in the reported number of couples using contraception between 1965 and 1970. By the end of 1970 over 780 000 IUDs had been inserted, 150 000 women had accepted Pills and 50 000 men used condoms.[16,17]

As usual the IUD data, because they are based upon clinical family planning services, have been analysed in almost excessive detail, while the contribution that the commercial distribution of condoms and Pills makes, and the role of abortion, are less understood. It is known that only slightly over 250 000 of the first 600 000 IUDs inserted were still in place in 1969.

Theoretical considerations suggest that the use of contraceptives resulting from the national programme would account for an estimated decline in the birth rate from the known level of 36.6 per 1000 in 1963 to a theoretical level of 32.0 in 1969. In fact, the 1969 level was 27.7. The difference is because of the effect of the commercial distribution of contraceptives and of illegal abortion – the two factors most frequently overlooked in national programmes. Unfortunately, no effect has been made to partition these two factors but, as in Korea, information on induced abortion rates is available.

During the early 1960s, the abortion rate in the island rose. By the late 1960s, the urban and rural areas combined reported a rate previously found only in urban areas. Routine surveys of all aspects of family planning and specialised prospective surveys of fetal wastage show similar trends, although not all details match perfectly. Cernada estimates 35 000 induced abortions took place annually in the 1960s.[17]

Twelve per cent of a sample of 2713 women aged 20–39 from Taichung city in 1962[18] reported at least one induced abortion.

Island-wide surveys (sample sizes 5000 upwards, age bracket 20–44) found rates of 9 to 10 per cent in 1964 and 1965, respectively, and of 12.3 per cent in 1967. Another estimate[19] put the percentages at 7.7 in 1966–67 and 8.9 in 1968–69. As the possibility of controlling fertility in Taiwan has been turned into reality so the average desired family size has fallen. Married women in 1965 claimed to want an average of 4.02 children and in 1970 3.8.

Other contemporary examples

Abortion rates appear to be rising in several Moslem countries. Recently Tunisia has seen a slight fall in its high birth rate. Contraceptive usage only accounts for a minority part of the decline in birth rates that has taken place recently[20,21] (Table 30). Abortion has become increasingly available. Although the abortion legislation was interpreted cautiously until the late 1960s, the 2000 terminations performed in 1968 equal a quarter of the total number of pregnancies averted by contraceptive usage. By 1974 the number of legal abortions had reached 12400 (the same rate – 2.2 per 1000 of the population as found for resident English women in the same year). The criminal abortion rate has not been measured. It is probably low because the birth rate is high and the population largely rural. If the estimates of births averted in recent years are correct, then any rise in the illegal abortion rate seems to have been relatively small. The current liberalisation of Tunisia's abortion law (p. 436) has occurred early in the evolution of abortion practices in that country.

Egypt and Turkey are countries where birth rates are beginning to decline in urban areas. They have annual incomes *per capita* ranging from $200 to slightly over $300, and accelerating rates of urbanisation. There is evidence of rising abortion rates. Kamal *et al.*[22] found that in Cairo University Hospital, although the number of abortion admissions fell from 2056 in 1959 to 1620 ten years later, the number of septic abortions increased five-fold, the percentage diagnosed as incomplete rose from 16 to 21 per cent and those requiring blood transfusions from 9 to 14 per cent. Treatment of abortion consumed 50 per cent of the maternity hospital budget. Ozbay & Shorter[23] reported that the prevalence of induced abortion rose in Turkey during the mid-1960s. The annual rate of population growth, while still high, fell from 2.93 in 1960 to 2.55 in 1970. Fisek[24] confirmed the abortion rise in a nationwide probability sample of fertile couples when he found that the ratio of abortions to births

Table 30. *Legal abortion and contraceptive usage in Tunisia* (*1968*)

Population	4922000
Birth rate per 1000 of the population[a]	40.8
Total number contraceptive users	39246
Primary IUD insertions 1968	8969
New tubal legations 1968	2513
Estimated annual number of births averted by family planning programme by 1968	30000
Effect of rising age of marriage	12000
Effect of changing age structure of population	5000
Effect of contraceptive usage	9000
Legal abortions	2211
Rate per 100 births	1.17
Legal abortion rate per 1000 of the population	0.45

[a] Official statistics corrected by Vallin.[21]

in 1967–68 was 1.5 times higher than the ratio reported by women earlier in their married lives. The discrepancy was highest (2.5) in metropolitan areas.

Information from other countries is less detailed but nevertheless points in the same direction. India had the first government family planning policy in the world, and the family planning message is now widespread. In the Lady Hardings Hospital, New Delhi, admissions for abortion (spontaneous and induced) were 15.5 per cent of the total cases in 1950 and 31.8 per cent in 1962. Thirty-nine and a half abortions were reported per 100 deliveries.[25] Rising abortion admission rates are found in many parts of Latin America. At one hospital in Colombia, abortion admissions rose five-fold in the 1960s.[26] In the whole of Chile in 1946 there were 182878 hospital deliveries and 23619 abortion admissions – a ratio of 12.9 abortions to 100 midwifery cases. With improvements in the availability of hospital beds deliveries rose to 268233 in 1966 but abortion admissions rose even more rapidly to 62807 – 23.4 abortions to 100 deliveries. By 1968 the number of abortions had fallen very slightly and the ratio to deliveries was 21.2:100.[27] Similar patterns are evident in Venezuela and elsewhere.

The Chulalongkorn Hospital, Bangkok, Thailand, is one of the busiest maternity hospitals in the world. Between 1960 and 1969 the absolute number of abortion admissions climbed from around 500 a year to over 1200 and the ratio of abortions to deliveries rose from 4–5:100 to 9–10:100.[28] Between 1968 and 1971 the percentage of abortions judged to be criminal at the Sirriragi Hospital, Bangkok, rose from 10.7 to 14.1 of all abortion admissions.[29]

Of course, the limitations of hospital statistics as a guide to abortion rates must not be overlooked. The pace of urbanisation is accelerating so it is to be expected that hospital admissions in the great cities of the world will also rise. However, the marked differential between urban and rural abortion rates means that, although some of the women filling the hospital beds may be recent migrants to the towns, induced abortions are part of this new way of life and were not occurring before on anything like the present scale. Also, as noted, admission rates are modified by rising standards of medical care. To return to the example of Chile, the number of hospital beds approximately doubled ($\times 1.8$) between 1937 and 1960, but abortion admissions more than quadrupled (from 12963 to 57368).

Summarising, in Korea, Taiwan, Tunisia, Latin America and a number of other countries there is strong evidence that at the beginning of the demographic transition there has been a rapid rise in the abortion rate. Abortion becomes a significant, probably the most significant, factor in the demographic changes taking place.

Developed countries

Did developed countries go through a similar phase of rising abortion rates *and* increasing contraceptive practice at some stage of the demographic transition? The beginning of the organised family planning movement after World War I, epitomised by the work of Sanger in the USA and Stopes in the UK, probably coincided with a genuine increase in availability and use of contraceptives. However, the problem of abortion did not diminish and there is some evidence that it increased.[30] For example, in the Camberwell district of London, annual abortion admission to St Giles Hospital rose from 147 in 1924 to 293 in 1936 and over the same period the birth rate fell from 18.2 to 13.2 per 1000.[31]

Perhaps in other areas of the country the peak of abortions had come even earlier. In Birmingham Central Hospital the ratio of abortion admissions to deliveries did decline very slightly from 1:4.9

for the years 1911 to 1913 to 1 : 5.5 for the years 1924 to 1928 (Table 4, p. 84).

The work of the Kinsey group in the USA gave a particularly useful perspective, which was summed up by Kinsey himself when he wrote,

> A record of the number of induced abortions among the married women born in the various decades shows an interesting trend. It would indicate that the smallest number of induced abortions was in the generation born before 1890, and that the prevalence of such abortions increased among the women born in successive decades up to 1909, but among the women born in the decades 1910–1919 and 1920–1929 induced abortion decreased.[32]

Evidence from other countries is even more fragmentary but points in the same direction. Lindquist[33] analysed known abortions in Malmo, Sweden, and comparing 1913 and 1920 found a 10 per cent increase in deliveries and 27 per cent rise in abortions. In Vienna the ratio of recorded abortions to confinements jumped from 19 to 57 : 100 between 1898 and 1913.[34] Convictions for abortion in Austria rose from 55 in 1919, to 267 in 1921, to 619 in 1923.[35] In New York illegal abortions reported from hospitals and dispensaries rose from 1350 in 1926 to 5197 in 1933.[36] In Cincinnati a three-fold rise in abortions occurred in 1918 and 1932.[37] In Australia abortion admissions rose from 11 to 15 per cent of all female hospital admissions between 1928 and 1931.[38]

Situations where the use of contraception improves and the resort to abortion decreases

It seems unlikely that a woman will plan a pregnancy in order to enjoy an induced abortion. In situations where there is ready access to all methods of contraception and sterilisation, will an increase in contraceptive practice take place at the expense of induced abortion?

Whatever the factors controlling achieved family size may turn out to be, and to date they are only partly understood, they act with remarkable uniformity in various countries. The birth rates of most Western industrialised countries share a common pattern. At the time of the Depression, between the two world wars, the birth rates of the industrialised nations fell to a low level, often as low as, or lower than, that current today. Commonly the age of marriage was somewhat higher, but this factor alone does not account for the low fertility and it must be assumed that the total number of births averted (by combined use of contraceptives and abortion) was of the same order of magnitude in the later 1920s and 1930s as it is today. However, there can be no doubt that the availability, use and effectiveness of contraceptive methods, as well as the resort to sterilisation, have all increased considerably over the past 40 years. Therefore, abortion was probably a more important factor in fertility control than at the present time (see Chapters 3 and 5) or, to put it the other way round, the use of contraception appears to have improved at the expense of induced abortion in the last generation. For example even between 1952 and 1968 the number of married women *not* using contraception in Denmark declined from two-thirds to one-fifth.[39]

Countries with a long history of legal abortion allow the process, which logic indicates must have taken place in western Europe and the USA, to be mapped more easily. It should be noted that illegal abortion is more likely to be a threatening procedure from the user's point of view than a hospital termination. Therefore, if there are data to show a switch from induced abortion to contraceptive usage where liberal abortions laws apply, this strongly supports the existence of a similar trend where abortion is illegal. Japan and Hungary have the duration of legislation and the availability of survey data on legal abortion and on contraceptive practices to test the hypothesis in detail. The experience of legal abortion in New York as discussed on p. 138 is also very relevant to this discussion.

Japan

During more than 20 years of liberal abortion law, the registered terminations in Japan first plateaued at around 1 100 000 annually (1954–59) and then fell to three-quarters of a million annually in the late 1960s. The birth rate in the two periods was comparable, suggesting an improvement in contraceptive practice. Changes in the age of marriage and size of population of married women have also occurred. Allowing for all these factors, Nizard has reviewed the total problems at a time of critical change (Table 31). The measure of 'natural fertility' is difficult and Nizard has taken the work of Henry[40] as his base. Muramatsu[41, 42] has paid

Table 31. *Estimate of births averted in Japan for different years between 1950 and 1965*

Age (years)	1950, events per 1000 women				Number of abortions registered per birth averted			
	'Natural fertility'	Japan 1950	Estimated births averted	Abortions registered	1950	1955	1960	1965
20–24	435	386	49	42	0.86	1.74	1.74	1.69
25–29	407	301	106	37	0.35	0.65	0.62	0.50
30–34	371	207	164	49	0.30	0.47	0.31	0.24
35–39	298	124	174	55	0.32	0.40	0.27	0.16
40–44	152	43	109	38	0.34	0.38	0.25	0.17
45–49	22	3	19	6	0.31	0.35	0.23	0.14
Birth rate					28.1	19.4	17.2	18.5

Table 32. *Role of abortion and contraception in Japan (1955–65)*

	1955	1960	1965
	(Millions)		
Married women (15–49)	13.4	14.8	16.7
Live births	1.7	1.6	1.8
Estimated births averted:			
by all methods	3.8	4.8	5.4
by contraception	1.2	2.0	3.0
by abortion	2.7	3.0	2.7
Ratio of births prevented by contraception: abortion	100:256	100:180	100:104
Estimated number of abortions	3.1	3.6	3.1
Reported number of abortions	1.2	1.0	0.8

greater attention to the under-registration of Japanese abortions and has adopted a slightly different methodology, but also arrives at similar conclusions (Table 32).

On several occasions the Mainichi newspapers have carried out reliable surveys of contraceptive practice among the Japanese couples which show increasing contraceptive use during the 1960s. In

summary, there has been a marked and demonstrable improvement in contraceptive practices accounting for a significant *decline*
in terminations against the background of a liberal abortion law.
Family size is similar in all social classes, but the role of abortion
differs. Among women with nine years education the percentage
experiencing abortion rose from 12.2 to 32 between 1952 and 1965,
but among those with 13 years or more of education it declined from
36 to 32.[43]

Japanese women were only permitted the use of intrauterine
contraceptives in the 1970s. Oral contraceptives remain formally
illegal and sterilisations, while performed, are few in number (17 300
in 1969). Had these defects in the family planning services been
filled, the switch to contraception might well have been more
marked. Nevertheless progress is probably always slow, because
each new cohort of contraceptive users tends to learn by mistakes.

Hungary

Between the two world wars the advertisement of contraceptives in Hungary was forbidden and the National Health Council
regarded intrauterine and vaginal inclusive devices as harmful to
health as well as morals. After World War II contraceptives were
available but on prescription and then, after 1953, freely available.[44]
The next year an abortion law allowing social as well as medical
indications was passed.

The availability of contraception services remains poor. In Poland
the law requires that a doctor give contraceptive advice to every
women who is terminated, but in practice only 50–60 per cent of
women receive advice. Hungary is in a particularly unfavourable
position because it has had no government sponsored contraceptive
service. Advice is available from gynaecological departments in hospitals and the Red Cross and Hungarian Woman's Association have
tried to publicise contraceptive methods, but progress has been slow.
In the mid-1960s, 40 per cent of married women claimed they had
never received any information on contraception in their whole lives,
and doctors were a source of information for only one-quarter of
these. Today a single formal lecture on contraception has been introduced in the final year of medical training. Female sterilisation is
rarely used and vasectomy unknown (this is partly as a reaction to
the Nazi occupation).

Despite all these difficulties, which are reminiscent of many
contemporary western European countries and of Britain, Scandin-

avia and the USA a generation ago, over 60 per cent of Hungarian married women use some form of contraception. Szabady and his colleagues in the Demographic Section of the Hungarian Central Statistical Office have conducted excellent studies (1958, 1960, 1965/66) of birth control practices in their country.

The 1965/66 survey involved a carefully chosen nationwide sample of 8800 women (0.5 per cent of all fertile women) who were questioned on many aspects of fertility control.[45] It is one of the most useful and accurate fertility surveys in the world. The desired family size in Hungary is one of the smallest in the world (in 1958–60 it was 2.4; in 1965/66, 2.1). In the cross-section of the population covered in the survey, the achieved family size was 1.98 in 1960 and 1.86 in 1966. Some improvement in contraceptive usage is apparent in different age cohorts. In the 25–29 age-group, 70 per cent of women practised a method of contraception, while in the over 40–65 age group less than half the women did so. As in most European nations *coitus interruptus* is the commonest method and it is also relatively more frequent in the older age groups (75 per cent of couples where the wife is over 40 use this method).

The surveys in the first half of the 1960s cover the early experience of liberal abortion. Among married women as a whole there was some change in the contraceptive methods used, with an increase of *coitus interruptus* at the expense of the condom, but, among women who had borne children or had had an abortion, there was an increase in the use of mechanical methods (Table 33).

Szabady[44] believes that progress in adopting contraception has been slow because of the availability of legal abortion, but the rate of improvement in contraceptive usage in post-war Hungary may have been comparable to that which took place in Britain or the USA between the two world wars. Hungary was late in taking to the Pill. In the latter part of the 1960s a quantum leap forward took place with the introduction of Hungarian manufactured oral contraceptives (Table 34).

It is an interesting byway of history to recall that the Austrian physiologist Haberlandt[46] explored the possibility of manufacturing an oral contraceptive (under the trade name Infecundin) with a Hungarian pharmaceutical firm in 1927. Haberlandt had an accurate grasp of the physiological mechanisms that are the basis of current oral contraceptive therapy. Although his ideas might well have been too much for the biochemical abilities of the pharmaceutical industry

Table 33. *Contraceptive methods and abortion in Hungary* (*1960–64*)

	1960	1964
Coitus interruptus	54	44
Condom	17	25
Diaphragm	4	12
Douch	8	6
Rhythm method	2	2
Birth rate per 1000 of the population	14.7	13
Legal abortion rate per 1000 women aged 15–49	65	79

Table 34. *Contraceptive methods and abortion in Hungary* (1970)

Cycles of Pills (Infecundin) distributed

Jan. 1970	133053
June 1970	150974
Dec. 1970	174586

1969 usage = one third of usage in 1970.
More users (57.9 per cent) in age group 20–29.
Decline in induced abortion 1969/70 = 7 per cent

Users per 1000 married women

Age (years)		
17–19	19[a]	
20–24	177	
25–29	162	
30–34		88
35–39	99	
40–44		
45–49	12	

[a] Weighted averages.

of the time, the immediate reason his project was frustrated was because of lack of medical interest. If it had been otherwise, the abortion problem in all countries might have been much different today. A generation's experience in the use of oral contraceptives would have been gained and, more important, distribution would not have been limited to medical prescription of the Pill had it been developed earlier.

Chile

The rise in induced abortion in Chile, which took place until the mid-1960s, has been noted. In 1964, the year many public family planning programmes began, 55900 women were admitted to hospitals with incomplete abortions (mostly the result of illegal interference). The number peaked at 62200 in 1965 (29.8 admissions per 1000 women aged 15–49) and by 1973 had fallen to 51000 (20.2 per 1000 women aged 15–49) (Fig. 51). Some of this decline was probably the result of improved illegal abortion techniques, as well as a change in numbers. In the demographic transition in Chile, the abortion rate (as measured by hospital admissions for incomplete abortion) was highest as births fell from the lower 30s to the upper 20s.[47,48]

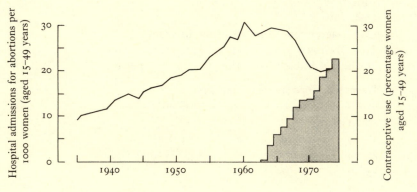

Fig. 51. Trends in illegal abortion and contraceptive practice (shaded) in Chile (1935–75).

Situations where abortion is the primary method of fertility control

As has been noted earlier, more induced abortions can be fitted into a unit interval of a fertile woman's lifetime than term deliveries. It has also been shown that the role of contraception is crucially important in extending the pregnancy interval and that, even when seldom used, greatly reduces the number of induced abortions necessary to achieve a desired goal of family size. If the availability of contraceptives within a community is very poor and any tradition of *coitus interruptus* weak, then the induced abortion rate can go to a very high level. A study in a Tokyo maternity hospital found that women not using any contraceptives had 1.1 abortions per year.[49] There is evidence that this has been the case in Romania and parts of the USSR during periods of liberal abortion legislation (see Chapter 3). Unfortunately, the statistics on abortion have not been published regularly and information on contraceptive practice is limited, so the scene remains more foggy than it might be otherwise.

The crude birth rate in Russia fell from 26.7 to 17.3 per 1000 between 1950 and 1968. There is a great deal of regional variation in the degree of fertility control. In the western USSR, abortion rates are thought to be rising and the statement by Russian authorities, that 'the increase in the supply of both control devices has not yet led to a decline in the intensity of abortions',[50] probably reflections the genuine experience of the country. As noted elsewhere, national statistics on abortion are not available, but, those available point to a high abortion rate. Sadvokasova[51] quoted by David,[52] found that 15 per cent of urban women and 16 per cent of rural women having an abortion had had a previous operation in the preceding year. Mehlan[53] reports on a sample of 1350 Russian women, 70 per cent of whom had had two or more previous abortions and 12 per cent six or more. Some women had had three abortions in one year, which can be expected to happen to some from a population that is not using *any* method of contraception.

The western European pattern of the nuclear family and relatively late marriage combined with a strong tradition of *coitus interruptus* did not extend to Romania or Bulgaria. Romania, especially, seems to follow the pattern of tending to use only abortion to control family size. During the period when abortion was available on request

(1957–66) the abortion rate rose *more* rapidly than the births fell. Tietze[54] calculates that it reached 60 per 1000 of the population by 1966. At the Filantropia, the largest gynaecological hospital in Bucharest, the ratio of deliveries to abortions altered from 1:6 in 1956 to 1:14 by 1962.[55] The high rates were the result of a lack of even a poor use of contraceptives, as much as a consequence of a low birth rate. No doubt the rate greatly taxed hospital services and the frequent repetition of the procedure may have affected the health of some women.

In 1966 the government restricted the abortion law. The birth rate rose dramatically and then fell, as illegal abortion networks were re-established (Chapter 4). Tragically, the government, unaware of the relationship between abortion and contraceptive practice, also clamped down on the availability of contraceptives – even though their use had been slight.

Patterns of contraception and abortion in different socio-economic classes

In some situations it is difficult to measure historical changes in abortion rates, but different social groups, at one instant in time, may recapitulate long-term trends in the evolution of abortion practices.

The study by Pearl,[1] mentioned at the beginning of this chapter, showed that reported abortions were most frequent among very poor white women and moderately wealthy black, but lowest in the very poor black and well-to-do whites (Table 35). That is, abortion was most frequent in those social groups which were well forward in the evolution of fertility control practices but had yet to reach the most advanced stage. Pearl commented upon his findings, 'they probably understate the true facts by a certain unknown amount. But on that account their significance as minimal values is enhanced.' Much subsequent data confirm Pearl's observations and his surmise was probably correct.

The Lebanon has a mixed Christian–Moslem population and a high birth rate, and abortion is illegal. Like Tunisia, it is also entering the demographic transition. Yaukey[56] has compared Moslem and Christian communities in urban and village settings. Sampling errors may be present and the rapport with the women was poor in some cases. Nevertheless the fertility histories, as

Table 35. *Contraceptive use and induced abortion* (Urban hospital obstetric records: $n = 22657$, 1931–32)

Socio-economic class	Contraceptive use (%)	Reported induced abortions per 100 pregnancies	
		Contraceptive users	Contraceptive non-users
Black			
total	19.7	1.0	0.4
very poor	16.5	1.1	0.5
moderately wealthy	38.4	2.4	0
White			
total	46.0	2.3	0.7
very poor	30.0	2.4	0.8
moderately wealthy	56.5	2.0	0.4
well-to-do	80.1	1.0	1.1

Table 36. *Reported abortions (per 100 completed pregnancies) and contraceptive use in various Lebanese communities*

	Abortions		Use of contraception by women married 10 years or more (%)
	Claimed spontaneous	Claimed induced	
Village			
Moslem	10.4	0.2	2
Christian	10.0	0.0	16
City uneducated			
Moslem	11.1	2.5	60
Christian	14.8	7.9	56
City educated			
Moslem	7.4	13.7	83
Christian	13.8	8.2	86

Table 37. *Birth control in Korea* ($n = 6372$, 1971)

	Percentage of ever married women (15–54) who have used specified method		
	Total	Urban	Rural
Abortion	24	34	17
Oral contraception	18	21	16
IUDs	19	18	20

recounted by the women themselves, demonstrate a rise in the induced abortion rate with urbanisation. This reaches its highest level amongst the educated and parallels a rising usage of contraceptives (Table 36). As in many societies beginning to use contraceptive techniques, *coitus interruptus* and the condom are the commonest methods in use, each being used at some time or other by 40–50 per cent of urban educated couples.

The rhythm method is used by 9 per cent of Moslems and 14 per cent of Christians in this same group. The raw data suggest that the Christian couples report a proportion of their induced abortions as spontaneous. Even where there may be serious under-reporting of induced abortions, especially in retrospective studies covering a fertile lifetime, the overall pattern is plain: in a country with a tradition of high fertility, the minority which has begun to have moderate to small families is achieving this goal by a mixture of contraception and induced abortion, and the usage of both is rising side by side. The example of Korea has already been used. The differential in urban and rural patterns of abortion and contraception is in the same direction as that in the Lebanon, although the government IUD programme has been particularly rigorous and has reversed the pattern in the use of this one method (Table 37).

Some of the most illuminating surveys of the incidence of induced abortion and contraceptive practice come from Latin America. Again the inaccuracies of studying illegal abortions are obvious, especially with retrospective studies. However, the CELADE studies of fertility control in selected large cities in Latin America show some important trends (Table 38).

Requena in 1970 has elaborated the hypothesis, based on studies

Table 38. *Contraception and abortion in Latin American cities*
(*1964*)

	Use of contraception (%)	Pregnancies per 1000 women per year	Average number of children	Abortions per 1000 women per year	Abortions per 1000 pregnancies
Mexico City	19.0	237	3.27	37	155
Bogota	31.3	226	3.16	26	117
San Jose	33.1	207	2.98	33	161
Caracas	34.8	207	2.97	34	163
Rio de Janeiro	—	147	2.25	21	141
Buenos Aires	52.3	84	1.49	21	246

carried out in Santiago, that 'the low socio-economic-cultural stratum of women is the one which shows a higher fertility, does not make use of abortion too often and makes practically no use of contraceptives. The medium stratum has an intermediate fertility, uses abortion often and begins to intensify the use of contraceptives. Finally, the high stratum shows the lowest fertility, makes less use of abortion and the most important factor is the contraceptive.'[57] Santiago is especially interesting because of the opportunity provided to study induced abortion in a community where the usage of efficient contraceptives (orals and IUDs) has risen from 0.4 per cent in 1963 to 11.2 per cent in 1967. During the period of increased contraceptive use, the induced-abortion rate, as measured by comparable techniques, increased from 44.9 to 56.2 per 1000 fertile women, and the abortion ratio from 15.5 to 20.1 abortions to 100 pregnancies. However, the maximum incidence of induced abortion moved down the social scale showing that, as contraceptive practices spread through a society, they are associated with first a rise on the frontier of the initiation of use and then a subsequent fall among the more experienced and effective users of contraception. A similar trend appears to be detectable in Russia in the 1920s, where the small towns had a moderate birth rate and the highest abortion rate (Fig. 26, p. 115).[58]

Studies of the individual
The contraceptive user and abortion

The usages of contraceptives and of induced abortion are intertwined even more closely when the individual rather than the community is surveyed. For example, in Korea a past history of induced abortion is twice as common in urban acceptors of IUDs, and over three times as high, as rural acceptors, as in the population at large. This pattern extends to all family planning methods and 45 per cent of women coming to a Seoul Health Centre for family

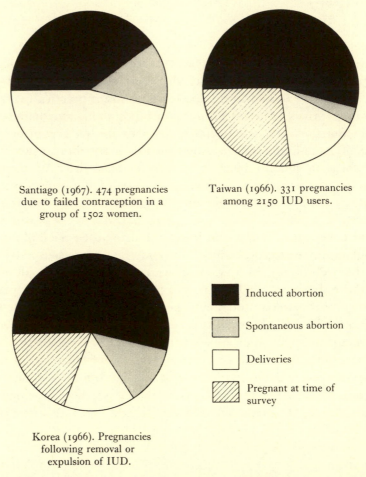

Santiago (1967). 474 pregnancies
due to failed contraception in a
group of 1502 women.

Taiwan (1966). 331 pregnancies
among 2150 IUD users.

Induced abortion

Spontaneous abortion

Deliveries

Pregnant at time of
survey

Korea (1966). Pregnancies
following removal or
expulsion of IUD.

Fig. 52. Pregnancy outcome during or following contraceptive use.

Table 39. *Percentage of women reporting one or more abortions in Rio de Janeiro, Brazil (n = 1734 married women)*

Contraceptive practice		
Currently or in the past		72.4
Always	40.9	
Occasionally	3.4	
Rarely	3.4	
Not currently	52.3	
Never		27.6

planning advice reported previous induced abortions in 1964, while in a random sample of the city's population in the same year only one-quarter reported induced abortions.

Amongst women who discontinue the use of an IUD for any reason, induced abortion is a common outcome of subsequent pregnancies (Fig. 52). In Korea 80 per cent of women discontinuing IUD use fell pregnant within six months, but immediately 54 per cent of pregnancies ended in induced abortions, 12 per cent in spontaneous abortions and only 44 per cent had gone to term or were extant at the time of follow-up. In a similar study of 562 ex-IUD users in Taiwan (a richer, more urbanised country with a lower birth rate), 10 per cent reported spontaneous abortions and 72 per cent induced abortions; only 18 per cent had gone to term or were pregnant at the time of interview. Following discontinuation of the Pill in Taiwan, 68 per cent of pregnancies ended in induced abortions. Taiwan also provides data concerning abortion before as well as after IUD insertion. Among 24984 pregnancies that took place before adopting the method, 8 per cent ended in induced abortions, while among 1576 occurring after discontinuing IUD use (or with an IUD in place) 51 per cent were deliberately terminated.[59]

The relationship appears to involve all contraceptive methods, even extending to Catholic women using the rhythm method. In a study from Colombia[60] it was found that, before adopting the rhythm method, 13 per cent of pregnancies ended in spontaneous or induced abortions, while 35 per cent of pregnancies that occurred after women adopted the method ended in abortions. In Brazil a

Table 40. *Relationship between contraceptive practice and induced abortion in Japan (1965)*

	Have had induced abortion (%)	No answer
Currently practising contraception	42.7	7.0
Previously practised contraception	47.2	8.3
Have not practised contraception	9.3	11.5

sample of 1734 women from Rio de Janeiro found a strong correlation between contraceptive practice and abortion (Table 39).[61]

Of particular interest is the group that used contraceptives in the past. As with IUD users in Korea, or Taiwan, so in Rio, the desire to control fertility sometimes lingers longer than the actual practice of contraception. In a Mexican study, 510 pregnancies out of 2016 (25.3 per cent) from a sample of family planning users ended in abortions, while only 156 out of 1882 (8.2 per cent) ended in abortions among a comparable group of non-users of contraception.[62] In Colombia, women admitted with induced abortions wanted smaller families than women admitted with spontaneous abortions.

The relationship can be found in many places. It is found in Japan (Table 40)[63] in Taiwan (Table 41) and India. In Delhi, Agarwala,[64] surveyed 2454 abortions (spontaneous and induced) among clinical records of an aggregate of 24065 pregnancies. The abortion ratio was slightly higher among those using contraceptives (11:100 pregnancies) than among those not using contraceptives (9:100 pregnancies). Earlier, the same author, pooling data from eight family planning clinics showed an abortion ratio of 19:100 live births in the 'contraceptive period of use' compared with 10.5 in the 'non-contraceptive period of use'. However, reporting may be subject to declining recall with time.

The large and carefully conducted study of a sample of 5375 Turkish households,[65] already referred to, allows the calculation of abortion rates for a number of contraceptive methods. Although spontaneous abortions dilute the relationship and certain tabula-

Table 41. *Relationship between contraceptive practice and induced abortion in Taiwan (1967)*

Percentage of women who had experienced induced abortion

Age (years)	Never used contraceptives	Ever used contraceptives
20–24	1.2	16.9
25–29	1.5	18.5
30–34	4.2	23.0
35–39	3.8	28.5
40–44	8.4	29.7
	3.5 ($n = 2921$)	24.8 ($n = 2048$)

Number of pregnancies	Never used contraceptives	Ever used contraceptives
1	0.3	5.6
2	0.2	3.2
3	1.7	8.3
4	1.6	14.5
5	2.7	22.4
6	5.9	32.1
7	10.0	30.7
8	12.6	48.8
9	14.3	41.1
10+	21.4	75.3
	3.5 ($n = 2911$)	24.8 ($n = 2068$)

Table 42. *Relationship between contraceptive practice and induced abortion (Turkey, 1968)*

Contraceptive method	Abortions per 1000 married women
None	50
Currently using	78
oral contraceptives	126
IUD[a]	264
condom	97
withdrawal	108

[a] 34 women, 9 abortions.

tions are based on small numbers, the broad relationship between contraceptive use and the resort to abortion is well established (Table 42).

At first sight the association of contraceptive use with a higher than usual probability of induced abortion seems to conflict with the frequently quoted evidence of non-users of contraceptives among women seeking induced abortions. However, pregnancies among contraceptive users are much less common than among non-users so that, numerically, abortions among non-users exceed abortions among contraceptive users.

The contraceptive non-user (and the unmarried)

Among over 16 000 women seeking abortions from the British Pregnancy Advisory Service, non-users accounted for 79 per cent of those who were sexual novices at the time of conception as well as 36 per cent of those who were sexually experienced. Non-use was inversely proportional to age, ranging from three out of five girls under 16 to only one in four among women aged 30–44.[66] Among 136 women who came for legal abortion under the National Health Service, 58 had not used any method of contraception prior to the unwanted pregnancy.[67] The correlation is not close and not limited to legal abortion. In Obeng's series of 300 women with illegal abortions, studied prior to the 1967 Act and coming mainly from social classes IV and V, 228 had used no method of contraception, 12 mechanical methods, 13 *coitus interruptus* and 25 rhythm.[68] In Colombia, at the University Hospital of San Vicente de Paul, Medellin, 55 per cent of women admitted with the consequences of illegal abortion knew of no method of contraception.

In a sample of over 1000 women questioned about contraception usage in the 12 months prior to having an abortion in New York, 54.4 per cent had used no contraceptive method.[69] Of those couples using a method, oral contraceptives were used by 36.4 per cent, condoms and spermicides by approximately 17 per cent, the rhythm method by 10 per cent, and withdrawal by only 8.5 per cent. (Compared with Europeans it seems that young Americans have lost the art of withdrawal!) The sample included married or engaged women and those with more casual relationships. Oral contraceptives were used by 30 per cent of married women and 43 per cent of those with a regular boyfriend, but by only 2 per cent of those with a casual boyfriend. Girls with a regular relationship were having coitus two to three times a week, but those with casual relationships less frequently, and there was a correlation between casual relation, low coital frequency and the use of condoms, rhythm and withdrawal. Women who discontinued using the method of contraception were more than usually likely to have had a change of relationship with their partners – in a minority of cases this involved the relationship becoming more close, e.g. they became engaged, but in the majority of cases the relationship was breaking down with separation, divorce or change of boyfriend. Roman Catholics were less likely than Protestants to use a regular method of contraception, but appeared equally likely to proceed to an abortion: indeed, 35 per cent of the sample were Roman Catholics.

A study of a more complex and interesting type was undertaken on a cohort of women who had given birth or had had abortions (but whose pregnancies would have come to term during the same interval) in Hawaii in 1971.[70] The 1579 women in the group were divided into 663 who planned to have a child and 916 who did not wish to become pregnant. Ninety-seven per cent of those planning to have a baby did not use a contraceptive method. Sixty-seven per cent of those not planning to have a baby did not use a contraceptive method. Of the latter group 68 per cent had a term delivery and 32 per cent had an abortion. Interestingly, amongst those who did not want a pregnancy but used birth control, 69 per cent had a delivery and 31 per cent an abortion: in other words, among women who had not planned to get pregnant the percentage choosing abortion was the same for those who used, and those who did not use, birth control methods. However, when the pooled data are dissected into those for the married and unmarried, and further divided into those for steady relationships and engaged couples, then correlation of abortion and contraceptive use reappears for certain groups.

It must be remembered, of course, that the non-users of contraception will fall pregnant more rapidly than users and, therefore, although the non-use rate in a particular population may be quite low, non-users will tend to swamp the statistics of women having abortions. Nevertheless contradictions appear to exist. Why?

They probably highlight the fact that abortion is most common early in the evolution of fertility control of a community, or subgroup within a community. The advancing edge of family planning is unstable and the attempt to use contraception may be characterised by numerous mistakes. They commonly occur with the break-up of a romance or marriage, events which may diminish or totally curtail the use of contraception.

In Novi Sad, Yugoslavia, Kaper-Stanulovic & Friedman (1974)[71] conducted a study of decision-making rather like the Hawaiian one quoted above. They followed an equal number of women (72) seeking abortion and attending a contraceptive clinic. The contraceptive-seeking women were somewhat older than the abortion seeking women, a higher percentage were married, and they had a history of half as many induced abortions. There were more rural women (43 per cent) in the abortion group than the contraceptive group (32 per cent) reinforcing the impression that abortion is most frequent among those groups adopting contraception. Similarly, students were over-represented in the abortion group. It may well be that efficient contraceptive practice takes two generations to be adopted. If this is the case, then it has important implications for family planning programmes in the developing world.

In the Yugoslavian study both groups ranked abortion twice as costly in emotional and social terms as the acquisition of contraception. Women using contraception had a greater sense of being able to control their destinies than those using abortion (Table 43), in particular women using contraception believed that the success of their marriage depended on their efforts.

It is the impression of some of those involved in the counselling of the young unmarried in industrialised nations that many of the non-users are women who intended to get contraceptive advice but were deterred by some minor hurdle: 'my sister was told off by the family doctor when she asked for the Pill', 'I'd made an appointment at the clinic but had to wait two weeks', 'I didn't want an "internal"'.

The young unmarried in industrialised nations are a subgroup of particular interest and importance. Patterns of premarital sexual behaviour are changing. Although the past generations may not have been as chaste as many would sometimes have believed, there is little doubt that in the USA, UK and Scandinavia the prevalence and duration of premarital intercourse has increased since World War II. A similar trend has occurred in eastern Europe slightly later and is just beginning to emerge in some developing countries. In some ways the young unmarried in developed countries are analogous to the married in underdeveloped countries, as a group initiating

Table 43. *Perception of the individuals' ability to control their lives* (*Novi Sad, 1973*)

Controllable factors	Women having abortion (%)	Women seeking contraception (%)
Who you marry	75	85
Happiness in marriage	51	88
Acquisition of money	70	97
Health/sickness	63	83
Friends/enemies	44	58
Number of children	61	82
Behaviour of children and adults	68	72

fertility regulation, and therefore using both abortion and contraception with increasing frequency.

The trend which it is postulated applies to the group, may be reinforced by only applying to the individual. Sexual behaviour, like car driving, requires practice, and mistakes are probably most common among late adolescents and those in their early 20s. The failure rate of most contraceptive methods can be demonstrated to decline with duration of use.[72] Part of this improvement will be related to the fact that motivation grows stronger as the desired number of children is achieved; part is no doubt due to individual and couple's own familiarity with their sexual needs and timings.

Developing the relationship between abortion and contraception

A major thesis of this chapter is that induced abortion is an inevitable correlate of the necessity to control human fertility. Early abortion is relatively simple and modern techniques enable it to be made available at the request of the woman in both developed and developing countries. The purpose of this next section is to explore ways in which society might assist the individual to combine the practices of abortion and contraception in the most advantageous way possible.

On the one hand, most rational combinations of abortion and

contraceptive practices would result in a low level of abortion. On the other hand, no practical scheme would dare set itself the unattainable goal of attempting to eliminate the resort to abortion. Therefore, the aims of those who assign considerable moral status to the embryo and of those who assign less moral significance largely overlap. Divergence of opinion only arises at the point where pressure for contraception alone might endanger the life of the woman, or cost society a significantly greater amount than the use of contraception and abortion together.

Availability, acceptability and aesthetics may be the most important factors determining contraceptive use. Nearly everywhere oral contraceptives, and possibly IUDs, could be made much more readily available. Pills would receive a boost in their use if the present medical restrictions on their distribution, especially to rural populations of developing countries, were lifted. The commercial distribution of spermicides and condoms is open to expansion, especially if they were more widely advertised and were, if necessary, subsidised in price. The rhythm method, because of the ability to teach it neighbour-to-neighbour without professional advice, could also find increased use in several countries. In many situations the use of *coitus interruptus* may spread further through society, particularly at the frontier of acceptance of contraceptive methods.

For many years into the future all the methods of fertility control mentioned will continue to play such an important role in family planning that it will be unwise to dispense with any one of them. If this conclusion is accepted then the important relationship between abortion and contraception appears in a new and more insistent way.

The limitations of contraceptive methods

With the possible exception of oral contraceptives, no reversible method of fertility control currently available is adequate to allow a large sample of users to control their fertility within the goals of family size that are now almost universal in industrialised nations, and that are hoped for in many developing countries. Using a computerised model population, Hulka[73] has shown that, if a reproductive period of 20 years is assumed and if three children are planned, then given average Western marriage ages, the woman is likely to achieve her desired family size while still in her 20s or early 30s and will then be faced with 12 to 15 years of fertile life, during

Table 44. *Percentage of legal abortions expected to be repeat abortions each year after legalisation of abortion*

Method	Assumed percentage effective-ness[a]	Percentage repeat abortions each year				
		1	2	3	5	10
Mechanical methods and IUDs	90	5.4	22.1	33.7	49.0	67.7
	95	2.8	12.7	20.8	33.1	51.9
Oral contra-ceptives	98	1.2	5.6	9.6	16.8	30.5
	99	0.6	2.9	5.1	9.2	18.1

[a] A 20 per cent monthly probability pregnancy in the absence of contraceptive practice is assumed – a fecundity characteristic of older women.

which she will be exposed to the risk of unplanned pregnancy. Hulka has calculated the number of unplanned births likely to occur during this interval given a contraceptive method which is 95 per cent effective during any cycle of exposure (for example the condom and diaphragm). Some 30 to 35 per cent of women will have one unplanned pregnancy, 46 to 56 per cent two or more unplanned pregnancies, and only 13 to 18 per cent of women will not exceed their desired family size. Using a very effective method, such as an IUD, there are still significant numbers of women who have one or more unwanted pregnancies. The estimates are difficult to make, and variation arises from the different assumptions that might be made concerning the spacing of the planned number of children.

Tietze[74] used a computer to investigate the same problem from another point of view. He asked how many repeated abortions can be expected if certain parameters of fertility and contraceptive effectiveness are assumed (Table 44). His theoretical conclusions fit reasonably well with observations on repeat abortions in New York[75] (a high degree of contraceptive effectiveness and 4 per cent repeat abortions after one year) and in Hungary (a lower, but still reasonable degree of contraceptive effectiveness, and 58–60 per cent repeat abortions after 10 years).

In the United States, Westoff & Ryder[76] have shown that, al-

Table 45. *Limitations of 'one-method' family planning*

Age of woman (years)	Additional births observed[a]		
	No family planning	IUDs[b]	Difference
22.5	7.14	6.48	0.66
32.5	3.10	2.24	0.86
42.5	0.38	0.13	0.25

[a] Based on programme data from Taiwan.
[b] Insertion and reinsertion in first pregnancy interval only.

though 90 per cent of couples use contraception, one-third of women admit that they have already had at least one unwanted child – even though at the time of the analysis the women in the sample had not yet reached the end of the fertile period of their lives. Potter[77] has spelt out the limitations of one-method family planning programmes using, in particular, the example of IUD use in Taiwan (Table 45).

The fact must be faced that with currently available methods of contraception communities can only control fertility to within the goals now set by a combination of abortion and contraception. The abortions may be legal or illegal, according to the attitude of the community. While thinking people may disagree upon the rate with which the nations of the world should approach zero population growth, there is a consensus of opinion that birth rates should be encouraged to fall. To deny the necessity for abortion in the control of fertility would be to advocate a *rise* in birth rates in both rich and poor countries.

Morbidity and mortality of fertility regulation

The options open to a couple planning a small- to medium-sized family are the prolonged use of oral contraceptives (or an IUD) with relatively few abortions, the use of less effective reversible methods combined with relatively many abortions, sterilisation soon after achieving the desired family size, or some combination of these. Each possibility has its merits and in a large community it is likely that all three will be used separately and often in sequence.

Each combination presents a small but measurable risk to life and health. Oral contraceptives, IUDs, and possibly even the practice of the rhythm method (p. 50), present risks to the women who use them. Sterilisation (especially of the woman) and abortion involve the dangers of any form of surgery. Simple reversible methods of contraception such as spermicides, condoms, the diaphragm and the use of *coitus interruptus* are without measurable mortality or morbidity but are less effective than the use of Pills or IUDs. All the risks involved are small and often difficult to measure. It seems reasonable to allow the risks associated with unplanned pregnancy to be an item in the arithmetic of mortality and morbidity associated with the control of human fertility.

Taking all these factors into account it is possible to set methods of fertility control in a ranking order of safety from the point of view of the couple using the method, although it would be misleading to press for the calculation of the risks in too great detail. Potts & Swyer attempted to lay out this perspective in 1970.[78,79] Tietze and his colleagues have recently set out the problem in more detail.[80] Part of the argument involves guesses about uncontrolled human fertility and judgements about the likely spacing of planned pregnancies. Some of the variables have changed significantly, even in the past five years. The risks of childbirth have continued to fall in developed countries. New information has been obtained on Pill and IUD risks, which has led to an upward revision of risks (especially among Pill users over the age of 40), while abortion induced early in pregnancy has proved even safer than was foreseen. It should also be noted that study of Pill risks and benefits is far from complete. Additional adverse effects may be discovered. Equally beneficial effects, which of their nature are more difficult to measure than adverse ones, may offset some or all of the harmful effects. In particular the effect of the Pill on breast disease (more common than thrombosis) is only beginning to emerge. So far it appears to be beneficial and the possibility of preventing some breast diseases with exogenous hormones is of great potential importance. But in contrast to the explicably, but unjustifiably, stormy history of understanding of the Pill and IUD, knowledge of abortion, because it is a surgical procedure with little potential for unpredictable long-term effects, is much more complete and secure.

In general a number of important conclusions are possible. First, in Western countries the risk associated with the use of oral contraceptives or IUDs is of the same order of magnitude as the

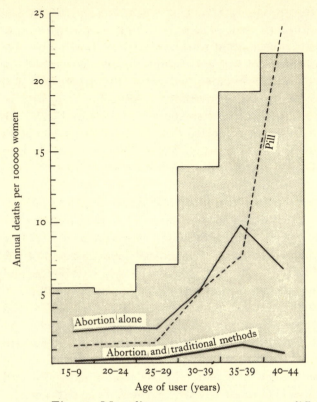

Fig. 53. Mortality rates consequent upon differing methods of fertility control compared. Total death rate resulting from pregnancy due to contraceptive non-use is shaded.

mortality due to the unplanned pregnancies likely to occur in the same unit interval of time as a result of the use of simpler but less effective methods, and both options are safer than repeated unwanted pregnancy (Fig. 53). The only apparent exception to this statement involves women over 40 on the Pill.

Secondly, repeated early legal abortion presents a comparable risk to life as the use of contraceptives. Indeed, for the older woman, where fertility is declining, the risk of death due to fertility and its control is less if the woman throws away her contraceptive Pills and relies on abortion when pregnancy occurs. Of course, in real life, the individual has a great many other factors to consider as well and the risk of death is so slight that it can be reasonably outweighed by aesthetic and convenience factors.

Thirdly, the use of legal abortion to deal with failures associated with the use of conventional methods of contraception, such as the condom, diaphragm and probably the use of *coitus interruptus*, is an order of magnitude safer than any other available choice. This time the differential between this and other options is such that it becomes necessary to consider it in counselling the individual couple and in planning nationwide family planning programmes.

Surgical sterilisation is nearly always a reasonable option. For the young couple who have achieved their desired family size, tubal sterilisation presents less overall risk to life than any contraceptive alternative in terms of mortality. The older woman may well risk her life less if she accepts repeated early legal abortion rather than a tubal ligation. Vasectomy, under local anaesthetic should be virtually without mortality and is always a clinically sound choice.

Therefore, just as abortion is an essential element in any consideration of the sociology of family planning practices, so it has proved to be an inescapable element in the clinical evaluation of birth control practices. And in both situations its inclusion is as creative as it is necessary. Family planning is immeasurably improved by including early legal abortion. It is more than a 'second best' or 'back up' or a 'long stop'. It is a crucial factor in most aspects of realistic family planning.

New options in family planning

Contraceptive development has sought a high degree of predictability in the prevention of pregnancy. But in biological terms, a method or device that is very effective as a contraceptive is also likely to produce tiresome side effects: a large IUD has a low pregnancy rate but produces a lot of bleeding; the combined oral contraceptive is virtually 100 per cent effective, partly because it has widespread systemic actions, blocking reproductive processes at several points and opening up the possibility of a range of side effects.

If, instead of contraceptives being regarded as taps that turn fertility on and off, they are seen as mechanisms to space out pregnancies (which in biological terms they are) and if they are used in conjunction with abortion (which in sociological terms they are already), then new and creative possibilities arise. Design can now concentrate on reducing side effects, even at the expense of some rise in the failure rate.

A method that gives priority to reducing a few of the existing side effects, rather than pregnancy rate, could lead to a greater degree of acceptability and therefore, in the long run, to fewer unwanted pregnancies. There are important consequences for ethics as well as for community health in the possibility that the total number of unwanted pregnancies and the total number of abortions (legal or illegal) might be reduced by openly guaranteeing legal abortions for contraceptive failures. The sticking point for the medical profession and family planning administrators has been to give the assurance that the unplanned pregnancy would be terminated.

Another constructive interaction between abortion and contraception could be in the field of contraceptive development. Oral contraceptives were first marketed in the USA in 1957, initially with 10 mg and later with 5 mg of progestational agent and a high oestrogen content. The dosages of both hormones were lowered subsequently and in 1969–70 the Committe for the Safety of Drugs in the UK recommended that Pills with 50μ g of oestrogen should be used when possible. Such an evolution of a pharmacological agent is the mirror image of normal development, where the principle has been to start with a low dose of the compound concerned and raise it until the desired end-point is achieved. In the case of contraception, because it was unacceptable to offer therapeutic abortion to women in trials of new agents, a high dose was slowly lowered as the years went by. Women died unnecessarily as a result of side effects and the method itself acquired an unjustifiably unpopular image. It is to be hoped that in the development of new forms of contraception rational thinking will prevail and those women who volunteer for trials will be offered termination, if they wish, when an experimental method fails.

However, the single most important consequence of developing a rational link between abortion and contraception would not be in public health or contraceptive development, but in the field of human behaviour.

Abortion as a turning point in contraceptive practice

It has been argued above that abortion is particularly common as a group, or an individual, first adopts artificial restraints on fertility and that the pressures that can push a couple towards or away from either contraception or abortion may be apparently quite trivial. In other words, abortion is most common when patterns of choice are most labile. If these hypotheses are correct, it might follow that the time of an abortion could be a turning point in patterns of fertility regulation.

Data on contraceptive use before and after an abortion are available from a number of localities, for both legal and illegal operations. Bernard, of the International Fertility Research Program, has developed the 'Christmas tree' device to show the extent of use before and after abortion (Fig. 55, p. 527). The trend is always in the same direction: overall contraceptive use improves and couples switch to more effective methods.[81] Experience is consistent whether it comes from centres where programmes of post-abortal contraceptive advice were being run or from situations where no special inputs had been engineered, although uptake is usually less. The profile of methods adopted may represent the opinions of the providers of service as much as the wishes of the users, but always there is a significant drop in the non-use of contraceptives.

The availability of abortion on request can increase the credibility of contraceptive methods for many users. As has been pointed out, those who use contraceptives are more likely than those who do not to resort to induced abortion; so also those who have abortions prove ready acceptors of contraception and have above-average continuation rates.

Few illegal abortionists provide adequate contraceptive advice. The most straightforward way to ensure such advice is given is for those interested in family planning to have the freedom to provide both the abortion service and the contraceptive service. It is a catchphrase of Preterm Inc., Washington D.C. that no woman should leave the clinic 'without a packet of pills in her hand or an IUD in her uterus'.

The Pill is best started on the day of operation.[82] Extensive clinical experience has been gained with IUD insertion after legal abortion,[82-86] and it has been demonstrated that use does not complicate recovery. Women with incomplete abortions often have uterine infections and for a long time there was an understandable reluctance to insert a foreign body into the uterus at the time of hospital curettage after illegal abortion. The studies of Goldsmith and his co-workers in Chile on the topic are remarkable for their importance and their clarity.[87,88] At the Felix Bulnes Hospital, Santiago, 584 women who chose to have an IUD inserted at the time of operation were randomly assigned to two groups. One group had Lippes loops inserted immediately, the other none. All were told to return in one month for a check and those who had not received the device had one inserted on this second visit. The allotment was double-blind so that the doctor assessing the woman's progress after the curettage and the doctor at the follow-up clinic did not know which women had devices *in situ*. No statistically significant difference was found between the two groups for any parameter concerned with intrauterine infection or other post-operative complication. Whereas only 20 per cent of women had returned to a follow-up clinic for an IUD insertion when the procedure was delayed, 80 per cent accepted the method when offered at the same time as operation. The surgeon also found insertion easy. IUD insertion at the time of curettage for incomplete abortion has been demonstrated to be equally successful in places as diverse as Uganda, Chile and Tunisia, and it is to be hoped that it will spread rapidly. In several places (see, for example, Ben Cheikh's work in Tunisia) it has been found that IUDs inserted post-abortion have a better continuation rate than those used in non-pregnant women.[89,90]

A great deal can also be done to extend contraceptive advice to women who have illegal abortions. Those women who are admitted to hospital with complications are usually pushed into the oldest and most overcrowded wards and discharged as rapidly as possible. The combination of outpatient vacuum aspiration[91] (often without any anaesthetic – because the cervix is usually partly open) and immediate IUD insertion is an attractive one to busy physicians and of immediate benefit to the many women. The International Planned Parenthood Federation Governing Body encouraged such care in 1972 when it unanimously passed a resolution urging member associations, 'In those countries in which abortion is illegal, to seek, where appropriate, to bring their influence to bear towards ensuring that adequate and socially humane services are available to treat incomplete abortions and other complications (of induced abortion) and that such services be linked with the provision of contraceptive services.'[92]

Abortion and family planning programmes

The best-informed global guess concerning the cost of fertility control was made by Robbins in 1973.[93] He estimated that for 1971 the world spent $3000 million. Half ($1485 million) went into abortion costs and half ($1545 million) into contraceptive programmes. The abortion costs were met partly from government funds (estimated world total $622 million) and partly through unorganised, commonly illegal, fees for service facilities. Seventy-three per cent of estimated abortion expenditure took place in developed countries.

An analysis of costs, however inaccurate, gives a picture of reality which is very different from the perceptions of most nations and often totally at variance with the political and cultural façade hiding abortion and contraceptive activity. Robbins estimated that the USSR spent $525 million on legal abortion services (35 per cent of the world total) and Latin America $140 million in unorganised illegal services. The estimate did not include the cost to the state of treating the consequences of illegal abortions admitted to hospital.

The starting point for any discussion, therefore, must be that abortion already consumes half the resources that the world devotes to fertility regulation. Is this the most responsible use of money? Would an alteration in the balance of contraception and abortion lead to a more cost effective use of resources? Can abortion services be made cheaper?

Some contraceptive programmes have been devised with the goal of cutting abortion rates. Such an undertaking seems possible but difficult and expensive.

The San Gregorio programme in Santiago is an example of a successful initiative.[94] San Gregorio is a working-class area of the city and has a centrally placed clinic within walking distance of all the dwellings. The family planning effort concentrated on women who had already had an abortion, wisely exploiting the proven desire to control fertility. One aspect of the programme was to place 'great emphasis...on the physical risks run by a woman who has an induced abortion, even mentioning the possibility of death'. Two random sample surveys, each of over 1250 women, were conducted in 1965 and 1967 to gauge the success of the contraceptive programme.[95] A 19.4 per cent decline in total fertility rate and a 39.4 per cent decline in the reported abortion rate ('spontaneous' and induced) occurred and the abortion:delivery ratio altered from 1:2 to 1:3. The age distribution of these changes show that the main decline in the age-specific fertility rate took place in the 30–39 age group while the abortion rate fell particularly in the 25–29 age group, possibly reflecting the situation where a rapidly changing community, eager to control its fertility and doing so at an increasingly earlier age, was suddenly and successfully offered above-average access to contraceptive services.

Unfortunately the San Gregorio area is an exception when compared with Santiago as a whole. Over the same years Monreal[95] found a significant increase in the abortion rate in other areas of the city between 1962 and 1966. In the lowest socio-economic groups fertility fell by 33 per cent, but the induced-abortion rate rose by 67.9 per cent. There appears to be a critical point in the provision of contraceptive services, above which they are associated with a fall in deliveries and induced abortions and below which they are associated with a fall in deliveries but a rise in induced abortions. In the San Gregorio area an estimated 16 per cent of women received contraceptive advice and the abortion rate fell, elsewhere the number of women protected was 8–10 per cent and the number of induced abortions rose.

The same trend can be discerned in a family planning programme in Japan in the 1950s, although the economic advancement of the country helped shift the balance of use towards contraceptive practive. Even so, Omran[96] represents some of Koya's data from Japan to good effect. Koya himself wrote, 'The decrease in induced abortions was not easily achieved. . . It was not until the fourth year of the program that the rate was brought down below the pre-guidance (family planning program) level and it took five years to achieve any really gratifying results.' (Korea, also, provides a similar example.)

In one study area, subjected to a great deal of education and the provision of simple contraceptive methods (from tablets, diaphragms, condoms and information on rhythm and withdrawal) the marital fertility fell by 38 per cent in two years (1963–64), while in a second area (which was merely exposed to the routine government programme) the marital fertility rate fell by only 13 per cent.[97] The relatively brief duration of the study tended to obscure the role of induced abortion, but the main reason for the lower fertility in the area, with the intense family planning inputs, appears to have been a better use of contraceptives rather than a more extensive use of abortion, or abortion plus contraception. The interval between the birth of the last child and the time of the interview was greater in those who used contraception and abortion (34.5 to 43.2 months) than in those who used contraception alone (27.1 to 27.3 months).

Unfortunately, the scale of the input necessary to achieve this result (one part-time physician and four nurse midwives for an estimated 1400 eligible couples) is more than could be supported nationwide. Nationwide, only 14 per cent of women visited a health centre in the years 1969–71.[98] In Korea 68 per cent of deliveries are attended by a relative, 11 per cent by a midwife, and only 5 per cent by a doctor. In 1964 the ratio of population to doctors was 1:2900 and the selected townships probably used more in money and skills for family planning than was available on average *for all* aspects of curative and preventive medicine. Even the control village, with the low family planning input, was more fortunate than the rural areas of most developing countries in the scale of its contraceptive services.

To use the example of another well-studied country, the national programme in Taiwan has cost about $8 per birth averted, and although this is a good investment for the money spent, it is unlikely that other, less prosperous, nations will achieve the scale of national programme to which Taiwan has been subjected. For example the *total* health budget *per capita* of many Asian and certain Latin-American countries is $1–$5. It must be recognised that the expense of teaching and services necessary to get from poor to good contraceptive use in one step, short-circuiting the problem of frequent abortion, is beyond attainment to a great many areas of moderate or high fertility. Therefore, the role of abortion in the demographic changes now occurring, or hoped for, in many developing countries seems likely to remain an important one and it would be deceptive to overlook it.

If it is accepted that the initiation of contraceptive usage is associated with increased resort to abortion, while later (as the success of contraceptive usage improves) there is a decline in induced abortion rates, then family planning programmes designed to raise contraceptive usage must also be expected to alter induced abortion rates. For example, when the Population Council instituted a post-partum contraceptive programme in 25 hospitals around the world, it discovered that 'The total number of abortion admissions during the operational months of the programme decreased by 26 per cent in the USA hospitals and by 12 per cent in the non-USA hospitals as compared with the twelve month period preceding this programme.'[99] Presumably the women responding to the contraceptive programme in the USA belonged to groups more than ready to accept contraceptive advice, while those in the other countries were less advanced in their fertility control patterns and the reduction in abortion rates was correspondingly less.

Conclusions

Sociological observation suggests that contraception and induced abortion are used to complement one another in the difficult task of controlling human fertility. Given a reasonable availability of contraceptives, there is no evidence that induced abortion and contraceptive practice compete. It appears unlikely that women become pregnant in order to have abortions, but it appears to be common practice that women will resort to abortion (whether legal or illegal) if the contraceptive method they are using fails. It seems that women who practise pre-conceptive methods of birth control are more likely to use post-conceptive methods if these let them down and, at the same time, those who use post-conceptive methods of family planning are also more likely to accept pre-conceptive methods when available; the two propositions are in no way logically exclusive.

Abortion and contraception are inextricably intertwined in their use. As the idea of family limitation spreads through a community there appears to be a rise in the incidence of induced abortion at the point where the community begins to initiate the use of contraceptives. There is evidence that abortion rates, as well as the use of contraceptives, are increasing in many developing countries. It may be predicted that in many places the rate may rise further before it falls. In developed countries, with the passage of time, the abortion rate has fallen in situations where contraceptive methods are known and available. Organised family planning services have an important contribution to make in accelerating the switch from induced abortion to contraceptive practice but two limitations have to be recognised. First, the reversible methods of contraception at present available are not sufficiently predictable, even when well and consistently used, to control fertility over a lifetime and meet the goals of family size set in modern industrialised nations, and therefore in the foreseeable future the resort to abortion cannot be eliminated. Secondly, the input necessary into a family planning service in order to achieve an immediate decline in birth rates from the high level found in developing countries, without any transitory rise in the abortion rate, is very much larger than has been contemplated in any national family planning programme. It may well represent a use of health resources which it would be difficult to justify if the overall needs of the community for health care are reviewed objectively.[100]

Abortion and contraception are also closely inter-related in their clinical consequences. In the total pattern of fertility control the use of induced abortion either alone or in combination with contraceptive methods produces profoundly different results. In certain circumstances, the combination of certain methods of contraception with legal abortion when failures occur can provide a safer option than any other pattern of fertility control. However, the non-quantifiable drawbacks of abortion commonly modify any considerations based purely on maternal mortality statistics.

These important inter-relationships between contraception and induced abortion are not widely recognised. Marie Stopes' reaction was noted at the beginning of this chapter. She began her influential book *Birth Control Today*,[101] 'This book deals with the *control* of conception solely. It does not discuss the destruction of the embryo after it has been formed, that is *abortion*, legally and physiologically quite a different process.' Stopes says she 'will not stop to scold her [*the woman who seeks an abortion*], for probably she will not trouble to read this, but she is a danger to the human race'. Semantically, Stopes was correct, practically she was wrong. History forced the early family planners to overemphasise the distinction between contraception and abortion. Unfortunately, the words preached by the birth control rebels of the 1930s have become the gospel of the establishment in the 60s and 70s. In 1971 the British Minister of Health and Social Security firmly rejected any notion that legal abortion might play a role in the two pilot family planning projects financed by the government.

The conflict between the clinical, sociological and economic facts of abortion, and the mythology with which it has been invested in the minds of most decision-makers, has had a crippling effect on family planning programmes. The malady is particularly difficult to cure because it has been partly invested by those interested in family planning. Each method of fertility control and each service programme has a particular political profile and therefore some methods and services have gained public respectability before others. In an attempt to further family planning, the more bland methods have been artificially separated and insulated from the most controversial – the trick that Marie Stopes was playing unconsciously. A moment's thought will show that some of the least effective programmes and methods are politically the most acceptable. For example, clinic-based contraceptive availability preceded community-based distribution, and maternal and child health-related programmes are easier to launch than, say, the social marketing of condoms. And abortion, which is almost universally acceptable, highly effective in meeting individual fertility goals, well understood scientifically and relatively easy for the community to provide, is proving the last method to surface in national and international family planning programmes.[102]

Predictably, the inter-governmental agencies, such as the United Nations Fund for Population Activities and the World Health Organisation are in an especially weak position to promote abortion services, although they command many of the available resources. The World Bank has a greater potential for action in the abortion service field but cannot move faster than recipient governments. Therefore, a particular responsibility falls on the non-governmental agencies; the Population Council and especially the International Planned Parenthood Federation. Fortunately, the resources needed to extend realistic abortion services into the poor, or at least into the urban, slums of the world are modest. Beyond, these large bodies, with their varying patterns of inbuilt restraints, are smaller active agencies such as The Pathfinder Fund, International Pregnancy Advisory Service and Population Services International.

Yet the epidemiological evidence that has been surveyed in this and preceding chapters points to the fact that induced abortion services are most needed by those adopting any form of fertility regulation. Abortion is the horse that pulls contraceptive practice into the community. If abortion is faced squarely, then contraceptive services fall into their right place. When abortion is omitted, then family planning programmes often lose direction. Money and man-power tend to go into so-called 'motivation' and policy makers attempt to obfuscate problems of service by talking of 'integrated' programmes. Unhappily, the lack of sensible abortion services in most national family planning programmes is a particular disservice to the most poor and underpriviledged in society.

In summary, an understanding of the advantages of abortion in fertility control, together with an appreciation of its political drawbacks, is essential if the public health and demographic problems related to family planning in the developing world are to be solved more rapidly and humanely than they were in the industrialised nations at a comparable stage in the demographic transition. It is a grave mistake to think of family planning programmes as just another form of development, like the building of a road or the introduction of a new strain of rice. In family planning, political constraints have forced the choice of the most uphill route clinically and the use of the lowest-yield programmes.

References

1 Pearl, R. (1939). *Natural History of Population*. Oxford University Press, Oxford.
2 Glass, D. V. (1940). *Population Policies and Movements in Europe*. Clarendon Press, Oxford.
3 Beebe, G. W. (1942). *Contraception and Fertility in the Southern Appalachians*. Williams & Wilkins, Baltimore.
4 Young, P. R. (1971). *Impact of Population Growth on Korean Economy*. Korean Institute for Family Planning, Seoul.
5 Ross, J. (1968). 'Women-years of use, cost of effectiveness and births prevented by the Korean National Programme.' Unpublished paper quoted by Berelson, B. (1970). *Studies in Family Planning*, May.
6 Hi Sup Chang (1969). *The Korean Family Planning Programme Achievements, Problems and Prospects*. Seoul.
7 Hong, S. B. (1966). *Induced Abortion in Seoul, Korea*. Dong-A Publishing Co., Seoul.
8 Ministry of Health and Social Affairs, Republic of Korea (1969). *Findings of the National Survey on Family Planning*, Seoul.
9 Hong, S. B. (1967). Induced abortion in rural Korea. *Korean Journal of Obstetrics and Gynaecology*, **10**, 275.
10 Hong, S. B. (1971). *Changing Patterns of Induced Abortion in Seoul, Korea*. Seoul.
11 Kap Suk Koh & Smith, D. P. (1970). *The Korean 1968 Fertility and Family Planning Survey*. Korean Institute for Family Planning, Seoul.
12 Smith, D. P. & Watson, W. B. (1972). 'Determination of targets for the Korean family planning program.' IPPF, London. (Duplicated document.)
13 Hong, S. B. & Watson, W. B. (1972). The role of induced abortion in fertility control in Korea. *Clinical Proceedings of IPPF SEOR Medical and Scientific Congress*. Australian and New Zealand Journal of Obstetrics and Gynaecology, p. 115.
14 Watson, W. B. (1971). Demographic problems confronting Korea's family planning program. In *The Proceedings of the National Family Planning Evaluation Seminar*, p. 138. Korean Institute for Family Planning, Seoul.
15 Freedman, R., Hermalin, A. & Sun, T. H. (1972). Fertility trends in Taiwan. *Population Index*, **38**, 141.
16 Chow, L. P. (1970). Family planning in Taiwan, Republic of China. Progress and prospects. *Population Studies, London*, **24**, 339.
17 Cernada, G. P. (ed.) (1970). *Taiwan Family Planning Reader*. The

Chinese Center for International Training in Family Planning, Taichung.

18 Chow, L. P., Huang, T. T. & Chang, M. C. (1968). 'Induced abortion in Taiwan, Republic of China.' IPPF, London. (Duplicated document.)

19 Sun, T. H. (1970). 'Induced abortion in Taiwan.' Ecumenical conference on abortion in Taiwan. IPPF, London. (Duplicated document.)

20 Lapham, R. J. (1970). Family planning and fertility in Tunisia. *Demography*, **7**.

21 Vallin, J. (1971). Limitation des naissances en Tunisie. *Population*, **26**, 181.

22 Kamal, I., Ghoneim, M., Tallat, M., Abdallah Eid, M. & Hamamsy, L. S. (1972). An attempt at estimating the magnitude and probable incidence of induced abortion in the UAR. In *Induced Abortion: A Hazard to Public Health?*, ed. I. R. Nazer, p. 130. IPPF, Beirut.

23 Özbay, F. & Shorter, F. C. (1970). Turkey: changes in birth control practices, 1963–1968. *Studies in Family Planning*, no. **51**, 1.

24 Fisek, N. H. (1972). Epidemiological study on abortion in Turkey. In *Induced Abortion: A Hazard to Public Health?*, ed. I. R. Nazer, p. 264. IPPF, Beirut.

25 Anard, D. (1965). Clinico-epidemiological study of abortion. *Indian Journal of Public Health*, **9**, 52.

26 Jubiz, A., Ochoa, G., Posalda, H., Morales, A., Espinosa, F. & Vergara, J. E. (1972). Aborto hospitalario. *Antioquia medica*, **22**, 35.

27 *Reportes de los Departamentos de Salud Pública y Medicina Social, Universidad de Chile, Facultad de Medicina* (1969).

28 Rosenfield, A. G. & Aree Somboonsuk (1971). 'An urban family planning centre.' IPPF, London. (Duplicated document.)

29 Suporn Koetsawang (1972). Personal communication.

30 Potts, M. (1972). Models for progress. In *New Concepts in Contraception*, ed. M. Potts & C. Wood, p. 213. Medical & Technical Publishing Co., Oxford & Lancaster.

31 Parish, T. N. (1935). A thousand cases of abortion. *Journal of Obstetrics and Gynaecology of the British Empire*, **42**, 1107.

32 Gebhard, P. H., Pomeroy, W. B., Martin, C. E. & Christenson, C. V. (1959). *Pregnancy, Birth and Abortion*. Heinemann, London.

33 Lindquist, E. (1931). Abortion in Malmo 1897 to 1927. *Acta Obstetricia et Gynaecologica Scandanavica*, **12**, Suppl. 1, 1.

34 Latzko, A. (1924). Quoted in Glass (1940); see note 2.

35 Peller, S. (1930). Quoted in Glass (1940); see note 2.

36 Taussig, F. J. (1936). *Abortion, Spontaneous and Induced: Medical and Social Aspects*. Kimpton, London.

37 Millar, W. M. (1931). Human abortion. *Human Biology*, **6**, 271.

38 Worral, R. (1933). Abortion. *Medical Journal of Australia*, **2**, 739.

39 Braestrup, A. (1971). Use of contraception by young mothers in Copenhagen. *Journal of Biosocial Science*, **3**, 43.

40 Henry, L. (1961). Some data on natural fertility. *Eugenics Quarterly*, **2**, 81.

41 Muramatsu, M. (1970). An analysis of factors in fertility control in Japan. *Bulletin of the Institute of Public Health, Tokyo*, **19**, 97.

42 Muramatsu, M. (1971). The abortion programme in Japan. Editorial. *Journal of Reproductive Medicine*, **7**(1), 30.

43 Figa-Talamanca, R. (1970). The relationship of contraception to abortion in Japan. *Genus*, **26**, 237.

44 Szabady, E. (1971). The legalizing of contraceptives and abortions. *Impact of Science on Society*, UNESCO, Paris, **21**, 265.

45 Szabady, E., Klinger, A. & Acsadi, G. (1966). The Hungarian fertility and family planning study of 1965–66. In *Preventive Medicine and Family Planning*, Proceedings of Fifth Conference of the Europe and Near East Region of the IPPF, p. 265. IPPF London.

46 Haberlandt, L. (1921). Über hormonale Sterilisierung des weiblichen Tierkörpers. *Münchener Medizinische Wochenschrift*, **68**, 1577.

47 Requena, M. B. (1969). 'The problem of induced abortion in Latin America.' IPPF, London. (Duplicated document.)

48 Monreal, T. (1976). 'Determinant factors affecting illegal abortion trends in Chile.' Pathfinder Conference, New Developments in Fertility Regulation. (Duplicated document.)

49 Muramatsu, M. (1970). Personal communication.

50 Valentei, D., Arab-Ogly, E. & Briev, B. (1967). *Narodonasselenye i ekonomika*, Moscow.

51 Sadvokasova, E. A. (1963). Nekotorye sotsial no-gigienicheskie aspekty izucheniya aborta. *Sovetskoe Zdravookhranenie*, **22**(3).

52 David, H. P. (1970). *Family Planning and Abortion in the Socialist Countries of Central and Eastern Europe*. Population Council, New York.

52 Mehlan, K.-H. (1970). Abortion in Eastern Europe. In *Abortion in a Changing World*, vol. **1**, ed R. E. Hall, p. 302. Columbia University Press, New York.

54 Tietze, C. (1969). 'Legal abortion in industrialised countries.' International Family Planning Conference, Dacca. (Duplicated document.)

55 Gheorghui, N. N., Coteata, V.-N. & Topa-Tudose, E. (1963). Observations on immediate and late complications in legal abortion at the Filantropia Hospital. *Obstetrica şi Ginecologia Buchuresti*, **3**, 229.

56 Yaukey, D. (1961). *Fertility Differences in a Modernizing Country*. Princeton University Press, Princeton, N.J.

57 Requena, M. (1970). Abortion in Latin America. In *Abortion in a Changing World*, ed. R. E. Hall, vol. **1**, p. 338. Columbia University Press, New York.

58 Peller, S. (1929). Statistics on abortion. *Zentralblatt für Gynäkologie*, **53**, 861, 2216.

59 Sun, T. H. (1973). 'The impact on fertility of Taiwan's family planning program.' IPPF, London. (Duplicated document.)

60 Jaramillo-Gomez, M. & Londono, J. B. (1968). Rhythm: a hazardous contraceptive method. *Demography*, **5**, 433.

61 Hutchinson, B. (1964). Induced abortion in Brazilian married women. *America Latina*, **7**, 21.

62 Janmejai, K. (1963). Socio-economic aspects of abortion. *Family Planning News, India*, **4**, 55.

63 Wagatsuma, T. (1971). The abortion program in Japan. *Journal of Reproductive Medicine*, **7**(1), 30.

64 Agarwala, S. N. (1962). Abortion rate among a section of Delhi's population. *Bombay Medical Digest*, **30**, no. 1.

65 Fisek, N. H. (1972). Epidemiological study of abortion in Turkey. In *Induced Abortion: A Hazard to Public Health?*, ed. I. R. Nazer, p. 264. IPPF, Beirut.

66 British Pregnancy Advisory Service (1973). *Client Statistics for 1971 with Commentary*. BPAS, Birmingham.

67 Pare, C. B. & Raven, H. (1970). Follow-up of patients referred for termination of pregnancy. *Lancet*, **i**, 635.

68 Obeng, B. (1967). 500 consecutive cases of abortion. Ph.D. thesis, University of London.

69 Bracken, M. B., Grossman, G. & Hachamovitch, M. (1973). Contraceptive practice amongst New York abortion patients. *American Journal of Obstetrics and Gynecology*, **114**, 967.

70 Diamond, M., Steinhoff, P. G., Palmore, P. A. & Smith, R. C. (1973). Sexuality, birth control and abortion: a decision making sequence. *Journal of Biosocial Science*, **5**, 347.

71 Kaper-Stanulovic, N. & Friedman, H. L. (1974). 'Abortion and contraception in Novi Sad, Yugoslavia: determinants of choice.' IPPF, London. (Duplicated document.)

72 Westoff, C. F., Potter, R. G. & Sage, P. C. (1963). *The Third Child*. Princeton University Press, Princeton, N.J.

73 Hulka, J. (1969). A mathematical model study of contraceptive efficiency and unplanned pregnancies. *American Journal of Obstetrics and Gynecology*, **104**, 443.

74 Tietze, C. (1974). The 'problem' of repeat abortions. *Family Planning Perspectives*, **6**, 148.

75 Daily, E. F., Nicholas, N., Nelson, F. & Pakter, K. (1973). Repeat abortions in New York City, 1970–1972. *Family Planning Perspectives*, **5**, 89.

76 Westoff, C. F. & Ryder, M. B. (1969). Family limitation in the United States. *International Population Conference*, vol. **2**, p. 1301. IUSSP, London.

77 Potter, R. G. (1971). Inadequacy of a one-method family-planning program. *Social Biology*, **18**, 1.

78 Potts, D. M. & Swyer, G. I. M. (1970). Effectiveness and risks of birth-control methods. *British Medical Bulletin*, **26**, 26.

79 Potts, D. M. (1971). The effectiveness and risks of birth-control methods. *British Medical Abstracts*, March, 5.

80 Tietze, C. (1969). Mortality with contraception and induced abortion. *Studies in Family Planning*, no. **45**, 6.

81 Tietze, C., Bongaarts, J. & Schearer, B. (1976). Mortality associated with the control of fertility. *Family Planning Perspectives*, **8**, 6.

82 Goldsmith, A., Edelman, D. A. & Brenner, W. E. (1974). 'Contraception immediately after abortion.' IFRP paper presented at twelfth annual meeting of the American Association of Planned Parenthood Physicians. (Duplicated document.)

83 Andolšek, L. (1967). Insertion of IUDs after abortion – preliminary report. In *Proceedings of the 8th IPPF Conference, Chile*, p. 285. IPPF, London.

84 Andolšek, L. (1972). Experience with immediate post-abortion insertions of the IUD. In *Family Planning Research Conference*, ed. A. Goldsmith & R. Snowden, p. 55. Excerpta Medica, Amsterdam.

85 Nygren, K.-G. & Johansson, E. D. B. (1973). Insertion of the endouterine Copper-T (TCn 200) immediately after first trimester legal abortion. *Contraception*, **7**, 299.

86 Hue, K., Kwon, H. Y., Michael, P. H. & Watson, W. B. (1974). A comparative study of the safety and efficiency of postabortal intrauterine contraceptive device insertion. *American Journal of Obstetrics and Gynecology*, **118**, 975.

87 Goldsmith, A., Goldberg, R., Eyzaguirre, M. & Lizana, L. (1972). IUD insertion immediately after incomplete abortion. *IPPF Medical Bulletin*, **6**(2), 1.

88 Goldsmith, A., Goldberg, R., Eyzaguirre, H., Lucero, S. & Lizana, L. (1972). IUD insertion in the immediate postabortal period. In *Family Planning Research Conference*, ed. A. Goldsmith & R. Snowden, p. 59. Excerpta Medica, Amsterdam.

89 Ben Cheikh, T. B. (1970). 'Comparative study of 1,000 cases of IUD insertions immediately after abortion with 1,000 cases of IUD insertions under normal conditions'. 3rd Seminar on Family Planning. IPPF, London. (Duplicated document.)

90 Ben Cheikh, T. B. (1970). Étude comparative de 1000 cas d'insertion de sterilet dans le post-abortum immediate et de 1000 cas d'insertion de sterilet dans les conditions normales. *Journal des Études Medicales sur le planning familial*, **3**, 50.

91 Peterson, W. F. (1974). Contraceptive therapy following therapeutic abortion. *Obstetrics and Gynecology, NY*, **44**, 853.

92 Kleinman, R. L. (ed.) (1972). *Induced Abortion*, IPPF, London.

93 Robbins, K. (1973). 'Estimated total cost of fertility control.' IPPF International Conference on Unmet Needs in Family Planning, Brighton. (Duplicated document.)

94 Faundes, A., Rodriguez-Galant, G. & Avendano, O. (1968). The San Gregorio experimental family planning program: changes observed in fertility and abortion rates. *Demography*, **5**, 836.

95 Monreal, T. & Armijo, R. (1968). Evaluation of the programme for the prevention of induced abortion and for family planning in the City of Santiago. *Revista Médica de Chile*, **96**, 605.

96 Omran, A. R. (1972). Epidemiological and sociological aspects of abortion. In *Induced Abortion: A Hazard to Public Health?*, ed. I. R. Nazer, p. 20. IPPF, Beirut.

97 Koya, Y. (1962). Why induced abortions in Japan remain high. In *Research in Family Planning*, ed. C. V. Kiser, p. 103. Princeton University Press, Princeton, New Jersey.

98 Sook Bang (1968). Comparative study of the effectiveness of a family planning program in rural Korea. Ph.D. thesis, University of Michigan.

99 Watson, W. B. (1971). Demographic problems confronting Korea's Family Planning Program. In *Proceedings of the National Family Planning Evaluation Seminar*, p. 117. Korean Institute of Family Planning, Seoul.

100 Berelson, B. (1964). National family planning programmes: a guide. *Studies in Family Planning*. Population Council, New York.

101 Stopes, M. (1934). *Birth Control Today*, 12th edn, reprinted 1971.

102 Potts, M. (1976). The implementation of family planning programmes. In *Contraceptives of the Future*, ed. R. V. Short and D. T. Baird, Proceedings of the Royal Society, London, *B*, **195**, 213.

14

The unwanted pregnancy

Part of the controversy surrounding abortion stems from assumptions made about children who are unwanted by one or both parents at conception, birth or during childhood.

Embryos that are deliberately aborted were clearly unwanted to an unacceptable degree, but what of unwanted pregnancies that continue? It is often said that the parents become reconciled to the pregnancy as it progresses yet few serious attempts have been made to evaluate this possibility or the alternative of lingering resentment in one or both parents. An effort is made below to review the data on the scale of the problem of unwanted pregnancy, and on the adverse results, on the quality of family life, of denying abortion. Research in this field usually implies that the choice of abortion is an altruistic one, made because the child, if born, might not enjoy the sort of life most people would wish for it.

But an opposite hypothesis relating abortion to the quality of life is also possible. It can be held that individuals and communities that resort to abortion are showing a degree of selfishness and lack of moral principle, which suggests they are likely to neglect, ill-treat or deprive their children.

Unfortunately there is more speculation than there are firm data in both these areas. Nevertheless the two hypotheses are so far apart that even the limited information available for review may be sufficient to distinguish between them.

Definitions and scale
The subject of unplanned and unwanted pregnancy is easy prey for semantic confusion. Short definitions of 'unwanted' in this

context are always inadequate, yet everyone knows what is meant by the term. Pohlman & Pohlman[1] have discussed 'unwantedness' in relation to time of birth, sex of child and other factors. Usually a planned pregnancy is a wanted pregnancy, but not all unplanned pregnancies are unwanted. Bearing in mind the inefficient contraception methods available to our parents, many of us could, in truth, be described as more or less happy accidents.

Unwanted pregnancies are a world problem. As a starting point, data from England and Wales for the year 1970 will be considered. The size of the problem can be assessed by the study of available statistics, or by retrospective questioning. When national statistics are used, a great deal of simplification is inevitable. Figures are available on the number of legally induced abortions, illegitimate births, premarital conceptions, adoptions and children taken into the care of local authorities for various reasons. It is obvious that there will be other conceptions, pregnancies and children, who are unwanted but never reach these categories, and the problem must necessarily be larger than such data suggest.

Any woman who seeks abortion for other than health or eugenic indications clearly demonstrates that her pregnancy is unwanted. From this point of view, there are three types of abortion that are relevant: namely illegal abortion, therapeutic abortion and unsuccessfully attempted self-abortion. The incidence of induced abortion in various countries has been discussed earlier. In England and Wales only 2.1 per cent of registered legal abortions are categorised by the operating doctor as cases presenting high risk to the mother's life, or involving possible fetal abnormality. The remaining 107000 operations are performed for mixed medico-social reasons, which generally means, in plain language that the pregnancy was unplanned, is unwanted and is resented to such a degree that the woman feels the emotional and physical costs of an abortion to be less than those of continuing pregnancy.

The illegal abortion rate in Britain after the 1967 Act is as difficult to estimate as it was prior to the change in the law. If our figures for criminal abortions are uncertain, we know even less about the number of women who try unsuccessfully to induce an abortion; but the woman who confesses to such an attempt, and who seeks reassurance that her fetus has not been damaged by the drugs that she took, is often met in antenatal clinics. Every year large quantities of drugs are still bought by desperate women in the pathetic belief that they will act as abortifacients, and observations on this trade have been presented earlier.

In 1970 there were 64744 illegitimate babies born in England and Wales. Not every illegitimate baby is an unwanted baby, but in an attempt to assess how many of these illegitimate children were unwanted and whose pregnancies were certainly unplanned, it is relevant to consider that the figure for adoptions in 1969 was 22500 (compared, incidentally, with only 15099 adoptions in 1960 – adoptions on the whole have risen in numbers in recent years). In addition a number of illegitimate children end up in care because their mothers are unable to look after them. In 1969 the number totalled 3302. Overall it may be reasonable to assume that slightly fewer than two-thirds of these illegitimate children resulted from unwanted pregnancies, say 45000 in total.

The Registrar General gives figures of deliveries within seven months of marriage that we can take broadly to be premarital conceptions. The figure for 1970 is 65121. Forced marriages are often far from happy marriages and, statistically, it can be shown that the fate of these forced marriages is significantly worse than the general run of marriages. It is fair to estimate that at least half such premarital conceptions were unwanted and we will assume a figure of 32500 for 1970. Even on these data of illegitimate and premaritally conceived pregnancies, a total of 77500 unwanted pregnancies in the year 1970 seems very likely and during this year there were 784486 total births.

A second method of assessing the problem of the unwanted pregnancy is by retrospective sample questioning. Lewis-Faning[2] in his report to the Royal Commission on Population, found that amongst 1000 women who had been married for 12 years or more, 243 reported at least one unwanted child. Similar studies have been carried out in the USA and it is interesting that Whelpton, Campbell & Patterson[3] have shown that among women married for at least ten years exactly the same proportion, namely 24 per cent, reports a minimum of one unwanted child. These authors have also shown that the incidence of unplanned pregnancy rises with parity and falls with the educational achievements of the mother and with the family income. The desired family size in the USA among poorer social groups is about the same, or sometimes even smaller, than among the most wealthy and better educated. This is equally true of recently married couples in contemporary Britain.[4] Unfortunately excess fertility is more common among the poor because contraception is begun at a relatively later stage in the partnership, and is used less efficiently. In 1968, Frazer & Watson surveyed 1500 women delivered consecutively in the London area.[5] They found that, of their sample, approximately half the deliveries involved unplanned pregnancies and they were able to demonstrate that there was a marked differential in the number of unplanned pregnancies between contraceptive users and non-users. They also compared 933 cases where contraception had been used and then stopped – circumstantial evidence of a wanted conception – with 992 cases where contraception was reported to have failed. The former group admitted to 9.5 per cent and the latter 18 per cent total abortions.

The unwanted child
Child and cruelty

Much has been written about the attitude of doctors, lawyers, theologians and politicians towards abortion. Something is known about the response of pregnant women to the problem, but little thought and study has been devoted to the effect of being an unplanned conception or an unwanted birth upon the subsequent life of the child.

A simple hypothesis can be considered that the child of an unplanned pregnancy may be adversely affected by its parent(s)' conscious or subconscious attitudes towards it. To some 'research to show a correlation between unwanted conception and child abuse may seem like an attempt to document the obvious'.[1] To others the question itself is unacceptable because the use of contraception and abortion, even to avert an evil, cannot be justified. Like the story of Ivan Mighthavebeen – the twelfth-century genius, twelfth child of poor Siberian peasant stock, who would have invented the aeroplane, movable type and the steam engine but for the fact that he was aborted by his mother at 10 weeks – the case of the battered baby who would have been better off aborted than born, has certain philosophical limitations. The problem needs to be posed more carefully.

All communities control their fertility, and abortion is almost invariably one of the methods used. The desire to control fertility is greatest where there are high spots of real or perceived hardship. Changes in communal attitudes such as a suddenly increased acceptance of abortion may, like a seasonal change in the snow line, bring a particular peak of human need into the open, and a woman will have an abortion rather than continue with the pregnancy. What we have to ask is, 'would the child, if born, have been at a particularly high risk of parental neglect or ill-use?' Child cruelty can provide the most dramatic evidence of parental rejection and some of the most powerful evidence of the need for improved birth control. However, as it is such a strongly emotive subject, it is a social testimony that must be viewed with caution. Cruelty is not confined to children who were unwanted at birth, unplanned at conception, or whose mothers may have sought an abortion. Any analysis of possible inter-relationships with abortion must avoid certain pitfalls. If, as is argued elsewhere, one of the major effects of more liberal abortion laws has been to transfer would-be backstreet abortions to the care of doctors, then the potential of liberal abortion legislation to cut down cases of child abuse seems limited. Conversely, one could regard illegal abortion as an important factor without which the child cruelty rate would rise. It is also possible to argue that the group of conceptions aborted under a liberal law, but who might be born under a restrictive law, are particularly at risk as targets of parental rejection. For example, the number of premarital conceptions ending in induced abortion appears to rise whenever the law is liberalised and such conceptions are over-represented among cases of cruelty to children.

Clearly the possibility of abortion may be totally irrelevant in certain cases. One or both parents may simply be manifesting a psychiatric condition which is temporary, or which may have developed after the birth of the child, who then suffers the physical or mental cruelty. A child of a different sex may not have been subject to the ill-treatment. A child may have been the wanted child of one set of parents, but be rejected following the establishment of a fresh union with a step-partner. A child may have been unwanted at conception, but the mother may still not have a sought a termination, however freely available. She may even have accepted the child as a 'punishment'. The child may be labelled 'unwanted' only in retrospect as the parents cast around to avoid guilt at their own behaviour.

A great deal is still unknown concerning patterns of parental cruelty. The condition is not always recognised by the outside world, definition is difficult and the true incidence is unknown. The fact that the child concerned is often unwanted is certainly significant, but, equally, there may be other known and unknown forces at play. Violence to children is most likely where some physical restraints of children are socially acceptable. For example, corporal punishment is found in 50 per cent of American working-class homes,[6] but only in 10 per cent of middle-class homes, and in a series of children who were violently ill-treated, over half came from that 25 per cent of American families whose earnings totalled less than $5000 per year.[7] Those who physically abuse children most frequently have a history of psychiatric disease and, at the time of the abuse may be subject to unusual environmental stress such as unemployment.

The phenomenon that is now universally known as the 'battered baby syndrome' exemplifies these problems. Recognition of the condition was exceedingly slow. The first description is probably that of West[8] who wrote in 1888 about 'Acute periosteal swelling in several young infants in the same family, probably rickety in nature' – and may well refer to a family over-burdened by fertility. The syndrome of multiple fractures and subdural haematomata was described in the 1940s, but the role of parental violence in the condition was not brought out until Silverman published his findings in 1953,[9] and the term 'battered baby' only entered the literature in 1962 when the Colorado paediatrician Henry Kempe and his colleagues assembled a series of 750 cases.[10] In recent years almost one article a week on the condition has been published in medical journals, and it has also received wide coverage in the lay press. However, the incidence is unknown because in many cases professional help may not be sought or, when it is sought, the true condition may not be diagnosed, the injuries being falsely ascribed to accidental causes.[11] Socio-medical studies have been carried out and some controlling factors have been identified but many remain unknown.

The battered child is usually under the age of four years, slightly more often a boy than a girl, frequently materially quite well cared for and adequately supplied with clothes and toys. The child may well have been fractious and have cried a lot before the violence began. The child is subject to unreasonable and repeated violence, often producing marked bruising, multiple fractures, dislocations and subperiosteal bleeding, subdural haematomata and visceral injuries. Rupture of the liver or of other abdominal organs can follow violence to the soft abdominal wall and cerebral damage follows blows to the head; either may be fatal. The parents will commonly seek medical advice, although often after several hours' delay, alleging that the child fell out of its cot, fell downstairs or that some other incident occurred, but the nature of the injuries is usually inconsistent with the history given by the parents. If one parent is involved, the other is generally aware of what has been happening. At least 60 per cent of battered children seen by physicians are at risk of further violence if the condition is not recognised immediately.

From the limited epidemiological evidence available, it has been inferred that no particular ethnic group predominates and that the condition is present among all socio-economic classes. However, lower income groups are over-represented and financial and housing conditions are correlated with the condition.[12] The father often has a criminal record or is unemployed.[13] The attitudes of the parents towards the conception, pregnancy or the child is critically important in relation to the possibility of the availability of abortion cutting down cases of child cruelty. Not only is the final attitude important, but also the time at which it became fixed. Fairbairn & Hunt[14] suggest that in many cases the rejection dates from the first recognition of pregnancy, but sometimes attitudes may have taken root only at delivery or even in the puerperium. It is significant that the premarital conception (possibly also extramarital conceptions) and last-born children are particularly at risk. In a study of 180 children subject to ill-treatment in 115 Massachusetts families, Merrill[15] found that just under half were premarital conceptions. Eighty eight per cent of all cases surveyed by Fontana *et al.*[16] were first or last-born children and these categories are, of course, also over-represented among women seeking abortion in the Western world. In cases of child cruelty, the woman is often pregnant again by the time the condition comes to light and thus, potentially, birth control and abortion have a double role in preventing child cruelty.

Shaw showed that about 4000 cases per year came to the attention of the New York Courts during the early 1960s, and he suggested that parental abuse and neglect may be one of the commonest causes of death in childhood in contemporary America.[17] Just as the control of fertility has played an important role in reducing maternal mortality in recent decades, so the effect of birth control practices upon infant and child mortality and morbidity rates is becoming increasingly significant.

The original 1962 paper by Kempe on 'battered babies' led to legislation in every state of the USA to enforce the reporting of child cruelty. In 1967 and 1968, this system of reporting was used as the foundation for a $500000 survey of the problem of the Department of Health, Education and Welfare. A sample of 1380 certifiable cases of ill-treatment, from over 12500 reported in the two years, was followed up. Reported incidence represented a rate of 849 cases of physical abuse per 100000 children under the age of 18 years in the USA. In 80 per cent of cases, the medical reports on the violence were available, 21 per cent required one week or more of hospitalisation and 3.4 per cent were fatal. Despite this high rate, cross-referencing with newspaper reports of deaths due to child abuse, showed that only 1 in 10 cases entered the survey and a good deal of under-reporting must be assumed. A sample survey of the USA carried out at the same time showed that 400 in every 100000 parents interviewed admitted physically injuring a child and 3000 in every 100000 interviewed knew of a family where this kind of incident had occurred. Only a fifth of the ill-treated children were under one year and the largest group were 3–9-year-olds.

The findings of the survey brought out a number of features that parallel much that is known about unwanted pregnancy and Gil,[7] who wrote the report, recommended 'comprehensive family planning programs *including the repeal of all legislation concerning medical abortion*' (italics added) as one component of any future solution. Mothers (or a mother substitute) were responsible for the assault in 47.6 per cent of cases and fathers (or a father substitute) in 39.2 per cent. Over 29 per cent of children lived in homes without a father, or father substitute. Ten per cent of the mothers were single and 20 per cent widowed, separated or divorced. Serious injuries were most likely to be committed by parents under the age of 25. The sample contained proportionately more children from large families than is found in America as a whole. The socially disadvantaged groups predominated but religious affiliations did not show any unusual bias.

The battered baby is only one in a series of child cruelty situations, some or all of which are partially related to unwanted pregnancy and therefore fall into an area overlapping the medico-sociological consequences of induced abortion. At one level is the neglected child, underweight, dirty, with severe nappy rash, often the product of an inadequate home and of inadequate fertility control. At the next level is physical abuse, which it is unreasonable to label as criminal but it is likely to have an adverse effect on the development of the child. It may be selective and limited to one child in a family. At the most extreme level are the overt examples of cruelty, where the child is beaten, burned or otherwise sadistically treated or even killed. Cases are usually dealt with by the criminal courts and are even less the object of rational analysis than are battered babies.

Infanticide is an extreme category of child abuse, normally involving the mother. (Child murder is the only crime of violence more commonly committed by women than men.) The child is smothered, drowned, or sometimes killed by more violent methods. Police prosecutions may not reflect the exact incidence of this type of social pathology, but statistics from Poland appear to demonstrate a genuine and marked decline in cases brought before the courts since the war. This has occurred since the liberalisation of abortion legislation. In the 1920s and 30s the annual number was around 1000, today it is between 20 and 50.[18] Part of this decline is probably also the result of improved living conditions, but it seems reasonable to assign a portion of the credit to the ability of women to resort readily to abortion. However, if the argument given elsewhere, that the main effect of the eastern European legislation has been to transfer would-be backstreet abortions to hospitals is correct, then this factor should not be over-rated.

Other aspects of child rearing

There is some danger of confusing unplanned with unwanted children. The mind readily forms stereotypes of unplanned, unwanted, neglected children as opposed to planned, welcomed and cared-for children. We shall attempt to show that such factors are statistically important but they should not be applied in individual cases, for deeper consideration reveals that within the human family situation, motivation and actions are seldom logically planned in detail. There is a wide no-man's land between the tiny minority of couples who ill-treat their children and the vast majority whose children have been happily accepted and loved. Within this no-man's land fall many children who are unplanned and unwanted and have never been accepted. There is a correlation between such factors and high parity. It is not intended to suggest that later children in all large families were unwanted or that all children in small families were wanted, but it does seem likely that the percentage of planning errors are higher in large families. Up to the present time data on this subject are deficient. It would seem that since a child's birth order is easily determined, this could be correlated with certain objective parameters of health and progress, once subjected to analysis. Such work would be particularly valuable because this is a subject where much is difficult to measure and we often lack objective criteria, even though we recognise that the growing child is susceptible to very subtle and slight changes in its environment.

There is also the 'unwanted' child who is subject to the mirror image of cruelty – obsessive care and attention – which may be almost as damaging.

Finally there is a relationship between accidental pregnancies and 'accidents' to children. An ingenious analysis of the effects of unplanned pregnancy on an easily defined measure of child suffering has been carried out by Martin,[19] at the Hospital for Sick Children, London. She studied, by interview with both child and family, 50 children admitted to the Burns Unit and a control group of 41 fit children matched from public health records. Most children who received burns had not been unattended at the time of the accident, but often a sibling, and in over half the cases an adult, was present. It emerged, however, that the adult, especially if it was the mother, usually acknowledged being preoccupied. Eight mothers were pregnant at the time with unplanned pregnancies and there was a raised incidence of unplanned pregnancies among the mothers with burned children.

Children born to women who sought abortion

In 1954 Caplan observed that a group of children receiving psychiatric treatment had all been born to mothers who had attempted, though unsuccessfully, to interrupt the pregnancy of the child concerned.[20] Beck[21] and David[22] have reviewed the more recent literature dealing with children born to mothers who did not want the pregnancy when it started. There are sufficient data[23-25] to suggest that the child who is unwanted in pregnancy has a greater than average chance of being consciously or unconsciously rejected after birth but to date only two studies have been devised to test this hypothesis in detail. The long history of the partial availability of therapeutic abortion in Sweden enabled Hans Forssman and Inger Thuwe to conduct a follow-up study of 120 children born to women *refused* termination and compare them with an equal number of controls. The study was a pioneer project and, rightly, is widely quoted. The matching of the controls has been criticised, and no doubt with hindsight some improvements in the study design might be made.

Forssman & Thuwe followed-up all the women refused application for abortion in Göteborg, Sweden's second largest city, between 1939 and 1941.[26] A third of the cases (68) had not taken the unwanted pregnancy to term and no doubt many interruptions were deliberate but illegal. In following-up the children that were born, the authors used civil and ecclesiastical registers, social agencies, school and military records and surveyed any contact with psychiatric departments. Criminal and drunken offences and various forms of public nuisance were also monitored.

Predictably, many of the 'unwanted' children were born into one parent families and their mothers, on average, were younger than the control groups. Not only was the relationship between the mother and her child under scrutiny but some aspects of the work may have measured societal attitudes to illegitimacy – which were more reactionary than in contemporary Sweden but more liberal than in much of the contemporary world. Forssman & Thuwe concluded:

> the unwanted children were worse off in every respect...the differences were often statistically significant, and, when they were not, they pointed in the same direction – to a worse lot for the unwanted children. One may assume that the children who were not born because their mothers got authorization for abortion would have had to face still greater disadvantages socially and medically.

Some of the criticisms of the Swedish study have been met in a more recent analysis of children born to women refused abortion, which was carried out in Czechoslovakia by Dytrych and his Czech and American co-workers.[27] It is based on 233 children born to women who had been refused legal abortion in Czechoslovakia in the years 1961–63. A control group of children was selectively matched for the school attended, sex, birth order, number of siblings, marital status of the mother and occupation of the father. The two groups were compared in over 400 different ways, involving physical and psycho-social factors (Fig. 54). Data were provided by (1) observers (who did not know to which group a child belonged), (2) school and medical records, and (3) evaluation by teachers,

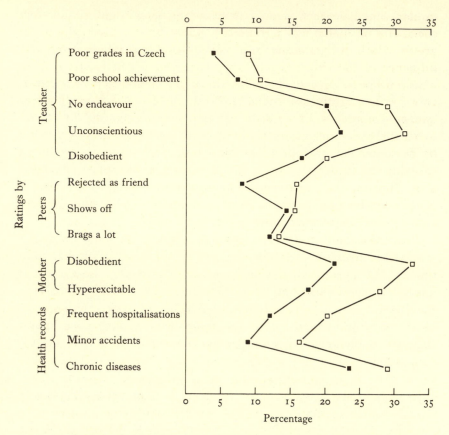

Fig. 54. Percentage manifestation of selected symptoms (as rated by mothers, teachers, peer groups and noted in health records) among children born to women twice refused legal abortions (□) and in a control group (■).

parents and the children's own peers. The authors conclude that the belief, 'that a child unwanted during pregnancy remains unwanted is not necessarily true. However the opposite notion,...that the birth of a child brings a complete change in attitude and that every woman who becomes a mother will love her child, is also untrue. The child of a mother denied an abortion is born in a potentially handicapped situation.'

There was no physical difference between the two groups during pregnancy and birth. The 'unwanted' children had a slightly greater number of acute illnesses than the control group, and school performance was marginally weaker in the study group. In particular, language proficiency (which is a good measure of a child's social environment) was significantly poorer in the case of the study group. Both the mothers and the children's teachers rated the diligence of the study group lower than that of the controls. The children's peers perceived children born to women who were refused abortion as slightly less sociable: for example, they were less frequently someone's 'best friend'.

All the differences were slight. No adverse characteristics could be predicted for an individual child born to a woman refused an abortion. Fortunately, family life is labile and children are adaptable. Indeed, the slight handicap measurable in the study group could even be a challenge to some individuals, and children in the study group were rated more highly for their 'sense of humour'.

This important study establishes that family planning enhances the quality of life for children as well as for parents. At the same time, to be the result of an unplanned or unwanted conception need not be an insuperable handicap. However, it should be noted that the Czech study was based on a small number of women refused an abortion out of 25000 who were granted an abortion, and, even among those who were refused, 47 per cent did not bear a live child, so that the mothers of the children involved probably had relatively slight reasons for seeking an end to the pregnancy.

In certain cases, the alternative to abortion is adoption. It is nearly always a painful solution for the mother. It can be a potentially humane solution for the child, but in practice results are often disappointing. While criminal statistics are only a very indirect measure of human health and happiness, they do suggest an area for concern. Adopted children are over-represented in juvenile courts, and for example, compulsive stealing is unusually common. However, it is possible that adoption processes could be improved if the average age of adoptive parents were brought down, if the religious barriers to adoption were eased, and if the 'blood relationships' were not preferred to strong emotional ties.[28] Unfortunately, the subject is one of speculation and conjecture with a dearth of reliable statistics.

Child cruelty and liberal abortion

Abortion involves the destruction of a fetus. Child cruelty is a form of partial physical or mental destruction. It is tempting to complete the equation and maintain that individuals, or communities, that adopt a liberal attitude towards abortion may also be those most likely to abuse the born child. This argument is implicit in much that is written or said about abortion. The passion aroused by abortion is partly a result of the clash between those who sincerely believe that abortion leads to the desirable goal that every child should be a wanted child and those who genuinely believe that it is the first precipitous step towards infanticide and the dissolution of all family ties. The resolution of this debate would do much to bring options closer, but, perhaps for the very reason that each assumption seems self-evident to those concerned and yet is the mirror image of the other, even less sociological research has been carried out to establish or refute the hypothesis of those opposed to abortion than that of those in favour of it.

There is, however, an assemblage of historical and geographical information that suggests that an important paradox obtains in this field. The assumption that legal abortion might lead to euthanasia and to the concentration camp flounders on observational data. In practice, the evidence of social history and the evaluation of contemporary cultures suggests that abortion is often outlawed and condemned in those cultures where the life and happiness of children is held in relatively low regard. Conversely, liberal abortion is being accepted increasingly in communities which endeavour to give maximum opportunities to the young.

Historical

In a precontraceptive era, celibacy and infanticide were virtually the only sure means of fertility control. Between 1750 and 1850 the population of Europe, which had previously been relatively stable, doubled and infanticide grew to startling proportions. Many of the leading countries made stringent laws against it but such laws were difficult to enforce and appear to have had little effect. The most popular methods of infanticide were dosing the baby with gin and/or opiates, strangulation, starvation and probably most common of all, smothering the infant that slept in bed with its parents. This latter event occurred so often that in some countries parents were forbidden by law to share the same bed with small children. Child cruelty and neglect were extreme.

Abandonment was a less objectionable method of dealing with the unwanted child, and in 1700 Thomas Coram, a sea captain living in Rotherhithe, was appalled at the plight of babies born in London. He petitioned King George II 'to prevent the frequent murders of poor miserable infants at their birth and to suppress the inhuman custom of exposing new born infants to perish in the streets'. As a result of his efforts, the London Foundling Hospital was opened in 1741. (It was in the Chapel of this hospital that Handel's *Messiah* was first performed.) All admissions were accepted and, in the early experience of this hospital, of 14 934 babies admitted 10 204 died. The hospital governors set up a subcommittee to study bills of mortality from London workhouses, and found that their own sad experiences were multiplied all over London. Between 1728 and 1757 they traced 468 081 christenings and 273 930 infants that died under the age of two in these workhouses.

Some years after its foundation, the Foundling Hospital came to establish a ballot system so that it did not admit more than 20 babies a day. Unfortunately, the desire of women to be rid of children was so great that precautions had to be taken to avoid 'children being dropped or other tricks being put upon the hospital'. The experience of the Foundling Hospital was repeated in all the large cities of Europe.

Disraeli, in his novel *Sybil* (1845) wrote 'Infanticide is practised as exclusively and as legally in England as it is on the banks of the Ganges.' The link between baby-farming and abortion in the nineteenth century has been noted in Chapter 5 (p. 163). Perhaps the many child murders at this time took place when children were left in the care of foster parents. The baby farmers often 'cared' for their charges by putting them to sleep with narcotics. So many infants died that the Infant Life Protection Society in London forced parliament to regulate baby farms in 1872.

The British experience was paralleled in France. Thirty-one per cent of the baptisms in Paris between 1770 and 1789 were of foundlings. In the late eighteenth century Napoleon, appalled at the problem of child murder in France, ordered that Foundling Hospitals should accept babies without questioning the parents, who could remain completely anonymous. The immediate effect of this Act was to treble the number of infants received into such hospitals, but their subsequent mortality remained high.

It is difficult to guess if the lot of many children deteriorated further in the nineteenth century or merely failed to improve.

Contemporary

Cruelty to children is exceptionally encountered in all countries, and in no country is it common. There are probably variations in the frequency of child cruelty between contemporary countries as there are in the historical sequences of any single society. It should perhaps be remembered that some of the less developed countries are only now going through some of the cultural and economic pressures experienced in the West at the time of the Industrial Revolution, together with the effects of the most massive migration in human history, namely from the traditional way of life in the villages to the urban slums. By the year 2000, the urban population of the developing world will be equal in size to the total population of the developing world in 1940. It is a migration which often weakens family bonds and leaves children to mature in an environment of horrendous deprivation. No one has more vividly portrayed the urban 'culture of poverty' than the late Oscar Lewis in retelling the daily lives of slum dwellers in Mexico City.[29]

It would be interesting to attempt a correlation between societal attitudes towards abortion and the prevalence of cruelty towards children in the same community or country. Where abortion is least likely to be liberalised, as in Mexico, a child's life is often harshest.

Currently, the only data are qualitative and not quantitative. In most developing countries infanticide certainly occurs. It may be more common than in the richer countries; certainly little is done when a baby's body is found on a refuse heap. In Bombay at least one hospital has a small cot at the entrance where a mother may come secretly at night and abandon her child. Sometimes mothers flee the maternity ward leaving their newborn infants behind as they have no prospects of supporting yet another child. An obstetrician from Manila tells of how a few years ago he was sitting with his wife when there was a thud outside his window as a small bundle was tossed into the courtyard. They found that it was a newborn baby, which one of the maids had delivered secretly. He had failed to notice who among his own staff was pregnant, and now she was literally throwing away her child. A maid in the Philippines earns about 300 pesos ($38) per month and her wages may well be essential support for her family back home in the countryside. Thus, if she kept her child she would have little choice but prostitution to support it. Church-run orphanages exist but they are overcrowded.

A speech by the President of Colombia, Carlos Resperpo, to the 1967 Inter-American Conference on Population is quoted by the British Catholic writer St John-Stevas as an example that those 'uneasy' about contraceptive programmes might accept as 'an argument that there are greater evils than contraception'. Resperpo said:

> I have visited the poorest slums of the Republic and I recommend the same visit to those people who examine the population above all from the moral point of view... What can we say of the frequent incest, of the primitive sexual experience, of the miserable treatment of children, of the terrible proliferation of prostitution of children of both sexes, of frequent abortion, of almost animal union because of alcoholic excesses? It is, in consequence, impossible for me to sit back and examine the morality or immorality of contraceptive practices without thinking at the same time of the immoral and frequently criminal conditions that the simple act of conception can produce in the course of time.

Apart from the fact that the argument could be used as a moral justification of legal abortion (although Resperpo and St John-Stevas would reject this), the description could have been written of Dickensian London.

The record of cruelty to children in Italy is worse than in many European countries. There is no state provision or supervision of orphanages and it is impossible to adopt a child without bribery. In 1971 an ex-Mayor of Rome, a member of parliament, the Director General of Public Assistance at the Ministry of Health and several other notables, were tried for misappropriating large sums from the State Agency ONMI, which supervises much of the money going into child welfare. An official investigation was established at the time of the scandal and reported that in over 100 orphanages, many of which were under the patronage of the local prelate, they had found children suffering from malnutrition, tied naked to their beds (in some cases the sheets were changed every 2 months), locked in rat-infested cellars for misbehaviour, used as free labour, tortured and sexually molested. The examples of the Philippines, Colombia and Italy have been chosen because they appear to be three of the countries that will take longest to adopt liberal abortion policies.

Conclusions

The previous chapters of this book have dealt with the prevalence of abortion, its role in fertility regulation, the public health implications of the choice between legal and illegal abortion and the politics of abortion legislation. In this chapter we have tried to explore the relationship between induced abortion and patterns of child-rearing. It is an area where intuitive feelings are often stronger than the available facts, but overall it seems that the children born to women refused abortion are slightly disadvantaged and that cases of child neglect and cruelty are more frequent in the case of unwanted pregnancies. At the same time, it has to be recognised that not all unwanted children are badly treated and that many children born to mothers refused abortion do exceedingly well. The reverse hypothesis, that a willingness to accept abortion is likely to be correlated with a low respect for life and poor-quality child-rearing, has no basis in historical or contemporary observation.

In broad terms, the eighteenth century in the West may be said to have been a century of institutionalised infanticide and the nineteenth century, when the birth rate first began to fall, one of a rising rate of abortion. But the nineteenth-century industrial nations such as Britain also made abortion illegal. The latter part of the twentieth century has seen the majority of the world adopt liberal abortion legislation. Often this change has occurred against a background of state concern and help for the sick and the weak, and for the status of women. Abortion reform in Britain, Scandinavia, USA and Australia all occurred in the same generation as major efforts to extend health care through state help. Tunisia is an example of a country with a record of legislation relating to women's rights that has also reformed its abortion legislation. Without getting side-tracked into political judgements on the details of the welfare legislation concerned, it seems reasonable to conclude that countries liberalising their abortion laws have had a more humane attitude to life than those where restrictive statutes were introduced.

It is possible that the twenty-first century will prove to be a time when adequate means of fertility regulation that fall outside the scope of any form of abortion legislation will become available. But for the present and foreseeable future we believe that the type of abortion law and the services for its implementation in a country are of profound significance for the health of women, the quality of family life and the ability of the community to meet its fertility goals. In the next chapter we draw these various threads together and discuss the problem of weighing the benefits of abortion to women and to society against the rights of the embryo.

References

1 Pohlman, E. M. & Pohlman, J. M. (1969). *Psychology of Birth Planning*. Schenkman, Cambridge, Mass.
2 Lewis-Faning, E. (1949). Family limitation and its influence on human fertility during the past fifty years. *Papers of the Royal Commission on Population*, vol. 1. HMSO, London.
3 Whelpton, P. K., Campbell, A. A. & Patterson, J. E. (1966). *Fertility and Family Planning in the United States*. Princeton University Press, Princeton, N.J.
4 Peel, J. & Carr, G. (1975). *Contraception and Family Design: A Study of Birth Planning in Contemporary Society*. Churchill Livingstone, Edinburgh.
5 Fraser, A. C. & Watson, P. S. (1968). Family planning – a myth? *Practitioner*, **201**, 351.
6 Miller, D. & Swanson, G. (1960). *Inner Conflict and Defence*. Holt, Rinehart & Winston, New York.
7 Gil, D. G. (1970). *Violence Against Children. Physical Child Abuse in the United States*. Harvard University Press, Cambridge, Mass.
8 West, S. (1888). *British Medical Journal*, **1**, 856.
9 Silverman, F. N. (1953). The Roentgen manifestations of unrecognized skeletal trauma in hospitals. *American Journal of Roentgenology*, **69**, 413.
10 Kempe, C. H., Silverman, F. N., Steele, B. F., Droegemueller, W. & Silver, H. K. (1962). *Journal of the American Medical Association*, **18**, 17.
11 Jackson, G. (1972). Child abuse syndrome: the cases we miss. *British Medical Journal*, **2**, 756.
12 Cameron, J. M. (1970). The battered baby. *British Journal of Hospital Medicine*, **4**, 769.
13 Skinner, A. E. & Castle, R. L. (1969). *78 Battered Children*. NSPCC, London.
14 Fairbairn, A. C. & Hunt, A. C. (1964). *Medicine, Science and Law*, **4**, 123.

15 Merrill, E. J. (1962). Physical abuse of children – an agency study. In *Protecting the Battered Child*, p. 1. American Human Association, Denver.

16 Fontana, V. J., Dononvan, D. & Wong, R. J. (1963). *New England Journal of Medicine*, **269**, 1389.

17 Shaw, A. (1963). *How to Help the Battered Child*. RISS, Dec. 70–104.

18 Wolinska, H. (1962). Przerwanie ciazy w swietle prawa karnego. In *Panstwowe Wydawnictwo Naukowe*, Warsaw.

19 Howell, C. (1972). Personal communication.

20 Caplan, D. (1954). The disturbance of mother–child relationship by unsuccessful attempts at abortion. *Mental Hygiene*, **38**, 67.

21 Beck, M. B. (1970). Abortion: the mental health consequences of unwantedness. *Seminars in Psychiatry*, **2**, 263.

22 David, H. P. (1973). Psychological studies in abortion. In *Psychological Aspects of Population*, ed. J. T. Fawcett. Basic Books Inc., New York.

23 Arén, P. & Amark, C. (1961). Prognosis in cases in which legal abortion has been granted but not carried out. *Acta Psychiatrica et Neurologica Scandinavica*, **36**, 203.

24 Holbein, R. (1960). Subsequent fate of mother and child after refused application for interruption of pregnancy. *Deutsche Gesundheit*, **15**, 188.

25 Hook, K. (1963). Referred abortion. A follow-up study of 249 women whose applications were refused by the Maternal Board of Health in Sweden. *Acta Psychiatrica et Neurologica Scandinavica*, **39**, Suppl. 168, 1.

26 Forssman, H. & Thuwe, I. (1966). One hundred and twenty children born after application for therapeutic abortion refused. *Acta Psychiatrica et Neurologica Scandinavica*, **42**, 71.

27 Dytrych, Z., Matejček, Z., Schüller, V., David, H. P. & Friedman, H. C. (1975). Children born to women denied abortion. *Family Planning Perspectives*, **7**, 165.

28 Editorial (1970). Adoption. *Lancet*, **ii**, 866.

29 Lewis, O. (1959). *Five Families*. Basic Books, New York.

15
A conspectus

The problem of abortion demands an answer. Restrictive abortion legislation has rarely, if ever, been effective in preventing induced abortions. Nations must either deal with the major public health hazard posed by illegal abortion, or create services to implement liberal laws and practices.

There are three main issues: the need to determine the role of abortion in the total pattern of fertility regulation; the need to reduce emotional tension, physical pain and risk to health presented by badly performed illegal abortions; and the need to balance the rights of the embryo against the rights of the mother.

Abortion discussions are all too often clouded by ignorance and fear – the worst of counsellors when important and difficult decisions have to be made. Fear arises from cultural indoctrination against abortion and from a reluctance to grant increased freedom to women or to a younger generation. It is the fear of the uncharted and the fear of change. The antidote to fear is knowledge, but ignorance on almost all aspects of abortion is widespread.

In the preceding chapters many biological, medical and sociological aspects have been discussed. The aim of this conspectus is to bring these various topics together and to offer the best judgements of which the authors are capable on the answers to the above problems.

The human right of a couple to control their fertility[1] was first asserted internationally at the United Nations Conference on Human Rights in Teheran (May 1968); 'parents have a basic human right to determine freely and responsibly the number and spacing of their children'. There was a deliberate avoidance of any mention of the means to regulate fertility and it is difficult to contend that it automatically includes abortion. Nevertheless, the philosophy of the couple's right, and above all the woman's right, to make the abortion decision has gained ground in many countries. Article 191 of the Federal Constitution of Yugoslavia states that it is a 'human right to decide on the birth of children. The right may only be restricted for reasons of health.' Here it is clearly intended to encompass induced abortion. The Republic of Slovenia in its Constitution explicitly states the obligations implied by the human right set out in the Federal Constitution: 'In connection with the realisation of the right, the social community guarantees the necessary education and appropriate social protection and medical help according to the law.'[2]

But in most places, as was shown in the World Population Conference in Bucharest in 1974, the role of abortion in fertility control is not faced squarely.

Abortion and contraception

The evidence presented earlier demonstrates that induced abortion is to be found in all societies. No developed country has brought down its birth rate without a considerable recourse to abortion and it appears unlikely that developing countries can ever hope to see any decline in their fertility without a massive resort to induced abortion – legal or illegal.

Over much of the world abortion appears to be becoming more common as the advantages of family planning gain wider acceptance. The difficulty of collecting data on induced abortion has been emphasised many times, but when information from many countries and social groups is analysed a common pattern can usually be discerned. Initially, as a community or group begins to control its fertility, couples attempt to space out pregnancies by adopting whatever contraceptive methods are available, but their first efforts in contraception are likely to be inefficient. Inevitably the first demographic effect of a nation becoming convinced of the benefits of birth control will commonly be an increase in abortion. Contraception and abortion are complementary not competitive methods of fertility regulation.

Given reasonable access to contraception, the resort to abortion declines as a society becomes more experienced in controlling its fertility, but it is never eliminated. A combination of abortion and

During month | | At abortion
of conception | | follow–up

Pittsburgh: 92 cases legal abortion (menstrual regulation). 1972–73

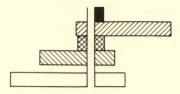

Bangkok: 166 cases illegal abortion admitted to hospital. 1973

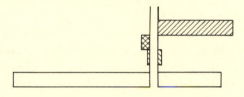

Washington: 1315 cases of legal abortion. 1972

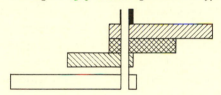

Singapore: 3152 cases of legal abortion. 1972

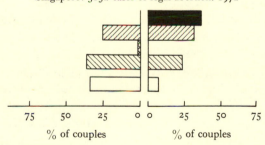

75   50   25   0   0   25   50   75

% of couples   % of couples

■ Sterilisation   ▨ Oral contraceptives

▨ IUDs   ▨ Other methods   ☐ No method

Fig. 55. Contraceptive usage before and after abortion in selected series of patients.

contraception remains the prime method of fertility regulation throughout the contemporary world. Unfortunately, the means of contraception available in the closing decades of the twentieth century, with few exceptions, remain incapable of meeting the goals of family size set and attained in developed countries and hoped for in developing countries. The exceptions are the statistically lucky minority who consistently use sophisticated methods, such as oral contraceptives, over long periods and those who choose, and are able, to be sterilised when they have attained their desired family size.

The relationship between abortion and contraception can be seen constructively. Usually, when abortion is accepted in the spectrum of fertility regulation procedures it is labelled a 'back-up', a 'long-stop', a 'last resort', or an 'unwelcome necessity'. But in reality the combination of abortion and contraception presents the least risk to life of the various options facing a couple seeking a reversible method of family planning and, unlike other methods, always allows a fully predictable control of fertility. As has been pointed out earlier, the combination of abortion and contraception may well present, in terms of professional skills and commodities, the least expensive way in which a society can fulfil its obligation to make the means of family planning available to all individuals. And in a world where medical resources are seriously overstretched this observation is one of some ethical significance.

Finally, if the combination of contraception and abortion comes to be fully accepted as the optimum choice for many individuals, then some consideration should be given to redesigning contraceptives, with an emphasis on reducing side effects and thereby improving continuation rates. This should be done even at the expense of effectiveness in preventing pregnancy because in the long run a combination of less effective contraceptives with better acceptance and continuation rates, combined with elective early abortion, will lead to less embryonic wastage than the present situation, where the two elements in the equation are separated, both at the level of contraceptive development and in the provision of family planning services.

Abortion services

The provision of services is the most straightforward of the problems posed by abortion, and the evidence for the way to proceed is clear.

The knowledge of how to provide early abortion cheaply with dignity, compassion and safety for women is available. Outpatient vacuum aspiration of the uterus is a simple, somewhat repetitive, well-tried technique. Undoubtedly women require an explanation of the operation. Most surgeons use a local anaesthetic, but some believe 'verbal anaesthetic' is sufficient. The operation takes five to ten minutes.

Outpatient abortions have even been conducted in such a way that the woman need not remove her street clothes; Yugoslavian women go home to their farms on a bus half an hour after the operation; girls used to fly to New York from the other side of the USA and return on the jumbo jet the same day; outpatient operations take place in Tunisia, India, Korea, Japan, the People's Republic of China and some English hospitals. In at least two US centres, nurses and midwives perform very early abortions. As the Lane Report suggested, it is certainly a general practitioner rather than a specialist operation.[3]

Some uncertainty inevitably surrounds the possible long-term consequences of abortion. The risks of subsequent sterility and psychological damage have been closely studied and are slight.

Unfortunately the clinical aspects of abortion have become the subject of emotional and political claims, as much as other aspects of this controversial subject. When moral arguments fail to deter women, the physical dangers are sometimes amplified. If a new long-term side effect is demonstrated, there are always those who are pleased to say 'I told you so'. Conversely, those who want the law to be liberalised will stress the hazards of illegal abortion and claim that hundreds, or thousands, of women die unnecessarily each year, when the actual number is far lower.

Basically, abortion is simple and safe when performed early, but, as with any common operation when it is carried out on a large enough scale, catastrophes do occur. Fortunately they are very rare. Neither must the obvious be forgotten – once a woman is pregnant she will have a delivery if she does not have an abortion and the continuation of the pregnancy is usually more dangerous in physical and mental health terms than is an early termination.

The wide differences in reported mortality and morbidity rates for legally induced abortions have been commented upon. Variations in complication rates are sometimes the result of the adoption of different criteria in different centres. What is 'haemorrhage', how is 'infection' to be defined? The assessment of mortality is much more certain. In the 1950s and 1960s mortality rates reported from Hungary and Japan were so low that they were disbelieved, but USA data have demonstrated even lower mortality levels, which are now being approached also in the UK. Cates has drawn a parallel between abortion as treatment (of an unwanted pregnancy) and the treatment of gonorrhoea.[4] There *is* a sense in which both the unwanted pregnancy and gonorrhoea can be regarded, like the common cold, as 'sexually transmitted diseases'. In the case of gonorrhoea the cure rate for a single injection of penicillin is about 90 per cent. In the case of termination of pregnancy a single uterine evacuation with a suction curette is successful in all but a few cases in a thousand. Similarly, in terms of mortality, for a single intramuscular injection of penicillin, the World Health Organisation estimates a death rate of 1.6 per 100000 injections, whilst first-trimester terminations carried out by vacuum aspiration currently carry a mortality rate of 1.7 per 100000 operations in the USA. The mortality of illegal abortion is more difficult to measure, but the International Planned Parenthood Federation Africa Region surveyed member countries in 1973 and recorded a death rate of up to 2000 per 100000 women admitted to hospital with incomplete abortions.[5] It may be argued that the less severely ill women did not reach hospital but equally many deaths occurred outside hospital. Whatever the limitations of the data, they confirm the gap between legal and illegal abortion in terms of maternal risk (see Table 46). Yet technically there is no reason why early abortion, if legal, should not prove almost as safe in Africa as in the USA. There need be no bottleneck in equipment, at least in urban areas and personnel could be found and trained to perform the work.

It must always be appreciated that if abortion is to be safe it must not only be legal but be performed early. To achieve this, decision-making must be simple and the advertisement of services unequivocal.

It is illuminating to consider the hypothetical situation where a global abortion service is designed to bring the world population to zero growth rate. Such a service is a fantasy, but it emphasises the

Table 46. *Legal and illegal abortion mortality*

		Deaths per 100 000 operations/admissions
Legal abortions		
First-trimester vacuum aspirations, USA (1972–76)		1.7
16–20 weeks (all methods), USA (1972–74)		18.3
Hospital admissions for incomplete abortions		
Ghana	1970	363
	1972	562
Nigeria	1970	2041
	1972	1020
Mauritius	1970	876
	1972	666
Uganda	1970	385
	1972	149
Sierra Leone	1970	1456
	1972	2459
Zaïre	1972	346

power and efficiency of abortion. The world's population is currently increasing by about 200 000 per day. It might require up to 300 000 abortions daily to avert this number of births – assuming that nothing is done to increase contraceptive usage. In order to carry this load we should require 10 000 trained abortionists, medical or lay. Most of these abortionists would work in the developing world and on an average they might each require to be paid about $5000 per year. Therefore the cost of running a global abortion service capable of reducing world population to zero growth would be in the order of $50–$100 million annually. (This figure would allow for supporting staff and the simple essential facilities.) The exact numbers could be debated, but so could the costs, because in practice a great many people would pay an economic rate for such a service if it were available. In Bombay the International Pregnancy Advisory Clinic charges an inclusive fee of less than $9 for a first-trimester abortion and actually makes a profit. In a world of 4000 million people these costs are almost incredibly small. The cost of running the hypothetical service is about the same as the budget of the International Planned Parenthood Federation, which is a non-governmental body and not as well financially supported as some other agencies in the field.

Global abortion on this scale would inevitably result in a few hundred deaths per year throughout the whole world, but this is about the same number as occurs at the present time solely as a result of illegal abortions in the single city of Bogota. Naturally we recognise that the establishment of such a service is not a current feasibility and that even if it were set up the motivation for the attainment of zero growth probably does not yet exist. There are, of course, cultural and economic factors that influence family size. Nevertheless it is rarely appreciated that we already have an exceptionally cost-effective, remarkably safe, easy to administer and apparently much sought-after method of fertility control, which could be made available immediately there is political will to do so.

A subsidiary effect of such a global abortion service would inevitably be an improvement in contraceptive usage. The same personnel would obviously be involved in both services. We have already shown that responsible abortion services promote realistic contraception.

The medical profession

The medical profession has played a key role in sustaining the paradox of community opposition to the rational and necessary individual need for abortion. Most abortion techniques require a trained person and doctors have exploited this logistic bottleneck to restrict the availability of the procedure. It is not just a fanciful interpretation of history to suggest that, if botanical reality had been otherwise and the ancient Greeks had discovered a herb which was common, harmless and could be self-administered, the legal and theological restraints on abortion would never have evolved. Or if man had evolved from a marsupial rather than a eutherian mammal, so that the greater part of gestation was completed in an external and accessible pouch, then the community would never have attempted to restrict abortion.

The admonition that the physician should heal himself is not likely to provide very wide clinical experience, but most doctors, nurses and paramedical workers do face the need for birth control. Indeed, physicians were among the first social groups to plan their families in the late nineteenth century. When *coitus interruptus* or the sheath failed, abortion was used. Those associated with medicine often have the easiest access to abortion. In one series of 1000 consecutive cases of legal termination, 15 per cent were doctors, doctors' wives, or nurses.[6] One of the numerous paradoxes of abortion is that those groups which are most opposed to the operation resort to it with above-average frequency.

Part of the medical profession's odd behaviour no doubt arose, and still arises, from the traditions of medical teaching. The incidence and significance of abortion has been underemphasised in the teaching of doctors and nurses. A decade ago the only ward into which students were not allowed to enter in one famous London teaching hospital was the ward admitting septic abortions. This biased teaching can be quantified for the time when many doctors now practising in Britain were trained. The Emergency Bed Service in London deals with cases general practitioners are unable to place. In March 1949, to take the example of a single month, the London Emergency Bed Service dealt with 235 women of fertile years and 88 were cases of abortion. It is indicative of medical attitudes towards abortion that teaching hospitals only accepted 4 out of the 88 cases although 58 requests were made to them. In total in that year 2160 abortion cases were admitted to 6 London regional hospitals and only 415 to teaching hospitals.[7]

Some doctors are opposed to abortion, strongly upholding the right of the embryo.[8,9] But the major issue that confuses them is not that they think abortion is murder – they usually vaguely remember sufficient embryology to ensure that it is not the case – but the fact that they are trained, and encouraged by society, to make paternalistic decisions. Many doctors are offended because in nearly all abortions the woman makes her own diagnosis and prescribes her own treatment, 'I am pregnant and I want it ended'. The operation is a simple one. These doctors perceive abortions as reducing them to 'mere technicians' and feel that the ritual of medicine is undermined. In the words of one distinguished gynaecologist, 'I don't like being told what to do by the patient.'

One important result of even moderate liberalisation of abortion laws is that the woman unwantedly pregnant is thereby encouraged to seek medical advice. Thus doctors are brought literally face to face with the previously concealed demand for abortion and this has had the possibly predictable result that thereafter they become as sympathetic as ordinary human beings and their authoritative paternalistic judgements are less often expressed.

The woman and the embryo

The problem of balancing the rights of the woman against the rights of the embryo remains. Induced abortion involves judgements about the value and quality and, indeed, the definition of life. On very rare occasions it involves the life of the woman, sometimes her health, usually the potential quality of her future role in society – and always the life of the fertilised ovum, embryo or fetus. The issue of life can become most confused by other factors at the very time when lucid, uncluttered thought is essential. Abortion discussion can all too easily become a political volley ball, an instrument used by the medical profession to score points in its competition with the rest of society, or an intellectual game of chess played by theologians in deep isolation from the realities of everyday life.

By definition, debate is impossible if either set of rights are accepted as absolute. There is a dangerous tendency to simplify abortion issues, sometimes out of ignorance, perhaps more commonly because many people are afraid to shoulder responsibility. The right-to-lifer, who does not know theology very deeply, or the woman's liberationist who will not listen to counter-arguments, can be equally at fault. If they preach the exclusive rights of the embryo, or of the mother, they automatically put an end to reasoned argument.

Those who look for simple, one-sentence, black-and-white rules will always be frustrated. Abortion extracts an unrelenting pragmatism from every situation. Each case demands an individual judgement.

The woman

Women seeking abortions are *not* a deviant minority, they are in fact a broadly representative sample of women in the childbearing years within the community to which they belong (Chapter 3). There may be a bias towards certain groups, for example the middle classes in South America or the Mediterranean, or the unmarried in the USA, Europe and Australia. But this does not abrogate the fact that induced abortion is found in all social, economic, educational, ethnic and religious groups. In fact, it is one of the few activities in which nearly any individual can become involved, yet which nearly all communities have sought, or still seek, to forbid.

There are several reasons for this paradox. The individual's need for abortion is unpredictable, one usually seen as someone else's problem. Many sincere and thinking individuals have maintained a forceful opposition to abortion until they, their wife or daughter, became involuntarily pregnant. And in extreme cases they may even revert to oppositions after a single unhappy, guilty episode that is rationalised as involving exceptional circumstances: my daughter was raped, or at least seduced, and should have a termination; my neighbour's daughter was promiscuous, or at least feckless, and should not. Each generation seems to have to learn to face the reality of abortion anew. Contemporary American teenagers are more conservative in their attitudes than older individuals.[10]

Attitudes and practice do not always coincide in the realm of birth control, and public policy on abortion and contraception can face in opposite ways at the same time. However, for the individual Westoff, Moore & Ryder have shown that liberal abortion attitudes and a positive stance on contraception are usually found in the same person and this relationship cuts across race and religion.[11] Conversely, in France it has been shown that opposition to abortion and to contraception often go together.[12] In a survey of over 2600 Australian women, 138 reported that they had either had or attempted to have an illegal abortion. Among the Catholics in the group, 10 (7 per cent of the total) refused contraceptive advice even after an illegal abortion.

Repeated abortions, at least as studied in Hungary, affect a woman's attitudes in several ways (Table 47). Most married women report that the relationship with their husbands became closer after pregnancy was established and while seeking an abortion. The willingness to have another abortion *increases* with each experience of abortion.

Women have only attained a reasonable degree of equality with men during the relatively recent decades of the twentieth century and in many countries still suffer discrimination backed by law or custom. The quip that Britain would have reformed abortions earlier if it had had a Parliament of Mothers, rather than the Mother of Parliaments, is not without foundation.

The emergence of the woman's right to have an abortion is a

Table 47. *Response to repeated legal abortions in Hungary* (*n* = 279, 1969)

Number of induced abortions	0	1	2	3+
Afraid of pregnancy at time of intercourse (%)	—	9.5	8.8	27.3
Intercourse at least twice a week (%)	38.0	33.8	36.7	37.9
Intercourse is often a pleasure (%)	35.2	40.5	51.5	34.9
Intercourse is never a pleasure (%)	2.8	1.4	—	4.5
Willing to have an abortion in the future (%)	43.1	54.9	56.3	72.7

new theme running through twentieth-century thought, and binding together Lenin who believed (1921) that women should have the right 'of deciding for themselves a fundamental issue of their lives' and the US Supreme Court, 52 years later, which concluded that 'the right of personal privacy includes the abortion decision'. Many would hold that such a 'right' over-rides the 'rights' of the early embryo. But an insistence that abortion is every woman's right is no different from the conviction that all abortions are murder: both are simplifications that arise because there is no clear alternative. Both mislead if pressed too far.

RISKS AND LEARNING

Abortion can be seen as a key in learning to regulate fertility. In all learning, practical acquaintance seems more important than pedagogic experience. Each generation appears to have to learn about human sexuality and the control of fertility, through its own mistakes and its own experience, as well as by the transmission of experience by peer groups, parents, books, films, discussions and school lavatory conversations. Learning the use of effective contraception is difficult for a number of reasons. Steinhoff and her colleagues[13-16] pointed out that it is more difficult to learn where the effect is remote rather than immediate. The couple who have unprotected intercourse are rather in the situation of the individual who smokes heavily. Each knows of the long-term risk, but the immediate gratification overcomes their inhibitions. Also, pregnancy has a probabilistic relationship with conception. Some women will get away with taking risks for some of the time and a few will get away with taking risks all the time. Probably nearly all girls are more concerned about whether their period will occur after their first unprotected intercourse than after any subsequent exposure to the risk of pregnancy. Indeed one in 23 women attending the British Pregnancy Advisory Service claimed that they had conceived on the first occasion ever on which they had had intercourse.[17]

To a greater or lesser extent almost all human being indulge in risk-taking. A parallel might be drawn with car driving. If all bad driving was inevitably associated with accidents people might not take so many risks, but like the risk of pregnancy following unprotected, or inadequately protected, intercourse many people get away with it. Furthermore, every so often a genuinely careful driver is involved in an accident, just as unwanted pregnancies sometimes occur among those conscientiously using contraceptives. This analogy is also interesting because, as all insurance companies know and all those who pay premiums are aware, young male drivers are at the greatest risk of being involved in accidents. This is partly due to lack of experience and partly to sexual aggressiveness. The same factors apply in sexual risk-taking, as after all, the male partner is an important variable in gambling sexually.

Steinhoff[14] refers to two other factors that make learning to control fertility difficult. The relationship between pregnancy and intercourse is unlike some other relationships in that one mistake can be disastrous. By contrast, an obese person trying to slim may yield to the temptation of one heavy meal without the irreversible destruction of his goal. But an unwanted pregnancy, when it occurs, cannot be undone by subsequent good behaviour.

Therefore, it is suggested that one constructive way of approaching the problem of abortion-seeking behaviour is to consider it as the outcome of a mistake in an important learning process – namely that of fertility regulation – which all normal adults go through. It is further suggested that there are certain aspects of the relationship between coitus and conception that make risk-taking common, especially in the young.

The fact that many women seeking abortion have not used any effective method of contraception has caused a great deal of comment. At one extreme such women have been labelled feckless. More commonly there is bewilderment among the onlookers. How are women seeking an abortion to be regarded? Do they really differ from other women? But, as noted, when parameters such as age, parity, social class and religion are measured they correspond very closely with those relating to women having babies. Perhaps the simplest hypothesis is not to look for differences, but to regard women who seek abortions as like other women, except that they have been unlucky.

To emphasise the commonality between those who seek abortions and the rest of mankind is not to exclude the possibility that certain subgroups are more than usually prone to risk-taking in relation to pregnancy, as in relation to other events in life. Some groups of people seem to find it unusually difficult to undertake any type of long-term planning, others appear to be compulsive risk-takers. No studies have been conducted to show if women who, for example, go to bingo every night or men repeatedly convicted of bad driving are more than usually likely to take pregnancy risks, but the hypothesis would seem a reasonable one.

MARRIED AND UNMARRIED

The consequences of sexual risk-taking are profoundly different among the married and the unmarried. Most married couples learn the difficult process of fertility regulation during the intervals of family building. Risk-taking either leads to a mistiming of a wanted pregnancy, or to a totally unplanned pregnancy. In the former case the penalty is slight; in the latter, circumstances often permit the conception to continue and there may be rapid parental rationalisation to the conclusion that it was indeed a wanted pregnancy.

Among the unmarried, errors in learnings are usually much more visible and the penalties heavier. On the one hand, the irregularities and unpredictability of premarital coitus makes birth planning more than usually difficult, on the other hand an unwanted pregnancy often leads to abortion, adoption or a 'shotgun marriage'.

For every sexually active woman who becomes involuntarily pregnant, there are probably several who have episodes of delayed menstruation and suffer what Steinhoff[14] calls a 'pregnancy scare'. Whether or not such a scare is ultimately associated with pregnancy, there is often a marked improvement in contraceptive usage after the event.

The embryo

Human development is almost miraculous in its complexity. The embryo is more than a lump of jelly. However, because it has the genetic potential to become a new human being, should each fertilised egg be afforded all the protection which society gives to a newborn child? Even after fertilisation when that potential is starting to develop it is important to understand those things that distinguish the embryo in early pregnancy from a newborn child. At three months it still only weighs 20 g, is 55 mm long and, although it may be said to have the outer form of a human being, the nervous system is in an early stage of differentiation, the brain has nothing of the size and complexity associated with the brain at term.

GENETIC UNIQUENESS

If embryonic development of itself is an unsatisfactory criterion for where society's protection of the unborn should commence, then so is the genetic uniqueness of that individual.[18] Teratomas are tumours which often have structural elements, such as teeth or hair, and can be genetically unique. They are found outside as well as within the reproductive tract, can occur before puberty and even develop in the male. The fertilised ovum, in about one in 2000 cases, gives rise to a mass of placental tissue (a hydatidiform mole) to the exclusion of embryonic tissue. It is not a 'potential human being', even though it is genetically unique.

The genetic uniqueness of the egg must be seen in the context of the richness of all biological processes. Every cell in the body contains all the genetic information required to create another person, just as each subscriber is provided with the whole telephone directory, even though only a few numbers will ever be used. The daily production of new blood cells in an adult person involves copying sufficient genetic information to provide blueprints for 50 times the world's present population. However, such 'cloned' individuals would be identical. In contrast, when sperm and eggs are produced they contain new combinations of genes, a result of the scrambling effect of genetic recombination and the production of mutants. Now not all of these new 'variations on a theme' are capable of producing viable human beings, and those which contain deleterious modifications are liable to elimination at some stage during their development. Many of these modifications are so harmful that they do not even yield functional sperm or eggs. After fertilisation has been completed, and throughout the subsequent development of the embryo, there is further elimination of embryos that are defective for genetic reasons, or as a result of errors of development.

DEVELOPMENTAL ERRORS

A healthy fertile man can have up to 30 per cent of his sperm showing microscopic abnormalities, that is, it is *normal* for a man to produce a high proportion of abnormal sperm.[19] Furthermore, of the millions of sperm deposited in the vagina, only a few thousand reach the egg and one alone will fertilise it. The female reproductive tract can be regarded as an obstacle course in which the cervical mucus and the anatomy of the tract eliminate all but first-rate sperm. Probably many eggs are faulty too, but they are more difficult to study and therefore data are scarce. As noted in Chapter 2, pathologist A. T. Hertig and obstetrician John Rock calculated that one in ten fertilised eggs failed to survive the few days of development (blastocyst stage), four out of ten failed to attach to the uterus (five days after fertilisation) and six out of ten were lost by 12 days after fertilisation.[20,21] In total, over half the fertilised eggs are aborted before the woman misses a period, and all the evidence suggests that they are aborted because they are abnormal. After the woman has missed a period and knows that she is pregnant, perhaps one in five recognised pregnancies will abort spontaneously. Again studies show most spontaneous abortion is an essential healing process, without which human reproduction would be a tragic succession of congenital errors.

Human development thus bears little resemblance to the Girl Guide campfire fable where a perfect little sperm always meets a perfect egg which goes on to produce a perfect baby nine months later. Evolution has opted for an alternative course. It appears that the production of a new human being is so complicated that, rather than attempt to produce impeccable blueprints at the egg and sperm stage and thus to develop a faultless embryo each time, large numbers of defectives are permitted and consequently there are frequent failures to produce healthy embryos. The somewhat clumsy, imperfect production that in reality takes place is combined with a mechanism of inspection and abortion of errors.

This enormous rejection of deleterious genetic novelties is not as wasteful as it may first appear, for every species needs a continual supply of genetic variation on which natural selection can subsequently act in order that the species may continue to evolve and adapt to changing environmental pressures. Unfortunately the mechanisms that produce such variation (recombination, or shuffling of the genes, and mutation) cannot differentiate between useless and useful novelty. Nature has solved this problem by having a rigorous system of quality control during those stages when the individual units likely to be rejected (sperm, eggs, and later embryos) represent relatively tiny amounts of biological investment.

If, rather naively, we regard spontaneous abortion as a quality control mechanism asking the question 'would this embryo develop into a normal, functioning human being?', then induced abortion can be viewed as a second mechanism with a similar function posing the question 'if this embryo develops into a human being, what quality of life will it and its parents have, and what effect will its birth and the birth of others like it have on the future of the human species?' The latter part of this question is not without relevance to a species, such as our own, faced with a continuously accelerating population size and dwindling resources of all kinds. Other animal species, much less sophisticated than man and thus without recourse to induced abortion, are known to resort to infanticide as a means of controlling their population size in a crisis. From a purely biological standpoint, induced abortion may be seen as an entirely natural human form of population control for a species as advanced as ours.

STAGES IN DEVELOPMENT

It is important to recognise that no single definition of when human life begins has ever been universally agreed and in the foreseeable future none will be. Some would take the stand that such a question is largely irrelevant in view of the continuity of life between generations provided by the sperm and the egg.

Biological knowledge about abortion and clinical techniques of termination have moved more rapidly than theology and legislation. Legal restrictions were introduced in early nineteenth-century America because of the demonstrable dangers of abortion. The lack of moralising at the time of the 1861 British Act or the 1866 New Zealand Act illustrates the same point. The theology relating to early pregnancy in all the great religions of the world was devised before the human egg had been seen, before the science of embryology was established and before the biological role of spontaneous abortion was understood.

The choice

It is unfortunate that there is no rubicon in human development, before which we can say, 'This is a lump of cells as trivial as a nail paring', and after which we can say, 'This is a human being'. Human reproduction is a continuum. It can be traced back to the point when primordial germ cells are first recognisable in the yolk cell endoderm (which in human development is about the twentieth day after fertilisation) and in a very real way the human reproductive process is still incomplete when a woman is caring for her infant *grand*children. If we accept that we are dealing with a continuous process are we left floundering, unable to distinguish between abortion, infanticide and murder? This is not the case and in many ways our judgement is more sound and less open to mistakes if we recognise that every decision on abortion must be made individually, weighing all the factors concerned and remembering that it is always in some part an arbitrary decision.

The reform and repeal of abortion laws was for long conducted on the assumption that abortion was a 'crime' – or if not a crime at least something of profound concern, from which the practitioner could only be exonerated in certain circumstances. Those seeking reform pointed to hard cases. Campaigns were fought around congenitally defective babies, pregnancy following rape or incest, and crippling social problems. Those opposing reform saw legal abortion as the thin end of a wedge leading to infanticide, euthanasia and the concentration camp. Experience has shown that most women seeking abortion are not hard cases but soft cases – the girl is unmarried; there has been a contraceptive failure in marriage; the couple cannot afford another child; the mother is healthy but the individuals involved have decided to limit their family and are prepared to go to considerable lengths to do so.

Abortion reform did indeed turn out to be the thin end of a wedge, but not in a way either side had foreseen. A disregard for human life did not follow. The American youth that protested about the war in Vietnam commonly supported abortion reform. The wedge was entirely within the context of abortion practices themselves. It proved to be virtually irresistible and had a radical effect.

The antithesis of the conventional Catholic attitude to abortion is to be found within the feminist movement, which has some of the revolutionary vigour the Church of Rome has lost. Like the early Christians, feminists currently see themselves as a persecuted group. They are sensitive to the feelings of other minorities, suspicious of government and of establishment and are a closely knit group offering warmth and security to each other – being capable of great altruism. Both Catholics and feminists have found the abortion issue an invaluable rallying point and the loyal disciples of each movement, although not necessarily the thinkers, have adopted simplistic inflexible theologies.

The worst ethical mistakes are often made by those who make what are really arbitrary judgements and then ask others to accept them as absolute. When an arbitrary choice is made, then the first thing is to recognise that it is, indeed, arbitrary. It is always open to debate; it may be changed in the light of new knowledge and new needs.

In practice we are forced to make many pragmatic and arbitrary judgements in human affairs. Society fixes a minimum age of marriage. Whether it should be 12 or 14, as in many countries, or in the 20s as in contemporary China is open to debate, but everyone would agree that it should not be as low as six or as high as 60. At what age should the vote be given in a democratic society? It is being brought down from 21 to 18 in many places. Should it go down to eight or be put up to 80? It is usually easy to exclude extremes in these arbitrary decisions but impossible to justify as absolutely correct the compromise finally accepted.

In the same way, at one extreme, it seems inappropriate to exclude an early abortion from the normal means of fertility regulation, at the other, most women and most doctors find abortion at 26 weeks deeply objectionable. The consensus that has arisen in many countries is for abortion on request up to 12 weeks of pregnancy, but only after increasingly careful, informed discussion in the second trimester of pregnancy.

We strongly believe in early abortion at the request of the woman, not because we believe she has an absolute right to dispose of the embryo, but because we believe she knows more about the situation in which she finds herself than is possible for anyone else. Unless she is incompetent, in the legal sense of the word, she is nearly always in the best position to make the necessary responsible choice. She may well wish to discuss the problem with other people and those who set up relevant services have an obligation to make sure she understands the nature and consequences of the operation. We also believe that society must make available adequate resources for adoption and for the support of one-parent families.

There seems to be a parallel between a woman's response to spontaneous abortion and the gravity with which she approaches induced abortion. Few women mourn a late period and none baptise, or in any other way ritualise, the disposal of menstrual towels. Similarly, there is a worldwide trade in medicines to induce menstruation. None work predictably, but when a pill for late periods is discovered it will have instant appeal. The surgical technique of 'menstrual regulation' is already being taken up in many countries. A spontaneous abortion early in pregnancy can be a messy and miserable process. In the case of a wanted pregnancy the woman resents the waste or fears for her future fertility, but she does not have that loss of reality and of individuality that she suffers if a child dies. Sjövall has summarised the normal woman's perception of pregnancy as divisible into three phases:

'My period is late'.

'I am pregnant.'

'I am going to have a baby.'

Termination in the first phase is acceptable to nearly all women. In the second phase – which corresponds to the first trimester, or possibly the interval prior to quickening – abortion elicits considerable thought, perhaps some anguish, but the decision should not be overdramatised. Abortion in the third phase invariably requires much stronger reasons.

Experience shows that individuals make sensible decisions over abortion and that alternative systems of decision-making have certain dangers. Women are much less likely to become involved in criminal activities than men, and female crimes of violence are especially rare. Yet a woman who really wants an abortion will go to extreme lengths to get it, whether it is legal or not. The irrelevance of abortion legislation to the incidence of induced abortion, all other considerations apart, is one of the strongest arguments for repealing or reforming restrictive laws. As pointed out earlier there may be as many provoked abortions in the single city of Santiago, where the procedure is illegal and the population Catholic, as in the whole of England, where abortion is legal and the population is largely agnostic or Protestant.

Individuals seek abortion regardless of religious teaching or of their stated convictions when not pregnant. In Britain, some Roman Catholics and nurses, both of whom have publicly criticised the 1967 Abortion Act, resort to it with above-average frequency.

Reconciling the irreconcilable

One of the most certain things that can be said about induced abortion is that opinions about it will remain divided. In many areas, particularly Christendom, the cleft is very deep: a significant number of people sincerely object to abortion, believe they would not have one themselves and genuinely wish to deter others in order to protect the embryo. Others, of equally strong conviction, fight for abortion on request as a human right. How should society frame legislation and set patterns of professional practice to encompass such profound differences?

Philosophically, it is not a new problem. The religious wars of sixteenth- and seventeenth-century Europe arose because society had divided into two groups with passionate, sincere and irreconcilable beliefs about religion, and therefore about the welfare of the human soul on this earth and throughout eternity. The only outcome, after great and sad turmoil, was the pragmatic discovery that a single belief could not be imposed. What appeared as an anticlimax after so much passion, eventually can be recognised as a noble theological and philosophical virtue – namely the ideal of tolerance in a pluralistic society.

Those striving to maintain restrictive abortion laws, or to reintroduce anti-abortion legislation are motivated by a strongly held conviction that society must do everything possible to protect the embryo and fetus, which they see as an unborn child. Some of those most deeply concerned about the problem, believe the developing embryo has an eternal soul. Unlike the religious wars of the sixteenth century, the abortion battle is fought with public demonstrations rather than armies, and leaflets rather than cannon. The proponents of abortion will say that murder is outlawed in every civilised society. The opponents will print that they do not advocate compulsory abortion. Like the prior historial analogies the only outcome, in a pluralistic society, of this irreconcilable clash of beliefs would seem to be the evolution of tolerance for those who seek legal abortion, and a realisation that restrictive legislation cannot be imposed.

Freedom and responsibility

But, if we leave early abortion purely to the choice of women, will they really throw away their contraceptives and will society step onto the Gadarene slope of child battery, infanticide, family break-up and sexual immorality?

The relationship between abortion and contraception has been discussed and no evidence found for the first supposition, although the opposite argument can be sustained. Again there is no evidence relating abortion to any adverse aspect of social living, but some to the contrary. England in 1967, when it reformed the abortion law, was by all reasonable standards a more humane country than England in 1861, when it imposed a restrictive abortion law, when it sent little boys up chimneys and down coal mines, flogged sailors, transported convicts to Australia and when tens of thousands of young prostitutes roamed around London.

In contemporary countries, prostitution, dual sexual standards for men and women and bad employment conditions for children are often worse in just those countries where abortion legislation is most firmly entrenched – for example, Latin America or Ethiopia.

Historically, the abortion decision seems to have been removd from women, either because the operation (as in the early nineteenth century) was then genuinely very dangerous, or more or less by accident. The lack of moral overtones and total absence of public comment on the 1861 Victorian Act has been emphasised.

In the late nineteenth century and throughout this century there have been moralists – nearly always men and often physicians – who pressed for and continue to seek repressive abortion laws. The most consistent of these were the Nazis who classified abortion with murder and treason as a capital crime. The few heads of state who, in addition to Hitler, have personally condemned abortion also have a questionable historical stature – one is ex-President Richard Nixon, another is President Idi Amin.

It is sometimes useful to turn a moral problem round. Murder, rape and theft are examples of human actions that are universally condemned. If we reverse the situation and say, 'What would happen if we could, by some magical process, eliminate these crimes?', then we have no difficulty in agreeing that the world would be a happier, healthier place. It is not so with abortion. What would happen if a pill were invented to cure all spontaneous abortions? Perhaps one in ten or even one in five babies would be seriously abnormal, not just hare lips and heart lesions, but shapeless, brainless monsters. Pregnancy would become a nightmare for every woman.

What would happen if all illegal abortions were eliminated? The already burgeoning population of the world would grow 50 per cent faster, the spectre of hunger would accelerate towards us, the painful growth of income *per capita* in many developing countries would halt, the slums of Manila, the *favellas* of Rio de Janeiro, the teenage prostitutes of Addis Ababa, the obscene social cancer of Calcutta would all worsen. To take a single quantitative example, the massive Indian family planning programme has perhaps prevented 13 million births in 20 years; yet the criminal abortionists in India are estimated to have averted at least 30 million births over the same interval. Abortion has the distinction of being the only 'crime' that is essential to the well-being of all developed societies and is a key element in dealing with the erosive effects of population growth on economic development and individual welfare in the Third World. In this respect it may ultimately be a factor in the very survival of the human species as we know it today.

In a world that is seriously concerned with curbing excessive rates of population growth and of achieving the most rapid improvement in maternal and child health, abortion would be seen as the central problem to be solved. In the world as it exists, society is unlikely to give abortion the priority which it deserves from the point of view of the individual in need. It is realistic to say that the quality of public health and family planning programmes can be judged by the realism or otherwise with which they approach this problem.

Induced abortion is one of the things which distinguishes man from animals. It is a uniquely human problem and it demands a fully human answer. Difficult and responsible decisions must be made if it is to be solved realistically, effectively and with compassion.

Table 48. *Population projections (millions) for the year 2050*

	Population in 1970	Population in 2050 if zero population growth attained by		
		1980	2000	2040
Developed	1 122	1482	1610	1853
Developing	2 530	4763	6525	11 591
Total world	3652	6245	8 135	13444

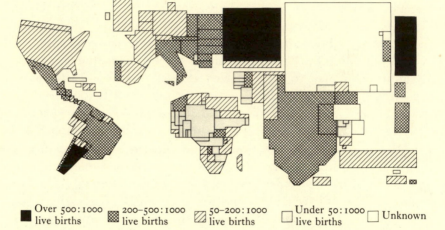

| ■ Over 500:1000 live births | ▨ 200–500:1000 live births | ▨ 50–200:1000 live births | □ Under 50:1000 live births | □ Unknown |

Fig. 56. Abortion ratios (combined legal and illegal).

References

1 Lee, L. T. (1973). Law, human rights and population: a strategy for action. *Virginia Journal of International Law*, **12**, 309.
2 Tomsic, V. (1974). 'Status of women, family planning and population dynamics.' Symposium on Law and Population, IPPF, London. (Duplicated document.)
3 *Report of the Committee on the Working of the Abortion Act* (1974). Chairman the Hon. Mrs Justice Lane, vols. **1**, **2** and **3**. HMSO, London.
4 Cates, D. (1976). Legal abortion in the United States: its effect on the health of women. In *New Developments in Fertility Regulation*, p. 143. Airlie House, Virginia.
5 Ampofo, D. A. (1976). 'Epidemiology of abortion in selected African countries.' IPPF, London. (Duplicated document.)
6 Diggory, P. L. C. (1969). Some experiences of therapeutic abortion. *Lancet*, **i**, 873.
7 Avery Jones, F., Bigby, A. M. & White, B. (1951). 'Memorandum on the admissions of abortions.' IPPF, London. (Duplicated document.)
8 Lo Sciuto, L., Balin, H. & Zahn, M. A. (1972). Physicians' attitudes towards abortion. Editorial. *Journal of Reproductive Medicine*, **9**, 70.
9 Knutson, A. L. (1967). When does human life begin? View points of public health professionals. *American Journal of Public Health*, **57**, 2163.
10 Zelnik, M. & Kantner, J. F. (1975). Attitudes of American teenagers towards abortion. *Family Planning Perspectives*, **7**, 89.
11 Westoff, C. F. Moore, E. L. & Ryder, N. B. (1969). The structure of attitudes towards abortion. *Milbank Memorial Fund Quarterly*, **47**, 11.
12 Girard, A. & Zucker, E. (1967). Une enquête auprès de public sur la structure familiale et la prévention des naissances. *Population*, **22**, 439.
13 Steinhoff, P. G., Smith, R. G. & Diamond, M. (1977). The characteristics and motivations of women receiving abortions. *Sociological Symposium*. (In press.)
14 Steinhoff, P. G. (1973). Contribution to Hawaii Menstrual Regulation Conference. (Duplicated document.)
15 Diamond, M., Steinhoff, P. G., Palmore, J. A. & Smith, R. G. (1973). Sexuality, birth control and abortion: a decision-making sequence. *Journal of Biosocial Science*, **5**, 347.
16 Smith, R. G. (1971). Abortion: risk and decision-making. *Pacific Health*, **4**, 13.
17 British Pregnancy Advisory Service (1971). *Sociomedical Breakdown and Report*. BPAS, Birmingham.
18 O'Mahony, P. J. & Potts, M. (1967). Abortion and the soul. *Month*, **38**, 45.
19 Eliasson, R. (1971). Standards for investigating human semen. *Andrologie*, **3**, 49.

20 Hertig, A. T. & Rock, J. (1949). A series of potentially abortive ova recovered from fertile women prior to the first missed menstrual period. *American Journal of Obstetrics and Gynecology*, **58**, 968.

21 Hertig, A. T., Rock, J., Adams, E. C. & Menkin, M. C. (1959). Thirty-four fertilized human ova, good, bad and indifferent, recovered from 210 women of known fertility. *Pediatrics, Springfield*, **23**, 202.

References to tables

Table 1 Potter, R. G. (1963). Birth intervals: structure and change. *Population Studies, London,* **17**, 172.

Table 2 Hathout, H. (1972). Looking at abortion material. In *Induced Abortion: A Hazard to Public Health?,* ed. I. R. Nazer, p. 216. IPPF, Beirut.

Table 3 Sokolova, N. S. (1970). Statistical analysis of the outcome of pregnancies. *Zdravookhranenie Rossiikoi Federatsii,* **14**, 38. Quoted by Steinhoff, P. G. (1972). Abortion data from the Soviet Union. *Abortion Research Notes,* November. Suppl. 1(3).

Table 4 Composite table from (1) Rongy, A. J. (1933). *Abortion: Legal and Illegal.* Vanguard Press, New York; (2) Whitehouse, B. (1929), in joint discussion on causes of early abortion and sterility – section of obstetrics and gynaecology and section on comparative medicine. *Proceedings of the Royal Society of Medicine,* **23**, 241; (3) *Interim Report of Departmental Committee on Maternal Mortality and Morbidity.*

Table 5 Obeng, B. (1967). 500 Consecutive cases of abortion. Ph.D. thesis, University of London.

Table 6 Gebhard, P. H., Pomeroy, W. B., Martin, C. E. & Christenson, C. V. (1959). *Pregnancy, Birth and Abortion.* Heinemann, London.

Table 7 Peled, T. (1974). Israel. In *Psychosocial Aspects of Abortion in Asia.* Proceedings of the Asian Regional Research Seminar in Psychosocial Aspects of Abortion, Katmandu, Nepal, November 1974, p. 53. Transnational Family Research Program, Washington D.C.

Table 8 Based on 'Induced abortion in Latin America'. (Duplicated document.) IPPF, Western Hemisphere (1970).

Table 9 Awan, A. K. (1969). *Provoked Abortion Amongst 1,447 Women.* Maternity and Child Health Association of Pakistan, Lahore.

Table 10 Larsen, T. B. (1972). Estimates of induced abortion in some Middle East countries. In *Induced Abortion: A Hazard to Public Health?,* ed. I. R. Nazer, p. 122. IPPF, Beirut.

Table 11 Simoneti, S. & Novak, F. (1972). 'Decline of birth rate and the influence of infant mortality.' IPPF, Western Hemisphere Region Meeting, Ottawa. (Duplicated document.)

Tables 12 and 13   Data supplied by B. M. Beric.

Table 14 Grzywo-Dabroski, quoted by Rongy, A. J. (1933). *Abortion: Legal and Illegal.* Vanguard Press, New York.

Table 15 Composite data from (1) Sklar, J. & Berkov, B. (1974). Teenage family formation in postwar America. *Family Planning Perspectives,* **6,** 80; (2) Soskice, D. (1973). 'The effect of the UK Abortion Act 1968 on the Birth Rate.' IPPF, London. (Duplicated document.)

Tables 16–18   Whitehead, J. (1847). *On the Causes and Treatment of Abortion and Sterility, The Result of an Inquiry into the Physiological and Morbid Conditions of the Uterus with Reference to Leucorrheal Affliction and the Diseases of Menstruation.* Churchill. London.

Table 19 Beric, B. M. & Kupresanin, M. (1971). Vacuum aspiration, using paracervical block, for legal abortion as an outpatient procedure up to the twelfth week of pregnancy. *Lancet,* **ii,** 619.

Table 20 Stallworthy, J. A., Moolgasker, A. S. & Walsh, J. J. (1971). Legal abortion: a critical assessment of its risks. *Lancet,* **ii,** 1245. Nathanson, B. M. (1972). Ambulatory abortion, experience with 26,000 cases. *New England Journal of Medicine,* **291,** 1189.

Table 21 United States National Academy of Sciences: Institute of Medicine (1975). *Legalized Abortion and the Public Health: Report of a Study by a Committee of the Institute of Medicine.* Washington D.C.

Table 22 Center for Disease Control, US Department of Health, Education and Welfare (1976). New Development in Fertility Regulation, Pathfinder Conference, Airlie House, New York. (Duplicated document.)

Table 23 (1) United States National Academy of Sciences: Institute of Medicine (1975). *Legalized Abortion and the Public Health: Report of a Study by a Committee of the Institute of Medicine.* Washington D.C.; (2) official UK statistics.

Table 24 Greer, H. S., Lal, S., Lewis, S. C., Belsey, E. M. & Beard, R. W. (1976). Psychological consequences of therapeutic abortion. King's termination study III. *British Journal of Psychiatry,* **128,** 74.

Table 25 Composite data from the (1) Registrar General's Quarterly Returns, *Hansard,* **887**(83), col. 154; (2) Godber, G. E. (1972). Abortion deaths. *British Medical Journal,* **3,** 424; (3) Lewis, E. M. (1975). The report on confidential enquiries into maternal deaths. England and Wales (1970–72). *Health Trends,* **9,** 51.

Table 26 Tietze, C., Pakter, C. J. & Berger, G. S. (1973). Mortality associated with legal abortion in New York City, 1970–72. *Journal of the American Medical Association,* **225,** 507.

Table 27 Ardwidsson, L. *et al.* (1968). A liberal abortion practice. *Lakartidningen Svensk Skotidning,* **65,** 4027.

Table 28 Official statistics. Analyses for the years 1969 and 1971 were first performed by P. Kestleman in 1972.

Table 29 Official statistics modified by Vallin. See Vallin, J. (1971). Limitation des naissances en Tunisie. *Population,* **26,** 181.

Table 30 Nizard, P. (1971). Official statistics. Analysis for the years 1969 and 1971 first performed by P. Kestleman in 1972. See Vallin, J. (1971). Limitation des naissances en Tunisie. *Population,* **26,** 181.

Table 31 Muramatsu, M. (1970). An analysis of factors in fertility control in Japan. *Bulletin of the Institute of Public Health, Tokyo*, **19**, 97.

Table 32 Modified from Klinger, A. (1969). Abortion programs. In *Family Planning and Population Programs*, ed. B. Berelson *et al.* University of Chicago Press, Chicago.

Table 33 Szabady, E. (1971). Personal communication.

Table 34 Szabady, E. (1971). Personal communication.

Table 35 Pearl, R. (1939). *Natural History of Population*. Oxford University Press, Oxford.

Table 36 Yaukey, D. (1961). *Fertility Differences in a Modernizing Country*. Princeton University Press, Princeton, N.J.

Table 37 1971 National fertility and abortion survey. Quoted by Watson, W. B. (1972). Demographic problems confronting Korea's family planning program. In *Proceedings of a National Family Planning Evaluation Seminar*, p. 117. Korean Institute for Family Planning, Seoul.

Table 38 Requena, M. B. (1971). The problem of induced abortion in Latin America. In *Proceedings of the International Population Conference of the IUSSP*, vol. **3**, IUSSP, Liège.

Table 39 Hutchinson, B. (1964). Induced abortion in Brazilian married women. *America Latina*, **7**, 21.

Table 40 Manichi Newspapers (1965). Quoted in Muramatsu, M. (ed.), *Japan's Experience in Family Planning – Past and Present*. Family Planning Federation of Japan, Tokyo.

Table 41 1967 Knowledge, Attitude and Practice Survey. Data supplied by L. P. Chow, 1971.

Table 42 Fisek, N. H. (1972). Epidemiological study of abortion in Turkey. In *Induced Abortion: A Hazard to Public Health?*, ed. I. R. Nazer, p. 264. IPPF, Beirut.

Table 43 Kaper-Stanulovic, N. & Friedman, H. L. (1974). 'Abortion and contraception in Novi Sad, Yugoslavia: determinants of choice.' IPPF, London. (Duplicated document.)

Table 44 Tietze, C. (1974). The 'problem' of repeat abortions. *Family Planning Perspectives*, **5**, 89.

Table 45 Potter, R. G. (1971). Inadequacy of a one-method family-planning program. *Social Biology*, **18**, 1.

Table 46 Derived from (1) Cates, D. (1976). 'Legal abortion in the United States: its effect on the health of women.' New Developments in Fertility Regulation, Pathfinder Conference, Airlie House, New York. (Duplicated document.) (2) Ampofo, D. A. (1976). 'Epidemiology of abortion in selected African countries.' IPPF, London. (Duplicated document.)

Table 47 Szabady, E. & Klinger, A. (1970). Pilot survey of repeated abortion seeking. In *Proceedings of the Conference on Psychosocial Factors in Transnational Family Planning Research*, ed. H. P. David & J. Bernheim, p. 31. Transnational Family Research Institute, Washington D.C.

Table 48 Population Council statistics.

References to Figures

Fig. 1   Potts, D. M. (1972). Limiting human reproductive potential. In
          Reproduction in Mammals, vol. **5**, *Artificial Control of Reproduction*, ed.
          C. R. Austin & R. V. Short, p. 32. Cambridge University Press,
          London.

Fig. 2   *Ibid.*, after Sauvy, A. (1969). *General Theory of Population*.
          Weidenfeld & Nicolson, London.

Figs. 3, 4 and 5 Original.   Data derived from Tietze, C. & Dawson, D. A.
          (1973). Induced abortion: a factbook. *Reports on Population/Family
          Planning*, **14** (first edition), 1.

Fig. 6.   Redrawn from Jongbloet, P. H. (1971). *Mental and Physical Handicaps
          in Connection with Over-ripeness Ovopathy*. Stenfert Kroese, Leyden.

Fig. 7   Redrawn from Shapiro, S., Levine, H. S. & Abramowicz, M. (1971).
          Factors associated with early and late fetal loss. *Advances in Planned
          Parenthood*, **6**, 45.

Figs. 8 and 9   Peel, J. & Potts, M. (1968). *Textbook of Contraceptive Practice*.
          Cambridge University Press, London.

Fig. 10   Hertig, A. T., Rock, J., Adams, E. C. & Menkin, M. C. (1959).
          Thirty-four fertilised human ova, good, bad and indifferent, recovered
          from 210 women of known fertility. *Pediatrics, Springfield*, **23**, 202.

Fig. 11   Drawn from statistics on Gens, A. (1930). The demand for abortion in
          Soviet Russia. In *Sexual Reform Congress*, ed. N. Haire, p. 143.
          Kegan Paul, London.

Figs. 12–17 and 19   Derived from the following: (1) David, H. P., Kalis, M. &
          Tietze, C. (1973). *Selected Abortion Statistics: An International
          Summary*. International Reference Center for Abortion Research,
          Bethesda, Maryland: (2) Tietze, C. & Murstein, M. C. (1975).
          Induced abortion: 1975 factbook. *Reports on Population/Family
          Planning*, **14** (second edition), 1; (3) *Le Mouvement Naturel de la
          Population dans le Monde de 1906 à 1936*. Les éditions de l'Institut
          National des Études Demographiques, Paris; (4) Kuczynski, R. R.
          (1931). *The Balance of Births and Deaths*, vol. **11**. The Brookings
          Institute, Washington D.C.; (5) *Demográfia Evkonyu* (1970). Kozponti
          Statiztika Hivatal, Budapest.

Fig. 18   Based on data in the following: (1) Tyler, C. W., Bourne, J. P., Conger, S. B. & Kahn, J. B. (1972). Reporting and surveillance of legal abortion in the United States, 1970. In *Abortion Techniques and Services*, ed. S. Lewit, p. 192. Excerpta Medica, Amsterdam; (2) Weinstock, E., Tietze, C., Jaffe, F. S. & Dryfoos, J. G. (1975). Legal abortions in the United States since the 1973 Supreme Court decisions. *Family Planning Perspectives*, **7**, 23.

Figs. 20, 21, 23 and 24   Tietze, C. & Murstein, M. C. (1975). Induced abortion: 1975 factbook. *Reports on Population/Family Planning*, **14** (second edition), 1.

Fig. 22   Official statistics for England and Wales (1969) as first set out by P. Kestleman.

Fig. 25   Gebhard, P. H., Pomeroy, W. B., Martin, C. E. & Christenson, C. V. (1959). *Pregnancy, Birth and Abortion*. Heinemann, London.

Fig. 26   Peller, S. (1967). *Qualitative Research in Human Biology and Medicine*. Wright, Bristol.

Fig. 27   Derived from the following: (1) Stamm, H. (1967) Statistiche Unterlagen zum Problem der Geburtenkontrolle unter der Familienplanung. *Ars Medici*, **11**, 748; (2) Hong, S. B. (1971) *Changing Patterns of Induced Abortion in Seoul, Korea*. Seoul; (3) Smith, R. G., Steinhoff, P. G., Pahmore, J. A. & Diamond, M. (1973) Abortion in Hawaii 1970–71. *Hawaii Medical Journal*, **32**, 213.

Fig. 28   *UN Demographic Year Book* (1970) UN, New York, and *General Survey of Family Planning in Okinawa* (1970) Okinawa Family Planning Association.

Fig. 29   Tietze, C. (1973). Two years' experience with a liberal abortion law: its impact on fertility trends in New York City. *Family Planning Perspectives*, **5**, 36.

Fig. 30   (1) David, H. P. & Wright, N. H. (1974). Restricting abortion: the Romanian experience. In *Abortion Research: International Experience*, ed. H. P. David, p. 217. Lexington Books, Lexington, Mass.; (2) Tietze, C. & Murstein, M. C. (1975). Induced abortion: 1975 factbook. *Reports on Population/Family Planning*, **14** (second edition), 1.

Fig. 31   Official statistics.

Fig. 34   Tietze, C. & Lewit, S. (1972). Joint program for the study of abortion (JPSA). *Studies in Family Planning*, **3**, 97.

Fig. 35   Hayashi, M. & Momose, K. (1966). Statistical observations on artificial abortion and sterility. In *Harmful Effects of Induced Abortion*, ed. Y. Koya. Family Planning Federation of Japan, Tokyo.

Fig. 36   Kessel, E. (1974). 'Menstrual Regulation in fertility control.' First Scientific Congress in Family Planning, Sri Lanka, IFRP. (Duplicated document.)

Fig. 37   Official statistics.

Fig. 38   Data compiled from official statistics. *Hansard*, and estimates by P. L. C. Diggory & M. Simms.

Figs. 39, 40 and 41   Based on data included in the Lane Committee report (see notes to Chapter 9).

Fig. 42   Official statistics.

Fig. 43   Tietze, C. & Dawson, D. A. (1973). Induced abortion: a factbook. *Reports on Population/Family Planning*, **14**, 1.

Fig. 44   (1) Tyler, C. W., Bourne, J. P., Conger, S. B. & Kahn, J. B. (1972). Reporting and surveillance of legal abortion in the United States, 1970. In *Abortion Techniques and Services*, ed. S. Lewit, p. 192. Excerpta Medica. Amsterdam; (2) Weinstock, E., Tietze, C., Jaffe, F. S. & Dryfoos, J. G. (1975). Legal abortions in the United States since the 1973 Supreme Court decisions. *Family Planning Perspectives*, **7**, 23.

Fig. 45   Zimmerman *et al.* (1976). Abortion law and practice: a status report. *Population Reports*, series E, no. 3.

Figs. 46 and 47   Data supplied by D. P. Smith and W. B. Watson.

Figs. 48 and 49   Derived from official statistics.

Fig. 50   Derived from references given in the text.

Fig. 51   Monreal, T. (1976). Determinant factors affecting illegal abortion trends in Chile. In *New Developments in Fertility Regulation*, p. 123. Airlie House, New York.

Fig. 52   Data for Santiago: T. Monreal, personal communication. Data for Taiwan: Taiwan Population Study Centre, 1976. Data for Korea: Han Su Shin (1967). IPPF Medical Bulletin, **1**, 3.

Fig. 53   Tietze, C., Bongaarts, J. & Schearer, B. (1976). Mortality associated with the control of fertility. *Family Planning Perspectives*, **8**, 6.

Fig. 54   Dytrch, Z., Matejček, Z., Schüller, V., David, H. P. & Friedman, H. C. (1975). Children born to women denied abortion. *Family Planning Perspectives*, **7**, 165.

Figs. 55 and 56   Compiled by the authors from a variety of sources.

INDEX